PROGRESS IN BRAIN RESEARCH

VOLUME 75

VISION WITHIN EXTRAGENICULO-STRIATE SYSTEMS

Recent volumes in PROGRESS IN BRAIN RESEARCH

Volume 56: Brain Phosphoproteins, Characterization and Function, by W. H. Gispen and A. Routtenberg (Eds.) – 1982

Volume 57: Descending Pathways to the Spinal cord, by H. G. J. M. Kuypers and G. F. Martin (Eds.) – 1982

Volume 58: Molecular and Cellular Interactions underlying Higher Brain Functions, by J.-P. Changeux, J. Glowinksi, M. Imbert and F. E. Bloom (Eds.) – 1983

Volume 59: Immunology of Nervous System Infections, by P. O. Behan, V. ter Meulen and F. Clifford Rose (Eds.) – 1983

Volume 60: The Neurohypophysis: Structure, Function and Control, by B. A. Cross and G. Leng (Eds.) – 1983

Volume 61: Sex Differences in the Brain: The Relation Between Structure and Function, by G. J. De Vries, J. P. C. De Bruin, H. B. M. Uylings and M. A. Corner (Eds.) – 1984

Volume 62: Brain Ischemia: Quantitative EEG and Imaging Techniques, by G. Pfurtscheller, E. J. Jonkman and F. H. Lopes da Silva (Eds.) – 1984

Volume 63: Molecular Mechanisms of Ischemic Brain Damage, by K. Kogure, K.-A. Hossmann, B. K. Siesjö and F. A. Welsh (Eds.) – 1985

Volume 64: The Oculomotor and Skeletalmotor Systems: Differences and Similarities, by H.-J. Freund, U. Büttner, B. Cohen and J. Noth (Eds.) – 1986

Volume 65: Psychiatric Disorders: Neurotransmitters and Neuropeptides, by J. M. Van Ree and S. Matthysse (Eds.) – 1986

Volume 66: Peptides and Neurological Disease, by P. C. Emson, M. N. Rossor and M. Tohyama (Eds.) – 1986

Volume 67: Visceral Sensation, by F. Cervero and J. F. B. Morrison (Eds.) – 1986

Volume 68: Coexistence of Neuronal Messengers – A New Principle in Chemical Transmission, by T. Hökfelt, K. Fuxe and B. Pernow (Eds.) – 1986

Volume 69: Phosphoproteins in Neuronal Function, by W. H. Gispen and A. Routtenberg (Eds.) – 1986

Volume 70: Aging of the Brain and Alzheimer's Disease, by D. F. Swaab, E. Fliers, M. Mirmiran, W. A. van Gool and F. van Haaren (Eds.) – 1986

Volume 71: Neuronal Regeneration, by F. J. Seil, E. Herbert and B. M. Carlson (Eds.) – 1987

Volume 72: Neuropeptides and Brain Function, by E. R. de Kloet, V. M. Wiegant and D. de Wied (Eds.) – 1987

Volume 73: Biochemical Basis of Functional Neuroteratology, by G. J. Boer, M. G. P. Feenstra, M. Mirmiran, D. F. Swaab and F. van Haaren (Eds.) – 1988

Volume 74: Transduction and Cellular Mechanisms in Sensory Receptors, by W. Hamann and A. Iggo (Eds.) – 1988

PROGRESS IN BRAIN RESEARCH

VOLUME 75

VISION WITHIN EXTRAGENICULO-STRIATE SYSTEMS

EDITED BY

T.P. HICKS

Department of Medical Physiology, Faculty of Medicine, The University of Calgary, 3330 Hospital Drive NW, Calgary, Alberta, Canada T2N 4N1

and

G. BENEDEK

Department of Physiology, University Medical School of Szeged, Dóm tér 10, H-6720 Szeged, Hungary

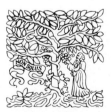

ELSEVIER
AMSTERDAM – NEW YORK – OXFORD
1988

ISBN 0-444-80972-4 (volume)
ISBN 0-444-80104-9 (series)

Published by:
Elsevier Science Publishers B.V. (Biomedical Division)
P.O. Box 211
1000 AE Amsterdam
The Netherlands

Sole distributors for the USA and Canada:
Elsevier Science Publishing Company, Inc.
52 Vanderbilt Avenue
New York, NY 10017
USA

Library of Congress Cataloging-in-Publication Data

Vision within extrageniculo-striate systems / edited by T.P. Hicks and
  G. Benedek.
        p. cm. -- (Progress in brain research ; v. 75)
    Proceedings of a satellite symposium held in 1987 in Szeged,
Hungary, in conjunction with the Second Congress of the
International Brain Research Organization.
    Includes bibliographies and index.
    ISBN (invalid) 0-444-80974-4 (U.S.)
    1. Visual pathways--Congresses.   2. Visual cortex--Congresses.
3. Optic nerve--Congresses.   I. Hicks, T. Philip.   II. Benedek, G.
III. International Brain Research Organization.   Congress (2nd :
1987 : Budapest, Hungary).   IV. Series.
    [DNLM: 1. Geniculate Bodies--anatomy & histology--congresses.
2. Visual Cortex--anatomy & histology--congresses.   3. Visual
Cortex--physiology--congresses.   W1 PR667J v. 75 / WL 307 V831
1987]
QP376.P7 vol. 75
[QP475]
612'.82 s--dc19
[612'.84]
DNLM/DLC
for Library of Congress   88-21212
                                                              CIP

Printed in The Netherlands

List of Contributors

B.P. Abramson, Department of Psychology and the Physiology Graduate Group, University of California, Davis, CA 95616, U.S.A.

B. Albowitz, Max-Planck-Institute for Biophysical Chemistry, Department of Neurobiology, Göttingen, F.R.G.

T. Awaji, Department of Physiology, Yamanashi Medical School, Tamaho, Nakakoma, Yamanashi 409-38, Japan

T. Bando, Department of Physiology, Faculty of Medicine, Niigata University, Niigata 951, Japan

P.P. Battaglini, Istituto di Fisiologia Umana, Università di Bologna, Piazza di Porta S. Donato 2, I-40127 Bologna, Italy

D.B. Bender, Department of Physiology, University at Buffalo, State University of New York, Buffalo, NY 14226, U.S.A.

G. Benedek, Department of Physiology, University Medical School, Dóm tér 10, H-6720 Szeged, Hungary

N. Berardi, Istituto di Neurofisiologia del C.N.R., Via S. Zeno 51, 56100 Pisa, Italy

D.M. Berson, Section of Neurobiology, Division of Biology and Medicine, Brown University, Providence, RI 02912, U.S.A.

S. Bisti, Istituto di Neurofisiologia del C.N.R., Via S. Zeno 51, 56100 Pisa, Italy

C. Blakemore, University Laboratory of Physiology, Parks Road, Oxford OX1 3PT, U.K.

C. Casanova, Department of Biological Sciences, University of Montreal, Montreal H3C 3J7, Canada

A. Cérat, Department of Biological Sciences, University of Montreal, Montreal H3C 3J7, Canada

L.M. Chapula, Department of Psychology and the Physiology Graduate Group, University of California, Davis, CA 95616, U.S.A.

O.D. Creutzfeldt, Department of Neurobiology, Max-Planck-Institute for Biophysical Chemistry, P.O. Box 2841, D-3400 Göttingen-Nikolausberg, F.R.G.

C.G. Cusick, Department of Anatomy, Tulane University Medical Center, 1430 Tulane Avenue, New Orleans, LA 70112, U.S.A.

P. Dean, Department of Psychology, University of Sheffield, Sheffield S10 2TN, U.K.

D. Emmans, Department of Psychology, University of Konstanz, P.O. Box 7733, D-7750 Konstanz, F.R.G.

A. Fiorentini, Istituto di Neurofisiologia del C.N.R., Via S. Zeno 51, 56100 Pisa, Italy

A.F. Fuchs, Regional Primate Research Center, University of Washington, Seattle, WA 98195, U.S.A.

C. Galletti, Cattedra di Fisiologia Generale, Università di Bologna, Piazza di Porta S. Donato 2, I-40127 Bologna, Italy

J.-P. Guillemot, Département de Kinanthropologie, Université du Québec, Montréal, Québec, H3C 3P8, Canada

W.O. Guldin, Institute of Physiology, Free University, Arnimallee 22, D-1000 Berlin 33, Germany

B. Gulyás, Laboratory for Neuro- and Psychophysiology, Faculty of Medicine, University of Leuven, Herestraat, B-3000 Leuven, Belgium

T.P. Hicks, Department of Medical Physiology, Faculty of Medicine, The University of Calgary, 3330 Hospital Drive N.W., Calgary, Alberta T2N 4N1, Canada

B. Hutchins, Department of Anatomy, Baylor College of Dentistry, Dallas, TX 75246, U.S.A.

C. Kaneko, Regional Primate Research Center, University of Washington, Seattle, WA 98195, U.S.A.

M. Katoh, Department of Anatomy, Fujita-Gakuen Health University, Toyoake, Aichi, 470-11, Japan

T.P. Lange, Regional Primate Research Center, University of Washington, Seattle, WA 98195, U.S.A.

F. Leporé, Département de Psychologie, Groupe de Recherche en Neuropsychologie Expérimentale, Centre de Recherche en Sciences Neurologiques, Université de Montréal, Montréal, Québec H2V 2S9, Canada

S. LeVay, Robert Bosch Vision Research Center, Salk Institute for Biological Studies, P.O. Box 85800, San Diego, CA 92138, U.S.A.

L. Maffei, Istituto di Neurofisiologia del C.N.R., Via S. Zeno 51, 56100 Pisa, Italy

M.G. Maioli, Istituto di Fisiologia Umana, Università di Bologna, Piazza di Porta S. Donato 2, I-40127 Bologna, Italy

H.J. Markowitsch, Department of Psychology, University of Konstanz, P.O. Box 7733, D-7750 Konstanz, F.R.G.

J.A. Matsubara, Department of Anatomy, Dalhousie University, Halifax, Nova Scotia B3H 4H7, Canada

I.J. Mitchell, Department of Psychology, University of Sheffield, Sheffield S10 2TN, U.K.

S. Molotchnikoff, Department of Biological Sciences, University of Montreal, Montreal H3C 3J7, Canada

L. Mucke, Max-Planck-Institute for Biophysical Chemistry, Department of Neurobiology, Göttingen, F.R.G.

M.J. Mustari, Regional Primate Research Center, University of Washington, Seattle, WA 98195, U.S.A.

M. Norita, Department of Anatomy, Fujita-Gakuen Health University, Toyoake, Aichi, 470-11, Japan

G.A. Orban, Laboratory for Neuro- and Psychophysiology, Faculty of Medicine, University of Leuven, Herestraat, B-3000 Leuven, Belgium

D.J. Price, Department of Zoology, University of California, Berkeley, CA 94720, U.S.A.

M. Ptito, Département de Psychologie, Groupe de Recherche en Neuropsychologie Expérimentale, Centre de Recherche en Sciences Neurologiques, Université de Montréal, Montréal, Québec H2V 2S9, Canada

J.P. Rauschecker, Max-Planck-Institut für biologische Kybernetik, D-7400 Tübingen, F.R.G.

P. Redgrave, Department of Psychology, University of Sheffield, Sheffield S10 2TN, U.K.

L. Richter, Département de Psychologie, Groupe de Recherche en Neuropsychologie Expérimentale, Centre de Recherche en Sciences Neurologiques, Université de Montréal, Montréal, Québec H2V 2S9, Canada

H. Sherk, Department of Biological Structure, University of Washington, Seattle, WA 98195, U.S.A.

P.D. Spear, Department of Psychology and Neurosciences Training Department, University of Wisconsin, Madison, WI 53706, U.S.A.

W. Spileers, Laboratory for Neuro- and Psychophysiology, Faculty of Medicine, University of Leuven, Herestraat, B-3000 Leuven, Belgium

S. Squatrito, Istituto di Fisiologia Umana, Università di Bologna, Piazza di Porta S. Donato 2, I-40127 Bologna, Italy

B.E. Stein, Department of Physiology, Medical College of Virginia, Virginia Commonwealth University, Richmond, VA 23298, U.S.A.

M. Sur, Department of Brain and Cognitive Sciences, Massachusetts Institute of Technology, Cambridge, MA 02135, U.S.A.

H. Toda, Department of Physiology, Yamanashi Medical School, Tamaho, Nakakoma, Yamanashi 409-38, Japan

B.V. Updyke, Department of Anatomy, Louisiana State University Medical Center, New Orleans, LA 70112, U.S.A.

J. Wallman, Department of Biology, CUNY, New York, NY 10031, U.S.A.

R.E. Weller, Department of Psychology, University of Alabama at Birmingham, 201 Campbell Hall, Birmingham, AL 35294, U.S.A.

T.J. Zumbroich, Department of Biology, B-022, University of California at San Diego, La Jolla, CA 92093, U.S.A.

Preface

This book contains the proceedings of a satellite symposium held in conjunction with the Second World Congress of Neuroscience under the auspices of the International Brain Research Organization. Each invited speaker was asked to contribute one chapter to the volume, one which should be based on a topic of current major interest in their field. Accordingly, the volume represents a thoroughly up-to-date account of research in extrageniculo-striate visual mechanisms.

The idea of holding a symposium on this topic arose from a similar meeting which had been held at the Society for Neuroscience meeting, at Dallas in 1986, organized by Drs. L.M. Chalupa and D.H. Robinson. At that one-day meeting, an obvious enthusiasm was evident, as expressed by the attendees. Since no publication emerged there, the present symposium seemed appropriate, especially in view of the venue of the 1987 IBRO Congress in Budapest.

Research in extrageniculate and extrastriate systems is currently undergoing a vigorous period, with important advances being made on an almost-monthly basis. It seemed particularly important therefore to attempt to bring together those individuals currently in the forefront of this research activity. Each speaker was selected carefully, to allow a balanced overview of areas such as those which would include: superior colliculus, tectal and pretectal nuclei, LP-pulvinar complex, cortical areas 18 and 19, lateral suprasylvian areas and finally, rostrally-located visual cortical areas. The topics covered a variety of species, ranging from rat and ferret to Old- and New-World primates. Anatomical accounts and physiological approaches dominated most sessions, although important contributions from behavioural and pharmacological experiments were made as well.

The idea of treating extrageniculo-striate mechanisms separately from the rest of the visual sciences may seem a little arbitrary to many, as it seems to imply that the extrageniculostriate pathways should in some sense be exclusive in nature; the name appears to establish that the pathways deal with everything that does not belong to geniculo-striate mechanisms. The title of the conference, however, may cover an especially well-delineated mechanism of vision that clearly is separable from the classical visual one which underlies geniculo-striate vision. The concept of two visual mechanisms that are sometimes called 'what' vision and 'where' vision is not yet entirely delineated; still, we hope that this conference at least will go some distance toward establishing this classification.

The warm, relaxed atmosphere within the Old-World, romantic setting of the famous Hungarian university town of Szeged was enjoyed greatly by all the delegates. Szeged, the host city of the satellite symposium, is a quiet, small city in the southern part of Hungary. It has played central roles in the history of the Hungarian nation over the centuries. In the recent past, several tragedies occurred, one of which was a devastating flood (1879) which swept away nearly all buildings, necessitating the rebuilding of the former small fishing and milling town into a city modern for its times. Szeged's academic development in this century began after the First World War, with the relocation to within its borders of the old university of Kolozsvár. In 1937, the Nobel prize for medicine and physiology was awarded to Albert Szent-Györgyi, who was the Chairman of the Department of Medical Chemistry of Szeged University.

The symposium took place in the House of Technique of Szeged that provided a good venue for the conference. The two and a half days of the meeting were punctuated by gastronomic and oenophilic delights which left the delegates with vows to renew their dietary efforts upon their return home. Therefore the participants, the food, and certainly not least, the scientific caliber of the conference, were of the highest quality. As Editors, we acknowledge with grateful thanks the co-operation of the speakers in making possible the rapid publication of this 'state of the art' account of extrageniculo-striate visual research through the prompt submissions of their manuscripts. Of course, the Publisher also is commended for having the book appear in timely fashion.

We must acknowledge the kind help of all those who made it possible for us to organize a conference in Szeged. The congress organization was made possible by the contributions of the researchers and technical assistants of the Department of Physiology of the University of Szeged as well as the Department of Medical Physiology of the University of Calgary. Professor Y. Kudo and Mrs. M. Nakai (Mitsubishi-Kasei Institute of Life Sciences, Tokyo) provided invaluable assistance in facilitating the production of the subject index and accordingly are due a hearty vote of thanks.

Luckily, not all the questions raised during the course of the conference were able to be answered − pointing the way for future scientific efforts and raising the likelihood of another similar meeting to advance yet further the frontiers of knowledge of the details of how integrated visual perception is manifested.

T.P. Hicks

Szeged, August 1987   G. Benedek

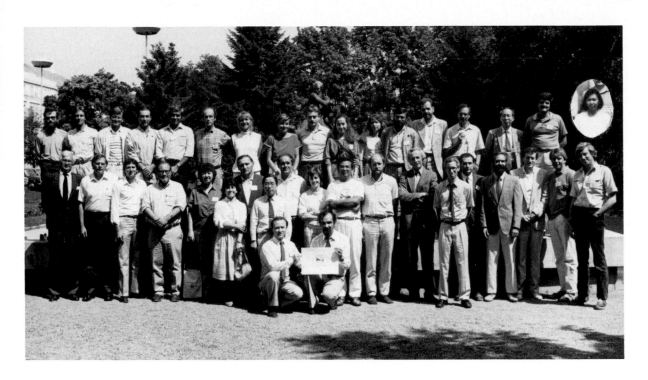

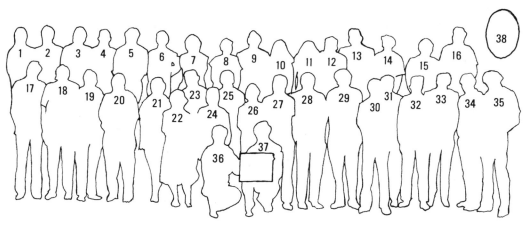

Upper row, in numerical sequence: **1** I.N. Pigarev, **2** C. Blakemore, **3** S. Molotchnikoff, **4** M. Ptito, **5** F. Leporé, **6** S. LeVay, **7** L. Krubitzer, **8** S. Bisti, **9** I. Bódis-Wollner, **10** E. Carvalho-Dias, **11** H. Sherk, **12** M. Sur, **13** I. Kappetér, **14** L. Maffei, **15** T. Bando, **16** W. McDaniel;
Lower row, **17** G.A. Orban, **18** M.J. Mustari, **19** B. Hutchins, **20** D. Bender, **21** C. Cusick, **22** R.E. Weller, **23** L.P. Simon, **24** T. Tsumoto, **25** J.P. Rauschecker, **26** M.-C. Wanet-Defalque, **27** M. Norita, **28** K.-P. Hoffman, **29** O.D. Creutzfeldt, **30** D.M. Berson, **31** S. Squatrito, **32** P.D. Spear, **33** B.E. Stein, **34** L.M. Chalupa, **35** P. Dean;
Bottom, **36** T.P. Hicks, **37** G. Benedek;
Inset, **38** J.A. Matsubara. *Missing from photo:* D. Emmans

List of Financial Supporters

Allergan Humphrey Canada, Ltd.
Aluép GT
Aluminiumszerkezetek Gyára
Bajai Épületasztalos és Faipari Vállalat
Bajai Lakberendezö, Épitö és Vas Ipari Szövetkezet
Chemical Works of Gedeon Richter Ltd., Budapest
Chemolimpex Hungarian Trading Co., Budapest
Csongrád m-i Tanácsi Épitöipari Vállalat
EGIS Pharmaceuticals, Budapest
High Oak Ranch Ltd., Ontario
Innisfree Electronics Ltd.
Kecskeméti Baromfifeldolgozó Vállalat, Szeged
Kendergép Leányvállalat, Szeged
Kiskunhalasi Baromfifeldolgozó Vállalat, Kiskunhalas
Malév, Hungarian Airlines
Medinvest Fövállalkozási Betéti Társaság, Szeged
Phylaxia Veterinary Biologicals Co., Budapest
Szegedi Kender és Müanyagfeldolgozó Vállalat
Szegedi Konzervgyár
Ujszegedi Szövöipari Vállalat, Szeged

Contents

T.P. Hicks and G. Benedek (Eds.)
Progress in Brain Research, Vol. 75
© 1988 Elsevier Science Publishers B.V. (Biomedical Division)

1

CHAPTER 1

Anatomical organization of the superior colliculus in monkeys: corticotectal pathways for visual and visuomotor functions

Catherine G. Cusick

Department of Anatomy, Tulane University Medical Center, 1430 Tulane Avenue, New Orleans, LA 70112, U.S.A.

Introduction

The superior colliculus has important links with systems for both visual perception and visuomotor functions. The anatomical basis for dual functions of the superior colliculus appears to lie in the well-documented connectional differences between the superficial and deep collicular compartments (see Huerta and Harting 1984; Kaas and Huerta 1987 for reviews). To date, most anatomical studies of the superior colliculus have concentrated on non-primates, in particular on cats. The goals of this paper are to discuss aspects of the anatomical organization of the superior colliculus in monkeys, and to attempt to relate dual collicular functions to afferents from cortical visual and visuomotor systems. New findings on visual corticotectal projections in squirrel monkeys will be presented.

Laminar organization of the superior colliculus: superficial and deep compartments

The usual layering scheme for the superior colliculus (Kanaseki and Sprague 1974) consists of alternating cell-dense and cell-poor layers, illustrated for a squirrel monkey in Fig. 1. The superficial layers (I – III) comprise, from superficial to deep, a thin, cell-poor stratum zonale (SZ), followed by a cellular layer about 300 μm thick, the stratum griseum superficiale (SGS), and finally an approximately 250 μm thick layer rich in fibers, the stratum opticum (SO). The superficial compartment of the superior colliculus is dominated by inputs from the retina and visual cortex (Wilson and Toyne 1970; Tigges and Tigges 1981). Its outputs, determined for macaque monkeys and squirrel monkeys, are primarily ascending to visual thalamic nuclei, the lateral geniculate nucleus and inferior and lateral pulvinar nuclei (Benevento and Fallon 1975; Benevento and Standage 1983; Harting et al. 1978, 1980; Huerta and Harting 1983). The superficial compartment thus appears to be concerned with the processing of visual information.

The deep compartment of the superior colliculus consists of the four remaining layers: an approximately 1 mm thick stratum griseum intermediale (SGI), followed by stratum album intermediale (SAI), and the two deep layers, stratum griseum profundum (SGP), and stratum album profundum (SAP). Although afferents of the deep compartment of the superior colliculus have not been completely studied in monkeys, these layers receive inputs from numerous sources within sensory and motor systems, including, for example, frontal, inferotemporal, somatosensory and auditory cortical areas (Fries 1984), the trigeminal and dorsal column nuclei, the inferior colliculus, ventral lateral geniculate nucleus, pretectum, substantia nigra, and mesencephalic and pontine reticular formations (see Kaas and Huerta 1987). The outputs of the deeper layers are similarly diverse, and include ascending projections to thalamic nuclei associated with control of eye movements and projecting to cortical oculomotor and polymodal areas, as well as descending projections to structures involved in controlling head and eye movements (see Harting 1977; Huerta and Harting 1984; Kaas and Huerta 1987). Thus, the deep collicular compartment appears to be concerned with visuomotor and polymodal functions.

Organization of extrastriate visual cortex in monkeys

Recent studies of visual cortex in primates have demonstrated the existence of a large number of extrastriate visual areas within the occipital and caudal temporal and parietal lobes. The most completely studied monkeys are Old World macaque monkeys and the New World owl monkey, and somewhat different schemes of organization have been proposed for these two groups (Kaas 1978; Van Essen 1985). In all primate species studied, three visual areas have been identified consistently:

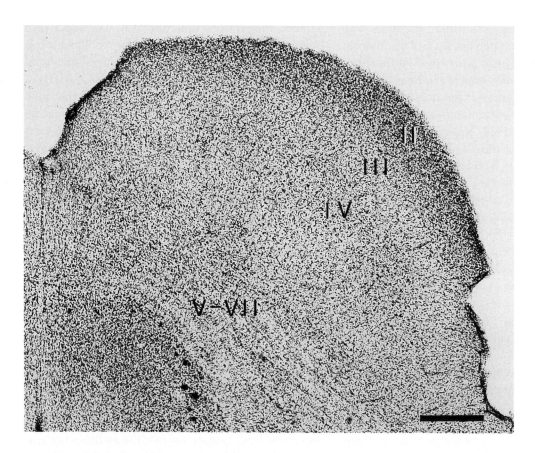

Fig. 1. Cytoarchitecture of the superior colliculus in a squirrel monkey. The collicular layers II – VII are indicated. Frontal section stained with cresyl violet. Medial is to the left. Scale = 0.5 mm.

area 17 (VI), VII (equivalent to area 18 in squirrel monkeys), and the middle temporal area, MT. The location of these areas on a lateral view of a squirrel monkey brain is shown in Fig. 2 (see Weller 1988, this volume). Although only VI and lateral VII have been mapped electrophysiologically in squirrel monkeys, it is highly probable that close homologies exist between owl monkeys and squirrel monkeys in the overall organization of visual areas, since they are both New World species (see Cusick et al. 1984). For this reason, we have adopted for squirrel monkeys the terminology used in studies of owl monkeys (Cusick 1987; Weller et al. 1987; Cusick and Kaas 1988). The dorsolateral area, DL, in squirrel monkeys thus includes cortex between MT rostrally and area 18 caudally (Fig. 2). The caudal half of this cortex occupies part of the region referred to as area 19 (Tigges et al. 1974, 1981). Cortical connections of VII are strong with the caudal portion of DL, DL_C, and minimal with the rostral portion of DL, DL_R (Tigges et al. 1974, 1981; Cusick 1987; Cusick and Kaas 1988; Fig. 2), supporting the concept that DL_R and DL_C are separate subdivisions within the dorsolateral area. DL_R has strong connections with a dorsomedial region of visual cortex that we refer to as the dorsal area, D (Weller et al. 1987; Cusick and Kaas 1988).

The visual cortex of monkeys appears to have segregated, in part, functions related to visual recognition and spatial localization. This view is supported by ablation studies in macaques, in which lesions in the inferior temporal lobe produce severe impairment on object recognition tasks, whereas lesions in the posterior parietal lobe produce impairments on a 'landmark' or visuospatial task. These results led to the proposal of 'two cortical visual systems,' one concerned with visuospatial tasks, and one with object vision (Ungerleider and Mishkin 1982; see Weller 1988, this volume). Visual information originating in area 17 is distributed along two major, multisynaptic corticocortical pathways, defined by terminations within the parietal or temporal lobes. Along the dorsal pathway, directed at parietal lobe areas, information is relayed from area 17 to MT, and from

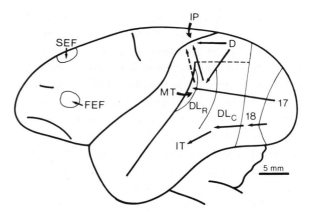

Fig. 2. Organization of cortical visual and visuomotor areas in squirrel monkeys. The arrows between areas indicate the flow of visual information from area 17 along separate pathways to the posterior parietal and inferotemporal cortex. Connections of DL_R and D appear mainly along pathways to parietal cortex (Cusick 1987; Weller et al. 1987). The dashed line between MT and IP indicates that the precise pathways between MT and parietal cortex are not known for squirrel monkeys. For further explanation, see text, and Weller (1988), this volume. D, dorsal area; DL_C, caudal dorsolateral area; DL_R, rostral dorsolateral area; FEF, frontal eye field; IP, intraparietal cortex; IT, inferotemporal cortex; MT, middle temporal area; SEF, supplementary eye field.

MT to the posterior parietal region. A further pathway involving a dorsal area, D, is available for transmission of information into the parietal lobe in squirrel monkeys (Cusick 1987; Weller et al. 1987). Along the ventral pathway directed towards the temporal lobe, information originating within area 17 is relayed to VII, from VII to DL (or V4 in macaque monkeys), and from DL or V4 to the caudal inferotemporal cortex, IT_C (Van Essen 1985; Weller and Kaas 1987; Weller 1988). The major pathways relaying visual information to the parietal and temporal lobes are illustrated in Fig. 2 for squirrel monkeys. Certain details in squirrel monkeys differ from the generally proposed scheme. For example, the precise relay from MT to the parietal lobe is not yet known for squirrel monkeys, and the relay from VII into the temporal lobe involves DL_C but not DL_R (Tigges et al. 1974; Cusick 1987).

In addition to visuosensory areas specialized for object vision and spatial analysis, a number of visuomotor areas have been identified in monkeys. Three eye movement-related areas are known: the traditional frontal eye field (FEF), posterior parietal cortex (postulated to be in the general location of intraparietal cortex, 'IP' in Fig. 2; area 7 in macaque monkeys), and the more recently identified supplementary eye field (SEF) that forms a rostral continuation of the supplementary motor area in macaques (Schlag and Schlag-Rey 1985, 1987), owl monkeys (Gould et al. 1986), and squirrel monkeys (Huerta et al. 1987). These areas are strongly interconnected with each other (Pandya and Kuypers 1969; Barbas and Mesulam 1981; Andersen et al. 1985; Huerta et al. 1987; Huerta and Kaas 1988). The FEF and IP areas project to the intermediate layers of the superior colliculus and have reciprocal connections with thalamic nuclei that are targets of deep collicular outputs (Lynch et al. 1985; Huerta et al. 1986; Asanuma et al. 1985).

Visual corticotectal pathways in monkeys

All visual areas identified in monkeys have been shown to project to the superior colliculus (Graham et al. 1979; Fries 1984). Corticotectal cells are found in layer V of all areas, and in layers V and VI of area 17 (Lund et al. 1975; Fries 1984). Most reports emphasize that visual areas of the occipital and caudal temporal and parietal lobes project to the superficial compartment of the superior colliculus. Projections from different areas distribute at different depths within the superficial layers, with area 17 and VII projections restricted to the outer portion of the superficial grey (Graham et al. 1979; Tigges and Tigges 1981; Graham 1982), and projections from MT extending through the complete depth of the SGS (Spatz and Tigges 1973; Graham et al. 1979; Ungerleider et al. 1984). In owl monkeys, the medial area (M), dorsomedial area (DM) and posterior parietal cortex (PP) all project to the deeper half of the SGS, with only DM involving the stratum opticum

(Graham et al. 1979). In squirrel monkeys, area 19 (or DL_C) also projects mainly to the deeper SGS (Tigges and Tigges 1981).

Thus, previous findings on laminar terminations suggest partial segregation of visual corticotectal pathways within the superficial grey. The apparent restriction of visual corticotectal projections to the superficial compartment is somewhat puzzling, however, in view of the visual responses within the deeper layers (Kadoya et al. 1971; Schiller and Koerner 1971; Cynader and Berman 1972; Wurtz and Goldberg 1972; Schiller et al. 1974; Updyke 1974; Mohler and Wurtz 1976; Mays and Sparks 1980) and the dependence of visual responses of the deeper layers on the visual cortex (Schiller et al. 1974). Visual input to the deeper layers may be conveyed from visuomotor areas, especially the frontal eye fields (e.g., Astruc 1971; Huerta et al. 1986; see also below for further refs.) and parietal areas (Lynch et al. 1985). However, for the frontal eye fields, only cells with movement-related activity, rather than strictly visual activity, appear to project to the superior colliculus (Segraves and Goldberg 1986).

In the present study, the sensitive anterograde anatomical tracer, wheat germ agglutinin conjugated to horseradish peroxidase (WGA-HRP), was injected into visual cortex in squirrel monkeys to demonstrate corticotectal projections from area 18 (VII; 3 cases: 2 single and one multiple-injection experiment), the caudal dorsolateral area, DL_C (3 experiments), the rostral dorsolateral area, DL_R (2 experiments), cortex near the DL_R/DL_C border (1 case) and the dorsal area, D (2 cases). Sections were cut parallel to the surface of flattened cortex and stained for HRP with tetramethyl benzidine (Mesulam 1978). Alternate sections were stained for cytochrome oxidase activity (Wong-Riley 1979) to identify architectonically the cortical areas injected. In one case, [^{3}H]proline was injected into DL_R, and the injection site and transported label were demonstrated autoradiographically (Cowan et al. 1972). The present results confirm the observations that occipital visual areas project to the superficial layers, and show in addition that each

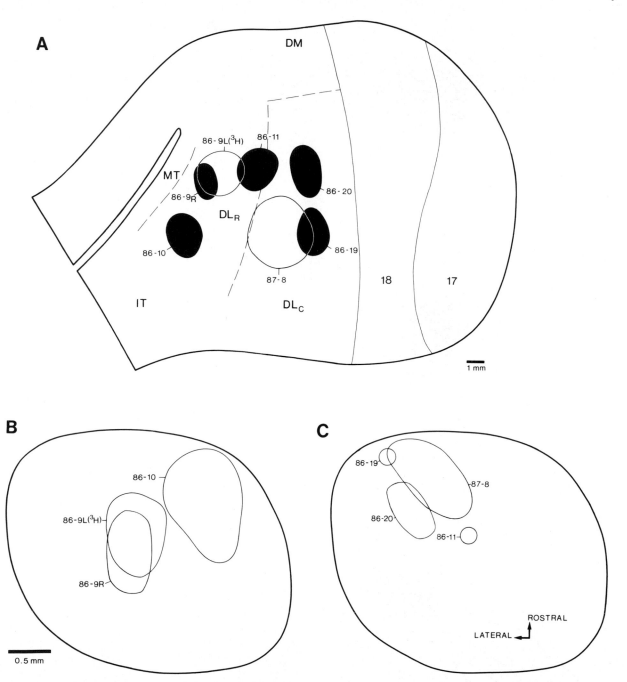

Fig. 3. Topographic patterns of corticotectal connections from DL_R and DL_C of squirrel monkeys. (A) Injection sites (black or open ovals) of WGA-HRP or [³H]proline are reconstructed onto a single tangential section of flattened cortex. (B) Dorsal view of the left superior colliculus showing labeled zones related to correspondingly numbered injections in DL_R. (C) Labeled zones related to injections in DL_C. Abbreviations as for Fig. 2. For (A), medial is toward the top and posterior to the right, and only the occipital and caudal temporal lobes are shown.

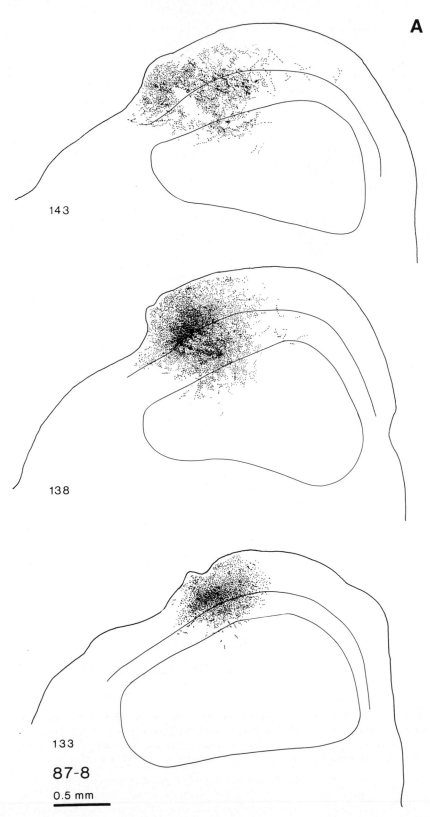

A

143

138

133

87-8

0.5 mm

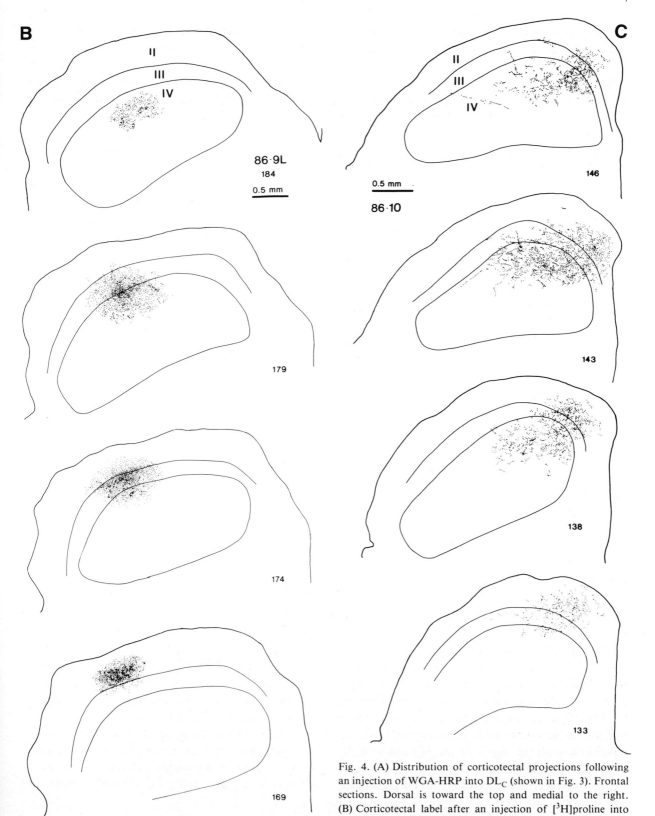

Fig. 4. (A) Distribution of corticotectal projections following an injection of WGA-HRP into DL_C (shown in Fig. 3). Frontal sections. Dorsal is toward the top and medial to the right. (B) Corticotectal label after an injection of [³H]proline into DL_R. (C) Corticotectal label from an injection of WGA-HRP within DL_R.

injected area provides at least a sparse input into the dorsal part of the intermediate grey layer.

Area 18 projections

In agreement with previous studies (Graham 1979; Tigges and Tigges 1981), fibers from area 18 distributed primarily in the outer half of the SGS. The SZ was relatively label-free. Numerous fibers occupied the SO, and a few fibers extended about 200 μm into the SGI.

Projections from the DL region

The injection sites of anatomical tracers within caudal and rostral DL are shown in Fig. 3A. As for all previous studies of visual corticotectal connections, the connections of DL_C and DL_R are organized topographically (Fig. 3B, C). The subdivisions DL_C and DL_R were defined initially, based on differences in cortical connections (Cusick 1987; Cusick and Kaas 1988). The corticotectal connections can be used to elucidate visual topography in DL_C and DL_R. Injection sites in DL_C presumed to be near central vision labeled, as expected, a rostrolateral part of the superior colliculus (cases 86-19, 87-8). More dorsally placed injections in cortex related to the lower visual quadrant produced label further into the lower field representation (case 86-20). Injection sites in DL_R labeled somewhat more peripheral visual field representations in the superior colliculus. Dorsal injections in DL_R labeled locations representing the lower field near the horizontal meridian (86-9R and L, and 86-11, near the DL_C/DL_R border), and a more ventral injection in DL_R labeled the paracentral upper field representation.

The laminar distribution of corticotectal label after injections in DL_C (Fig. 4A) was similar to that described previously by Tigges and Tigges (1981). The densest label was in the deeper half of the SGS. Sparser label extended into the outer SGS and did not involve the SZ. A few labeled fibers extended through the depth of the SO and into the outer 200 μm of the SGI.

The corticotectal projection from DL_R extended somewhat more deeply than the DL_C input (Fig. 4B and C). Again, the densest label was in the inner half of the SGS. Sparse label occupied the outer SGS, and the SO contained labeled fibers. The label in the SGI was generally denser than that seen following DL_C injections, and extended up to 500 μm from the lower border of the SO. SGI label in all cases was typically found in more rostral sections in locations directly below the SGS label. Thus, corticotectal projections occupied a radially aligned 'column' in the superficial layers and the outer SGI, providing a possible anatomical substrate for the alignment of the visual maps in the superficial and deep layers.

Projections from the dorsal area, D

Corticotectal projections were studied in 2 cases after injections that were largely within the dorsal area but which involved area 18 slightly. In both examples label occupied mainly the deeper part of the SGS and the SO and was less dense in the upper part of the SGS. Dense label also was in the upper SGI, directly below the superficial projection. In the case shown in Fig. 5, the projection extended mediolaterally for about 700 μm in the SGI compared with about 300 μm in the SGS.

Discussion: two visual corticotectal systems?

The 4 areas of visual cortex studied in squirrel monkeys project densely to the superficial compartment of the superior colliculus but also send a smaller component to the outer part of the deeper layers. The superficial and deep projections are in radial register, as are the visual maps in the superficial and deep compartments. In some cases, the deeper input was broader than the superficial, correlating with the larger visual receptive fields found in the deeper layers (Cynader and Berman 1972; Goldberg and Wurtz 1972). The laminar organization of visual corticotectal terminations is shown schematically in Fig. 6.

In squirrel monkeys, area 18 and DL_C are the two principal stations in the relay of information from area 17 to the caudal inferotemporal cortex (Tigges et al. 1974, 1981; Cusick 1987; Cusick and

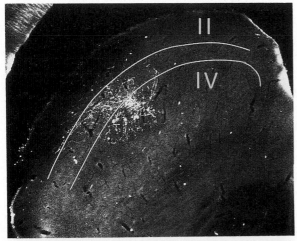
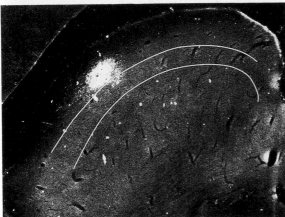
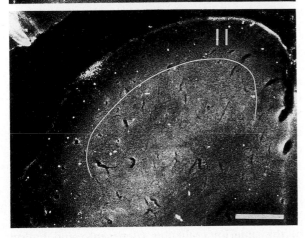

Fig. 5. Darkfield photomicrographs of corticotectal label after an injection of WGA-HRP into the dorsal area. Borders of the SO are indicated. Frontal sections spaced at 250 μm intervals, with the most rostral section at the top. Scale = 0.5 mm.

Kaas 1988). The first station, area 18, projects mainly to the outer SGS. Area 18 projections thus overlap the location of cell bodies in the superior colliculus projecting to both the dorsal lateral geniculate nucleus (in macaque and presumably also in squirrel monkeys; Benevento and Standage 1983) and the inferior and lateral pulvinar (Benevento and Standage 1983; Huerta and Harting 1983). DL_C terminations are mainly in the sublayer of the SGS projecting to the inferior and lateral pulvinar (as are projections from DL_R and D) (Huerta and Harting 1983).

For both area 18 and DL_C, fibers to the deeper layers are restricted to the upper 200 μm of the SGI. A minor projection to the deeper layers from

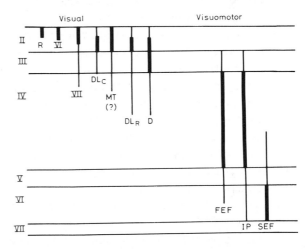

Fig. 6. Laminar depth of visual and visuomotor corticotectal projections in monkeys. The layers of the superior colliculus are shown at left. Sites of cortical projections are indicated as lines. Thicker lines indicate more dense projections, thinner lines, more sparse. Sparse input to layer IV from MT is based on Spatz and Tigges (1973) (for marmosets). The complete extents of projections (dense and sparse) shown for VII, DL_C, DL_R and D are based on the present report for squirrel monkeys. References for dense projections from visual cortex include: Graham et al. (1979) (areas VI, VII, and MT for owl monkeys); Tigges and Tigges (1981) (areas VI, VII, and 19 (or DL_C) and retinal input in squirrel monkeys); Graham (1982) (area 17 of macaque monkeys); and Ungerleider et al. (1984) (MT in macaque monkeys). The laminar extent of projections from visuomotor areas is based on Lynch et al. (1985) (FEF and IP cortex of macaque monkeys); Huerta et al. (1986) (FEF in owl, squirrel and macaque monkeys); and Huerta and Kaas (1988) (SEF in macaque monkeys). R = retina.

these areas is not surprising, in view of other anatomical evidence that area 18 and DL_C can participate in visuospatial or visuomotor processing. For example, both areas are interconnected with the frontal eye fields in squirrel monkeys (Tigges et al. 1981; Cusick and Kaas 1987; Cusick 1987). In addition, area 18 has direct connections with both MT and intraparietal cortex (Tigges et al. 1974, 1981; Cusick and Kaas 1987).

Both DL_R and D project to the deep collicular compartment and appear to terminate somewhat more deeply than area 18 and DL_C. Based on connections with parietal cortex, both DL_R and D appear to be stations for the relay of visuospatial information into the parietal lobe in squirrel monkeys (Cusick 1987; Weller et al. 1987). Thus, cortical areas along the dorsally projecting pathway may connect more strongly with deeper collicular layers than cortical areas along the pathway to inferotemporal cortex. Of course, data from more areas are needed to test this hypothesis, and critical information will come from studies of MT. Although a projection from MT terminating throughout the SGS (but mainly in the deeper half) has been described for owl monkeys (Graham et al. 1979) and macaque monkeys (Ungerleider et al. 1984), additional projections to the SGI have been described only in the New World marmoset (Spatz and Tigges 1973).

Interesting parallels to the present results can be found in the visual corticotectal pathways in cats. Areas 17, 18, and 19 in cats project mainly to the superficial compartment (Kawamura et al. 1974; Updyke 1977), but also send a small projection to the SGI (Kawamura et al. 1974). Lateral suprasylvian areas project both to the SGS and the intermediate gray (Kawamura et al. 1974; Segal and Beckstead 1984; Illing and Graybiel 1986). The dense projection to the superficial layers is sheet-like, while fibers to the SGI form patches that are not in register with the AChE-rich zones of the SGI (Illing and Graybiel 1986). Visual responses of neurons in the SGI are highly dependent on inputs from lateral suprasylvian cortex (Ogasawara et al. 1984). Illing and Graybiel (1986) suggest that single

lateral suprasylvian cortical fibers may project to both SGS and SGI in a column-like fashion, and could thus provide for the precise registry of the visual maps in the superficial and deep layers.

Corticotectal relations of temporal visual areas
The superior colliculus of macaque monkeys receives projections from a broad region of the temporal lobe that contains a number of functional subdivisions (Kuypers and Lawrence 1967; Fries 1984; Van Essen 1985). Inferotemporal cortex and areas within the superior temporal sulcus (STS) were labeled by HRP injections within the deeper layers of the superior colliculus (Fries 1984). Corticotectal projections from the inferotemporal and STS areas (with the exception of MT; Ungerleider et al. 1984) have not been studied with modern tracing techniques, and thus the precise laminar termination pattern is unknown. The information conveyed by caudal IT to the deeper layers of the superior colliculus is somewhat difficult to predict from the known physiological properties of the two regions. Neurons in IT show selectivity for stimulus form (Desimone et al. 1984), and the IT cortex appears to have an important role in analysis of visual patterns (Ungerleider and Mishkin 1982). Physiological studies of corticotectal cells in IT would be particularly interesting for revealing the contribution of IT to visuomotor functions of the superior colliculus.

The superior temporal polysensory area (STP) in macaques may be influenced by the outputs of the deep layers of the superior colliculus. Neurons in STP continue to respond to visual stimuli after striate cortex lesions, and visual responses in the contralateral hemifield are eliminated by lesions of the superior colliculus and striate cortex in the same hemisphere (Bruce et al. 1986). STP receives inputs from the medial pulvinar (Burton and Jones 1976), which is in turn a target of the deeper layers of the superior colliculus (Benevento and Fallon 1975; Harting et al. 1980; Benevento and Standage 1983). Thus, it seems reasonable to predict that STP would project most heavily to the deeper collicular layers and have a role in visuomotor functions as well as visual attention and orientation (see Bruce et al. 1986). Interestingly, STP also has strong connections with posterior parietal cortex (Mesulam et al. 1977), a region with important roles in visual attention and motor control (e.g. Mountcastle et al. 1975; Shibutani et al. 1984).

Visuomotor corticotectal projections

Frontal eye fields

The frontal eye fields, from which eye movements are evoked by low levels of electrical stimulation, have been identified in a range of primate species, including macaque monkeys (Ferrier 1875; Robinson and Fuchs 1969; Bruce et al. 1985), squirrel monkeys (Blum et al. 1982; Huerta et al. 1986), owl monkeys (Gould et al. 1986), and marmosets (Blum et al. 1982). The corticotectal projections of the frontal eye fields in macaque monkeys have been most extensively studied (Astruc 1971; Künzle et al. 1976; Künzle and Akert 1977; Leichnetz et al. 1981, 1986; Stanton et al. 1982; Komatsu and Suzuki 1985; Lynch et al. 1985; Huerta et al. 1986; Segraves and Goldberg 1986).

Recent efforts to define the frontal eye fields in macaque monkeys using microstimulation techniques (Bruce et al. 1985; Huerta et al. 1986) have demonstrated that the FEF occupies a restricted part of prearcuate cortex that has a variable relationship to surface landmarks. The greatest part of the FEF is located within the anterior bank of the arcuate sulcus. Studies of prearcuate corticotectal connections agree that the major terminations are in the SGI. The projection forms dense patches separated by small gaps with less label (Künzle et al. 1976; Lynch et al. 1985; Huerta et al. 1986). Descriptions of projections outside of the SGI vary in different studies (e.g. Künzle and Akert 1977; Lynch et al. 1985). In two studies that have reliably identified the location of the FEF by using microstimulation methods to define injection sites, projections were found to the SGI, with sparser inputs to the deep and superficial layers (Stanton et al. 1982; Huerta et al. 1986), as shown schematically in Fig. 6. The collicular projection

from physiologically identified frontal eye fields is topographically organized (Stanton et al. 1982; Komatsu and Suzuki 1985). Dorsomedial FEF sites that elicit large saccades project to the caudal superior colliculus where large saccades are represented, and the ventrolateral FEF, eliciting small saccades, projects to the rostrolateral SC, where small saccades are represented (Stanton et al. 1982).

Profound visuomotor deficits are produced by combined lesions of the frontal eye fields and superior colliculus, compared to the subtle deficits that follow destruction of either structure alone (Schiller et al. 1980). The frontal eye fields and superior colliculus thus form two channels for the control of visually guided eye movements. These channels are highly interconnected by the direct FEF corticotectal pathway and indirectly by many sets of visuomotor or oculomotor structures along the neuraxis (Huerta and Harting 1984; Huerta et al. 1986). For example, the deep layers of the superior colliculus project to several thalamic structures that connect with the frontal eye fields, especially the paralamellar mediodorsal nucleus and the magnocellular portion of the ventral anterior nucleus, VA_{mc} (Benevento and Fallon 1975; Harting et al. 1980; Barbas and Mesulam 1981; Stanton et al. 1982; Huerta et al. 1986). These nuclei are targets of the visuomotor-related lateral part of the substantia nigra pars reticulata (Carpenter et al. 1976; Ilinsky et al. 1985) that also projects to the deeper layers of the superior colliculus (Jayaraman et al. 1977; Beckstead et al. 1981). The deeper collicular layers and the frontal eye fields also have in common connections with the paracentral nucleus (PC), central lateral (CL), ventral lateral (VL), parafascicular, medial pulvinar, limitans, and suprageniculate nuclei (see Huerta et al. 1986, for review).

Projections from the SEF

The existence of an eye movement-related zone of cortex rostrally contiguous with the supplementary motor area has only recently been demonstrated in macaque monkeys, owl monkeys, and squirrel monkeys (Schlag and Schlag-Rey 1985, 1987; Gould et al. 1986; Huerta et al. 1987). The connections of this region have been examined in detail using microstimulation methods to identify the borders of SEF for restricting injections of anatomical tracers within this field. Corticotectal projections are mainly to the deep gray with sparser inputs to the intermediate gray (Huerta and Kaas 1988; shown diagrammatically in Fig. 6). The location of the SEF has major connections with the VA-VL complex of the thalamus, especially with VL_O and VL_M (Schell and Strick 1984). Interestingly, as for the FEF, connections exist with structures that receive inputs from the deeper layers of the superior colliculus, including paralamellar MD, PC, CL, and VA_{mc}.

Posterior parietal corticotectal relations

The inferior parietal lobule of macaque monkeys has been implicated in visuospatial functions, visual attention mechanisms, and visuomotor control (Hyvärinen and Poranen 1974; Mountcastle et al. 1975; Keating et al. 1983; Shibutani et al. 1984). However, the most studied part of this region, the convexity of the inferior parietal lobule, has at most sparse projections to the superior colliculus (Weber and Yin 1984; Lynch et al. 1985). Dense corticotectal projections arise instead from the inferior bank of the intraparietal sulcus and terminate densely within the intermediate and deep gray layers (Lynch et al. 1985). It is this sulcal cortex which has the stronger connections with the FEF (Barbas and Mesulam 1981; Andersen et al. 1985) and may have a greater role in oculomotor functions than the gyral cortex (Shibutani et al. 1984). The parietotectal pathway distributes more deeply within the superior colliculus compared to the pathway from the FEF (shown diagrammatically in Fig. 6; Lynch et al. 1985). Like the frontal eye field, posterior parietal cortex receives thalamic projections from targets of the deep layers of the superior colliculus, including the VA_{mc}, PC, CL, Pf, and suprageniculate-limitans complex (Kasdon and Jacobson 1978). Thus,

posterior parietal cortex may also share common functions with the deep collicular compartment.

Summary and conclusions

Evidence that occipital visual areas and visuomotor cortical areas in monkeys project to the superficial and deep compartments of the superior colliculus, respectively, was first found more than 20 years ago in a survey of corticotectal projections using silver degeneration techniques (Kuypers and Lawrence 1967). In this early study, an occipital projection to the upper portion of the SGI was recognized, in addition to the dense input to the superficial gray. Much progress has recently been made in our understanding of the numbers and interconnections of separate cortical areas, and more sensitive anatomical methods have permitted refinements in some of the observations on corticotectal projections. Thus, individual visual cortical areas project most densely to different depths within the SGS (Graham et al. 1979; Tigges and Tigges 1981). The present results show in addition that certain occipital visual areas in squirrel monkeys project to the upper portion of the SGI, the specific sublayer in which visual-motor interactions may occur within the deeper layers in macaque monkeys (Mohler and Wurtz 1976; Mays and Sparks 1980). Visual areas related to the 'dorsal' corticocortical pathway to the parietal lobe, DL_R and D, appear to project more strongly to the SGI than the 'ventrally-related' areas, DL_C and area 18. Projections of both posterior parietal and inferotemporal cortex appear to be mainly to the deeper layers, as are inputs from visuomotor areas of cortex. Thus, collicular visual and visuomotor compartments are closely linked with cortical perceptual and motor systems, respectively.

Acknowledgments

Supported by Biomedical Research Support Grant 2077R. Experiments on connections of the dorsal area were performed in collaboration with Dr. R.E. Weller. Drs. M.F. Huerta, B.V. Updyke,

R.E. Weller, and R.A. Hartwich-Young provided helpful comments on the manuscript. I thank Monique Gibson, Robin Palmer, and Cecily Stewart for technical assistance, and Debbie Lauff for typing the manuscript.

References

Andersen, R.A., Asanuma, C. and Cowan, W.M. (1985) Callosal and prefrontal associational projecting cell populations in area 7A of the macaque monkey: a study using retrogradely transported fluorescent dyes. *J. Comp. Neurol.,* 232: 443 – 455.

Asanuma, C., Andersen, R.A. and Cowan, W.M. (1985) The thalamic relations of the caudal inferior parietal lobule and the lateral prefrontal cortex in monkeys: divergent cortical projections from cell clusters in the medial pulvinar nucleus. *J. Comp. Neurol.,* 241: 357 – 381.

Astruc, J. (1971) Corticofugal connections of area 8 (frontal eye field) in *Macaca mulatta. Brain Res.,* 33: 241 – 256.

Barbas, H. and Mesulam, M.-M. (1981) Organization of afferent input to subdivisions of area 8 in the rhesus monkey. *J. Comp. Neurol.,* 200: 407 – 431.

Beckstead, R.M., Edwards, S.B. and Frankfurter, A. (1981) A comparison of the intranigral distribution of nigrotectal neurons labeled with horseradish peroxidase in the monkey, cat, and rat. *J. Neurosci.,* 1: 121 – 125.

Benevento, L.A. and Fallon, J.H. (1975) The ascending projection of the superior colliculus in the rhesus monkey. *J. Comp. Neurol.,* 160: 339 – 362.

Benevento, L.A. and Standage, G.P. (1983) The organization of projections of the retinorecipient and non-retinorecipient nuclei of the pretectal complex and layers of the superior colliculus to the lateral pulvinar and medial pulvinar in the macaque monkey. *J. Comp. Neurol.,* 217: 307 – 336.

Blum, B., Kulikowski, J.J., Carden, D. and Harwood, D. (1982) Eye movements induced by electrical stimulation of the frontal eye fields of marmosets and squirrel monkeys. *Brain Behav. Evol.,* 21: 34 – 41.

Bruce, C.J., Goldberg, M.E., Bushnell, M.C. and Stanton, G.B. (1985) Primate frontal eye fields. II. Physiological and anatomical correlates of electrically evoked eye movements. *J. Neurophysiol.,* 54: 714 – 734.

Bruce, C.J., Desimone, R. and Gross, C.G. (1986) Both striate cortex and superior colliculus contribute to visual properties of neurons in superior temporal polysensory area of macaque monkey. *J. Neurophysiol.,* 55: 1057 – 1075.

Burton, H. and Jones, E.G. (1976) The posterior thalamic region and its cortical projection in New World and Old World monkeys. *J. Comp. Neurol.,* 168: 249 – 302.

Carpenter, M.B., Nakano, N. and Kim, R. (1976) Nigrothalamic projections in the monkey demonstrated by autoradiographic technics. *J. Comp. Neurol.,* 165: 401 – 416.

Cowan, W.M., Gottlieb, D.I., Hendrickson, A.E., Price, T.E. and Woolsey, T.A. (1972) The autoradiographic demonstration of axonal connections in the central nervous system. *Brain Res.,* 37: 21 – 51.

Cusick, C.G. (1987) Evidence from patterns of cortical connections for subdivisions within the dorsolateral visual cortex of squirrel monkeys. *Neuroscience,* 22: S122.

Cusick, C.G. and Kaas, J.H. (1988) Cortical connections of area 18 and dorsolateral visual cortex in squirrel monkeys, *Visual Neurosci.,* in press.

Cusick, C.G., Gould, III, H.J. and Kaas, J.H. (1984) Interhemispheric connections of visual cortex in owl monkeys (*Aotus trivirgatus*), marmosets (*Callithrix jacchus*), and galagos (*Galago crassicaudatus*). *J. Comp. Neurol.,* 230: 311 – 336.

Cynader, M. and Berman, N. (1972) Receptive-field organization of monkey superior colliculus. *J. Neurophysiol.,* 35: 187 – 201.

Desimone, R., Albright, T.D., Gross, C.G. and Bruce, C. (1984) Stimulus selective properties of inferior temporal neurons in the macaque. *J. Neurosci.,* 4: 2051 – 2062.

Ferrier, D. (1875) Experiments on the brains of monkeys. No. 1. *Proc. R. Soc. Lond. (B),* 23: 409 – 430.

Fries, W. (1984) Cortical projections to the superior colliculus of the macaque monkey: a retrograde study using horseradish peroxidase. *J. Comp. Neurol.,* 230: 55 – 76.

Goldberg, M.E. and Wurtz, R.H. (1972) Activity of superior colliculus in behaving monkey. I. Visual receptive fields of single neurons. *J. Neurophysiol.,* 35: 542 – 559.

Graham, J. (1982) Some topographical connections of the striate cortex with subcortical structures in *Macaca fascicularis. Exp. Brain Res.,* 47: 1 – 14.

Graham, J., Lin, C.-S. and Kaas, J.H. (1979) Subcortical projections of six visual cortical areas in the owl monkey, *Aotus trivirgatus. J. Comp. Neurol.,* 187: 557 – 580.

Gould, III, H.J., Cusick, C.G., Pons, T.P. and Kaas, J.H. (1986) The relationship of corpus callosum connections to electrical stimulation maps of motor, supplementary motor, and the frontal eye fields in owl monkeys. *J. Comp. Neurol.,* 247: 297 – 325.

Harting, J.K. (1977) Descending pathways from the superior colliculus: an autoradiographic analysis in the rhesus monkey. *J. Comp. Neurol.,* 173: 583 – 612.

Harting, J.K., Casagrande, V.A. and Weber, J.T. (1978) The projection of the primate superior colliculus upon the dorsal lateral geniculate nucleus: autoradiographic demonstration of interlaminar distribution of tectogeniculate axons. *Brain Res.,* 150: 593 – 599.

Harting, J.K., Huerta, M.F., Frankfurter, A.J., Strominger, N.L. and Royce, G.T. (1980) Ascending pathways from the monkey superior colliculus: an autoradiographic analysis. *J. Comp. Neurol.,* 192: 853 – 882.

14

Huerta, M.F. and Harting, J.K. (1983) Sublamination within the superficial gray layer of the squirrel monkey: an analysis of the tectopulvinar projection using anterograde and retrograde transport methods. *Brain Res.*, 261: 119 – 126.

Huerta, M.F. and Harting, J.K. (1984) The mammalian superior colliculus: studies of its morphology and connections. In: H. Vanegas (Ed.), *Comparative Neurology of the Optic Tectum,* Plenum Press, New York, pp. 687 – 783.

Huerta, M.F. and Kaas, J.H. (1988) Connections of the Supplementary Eye Field (SEF) in macaque monkeys. *Soc. Neurosci. Abstr.,* 14, in press.

Huerta, M.F., Krubitzer, L.A. and Kaas, J.H. (1986) The frontal eye field as defined by intracortical microstimulation in squirrel monkeys, owl monkeys, and macaque monkeys. I. Subcortical connections. *J. Comp. Neurol.,* 253: 415 – 439.

Huerta, M.F., Krubitzer, L.A. and Kaas, J.H. (1987) The frontal eye field as defined by intracortical microstimulation in squirrel monkeys, owl monkeys, and macaque monkeys. II. Cortical connections. *J. Comp. Neurol.,* 265: 332 – 361.

Hyvärinen, J. and Poranen, A. (1974) Function of the parietal associative area 7 as revealed from cellular discharges in alert monkeys. *Brain,* 97: 673 – 692.

Ilinsky, I.A., Jouandet, M.L. and Goldman-Rakic, P.S. (1985) Organization of the nigrothalamocortical system in the rhesus monkey. *J. Comp. Neurol.,* 236: 315 – 330.

Illing, R.B. and Graybiel, A.M. (1986) Complementary and non-matching afferent compartments in the cat's superior colliculus: innervation of the acetylcholinesterase-poor domain of the intermediate gray layer. *Neuroscience,* 18: 373 – 394.

Jayaraman, A., Batton, R.R. and Carpenter, M.B. (1977) Nigrotectal projections in the monkey: an autoradiographic study. *Brain Res.,* 135: 147 – 152.

Kaas, J.H. (1978) The organization of visual cortex in primates. In: C.R. Noback (Ed.), *Sensory Systems of Primates,* Plenum Press, New York, pp. 151 – 179.

Kaas, J.H. and Huerta, M.F. (1987) The subcortical visual system of primates. *Adv. Primatol.,* in press.

Kadoya, S., Wolin, L.R. and Massopust, Jr., L.C. (1971) Photically evoked unit activity in the tectum opticum of the squirrel monkey. *J. Comp. Neurol.,* 142: 495 – 508.

Kasdon, D.L. and Jacobson, S. (1978) The thalamic afferents to the inferior parietal lobule of the rhesus monkey. *J. Comp. Neurol.,* 177: 685 – 706.

Kawamura, S., Sprague, J.M. and Niimi, K. (1974) Corticofugal projection from the visual cortices to the thalamus, pretectum and superior colliculus in the cat. *J. Comp. Neurol.,* 158: 339 – 362.

Keating, E.G., Grooley, S.G., Pratt, S.E. and Kelsey, J.E. (1983) Removing the superior colliculus silences eye movements normally evoked from stimulation of the parietal and occipital eye fields. *Brain Res.,* 269: 145 – 148.

Komatsu, H. and Suzuki, H. (1985) Projections from the functional subdivisions of the frontal eye field to the superior col-

liculus in the monkey. *Brain Res.,* 327: 324 – 327.

Künzle, H. and Akert, K. (1977) Efferent connections of cortical area 8 (frontal eye field) in *Macaca fascicularis.* A reinvestigation using the autoradiographic technique. *J. Comp. Neurol.,* 173: 147 – 164.

Künzle, H., Akert, K. and Wurtz, R.H. (1976) Projection of area 8 (frontal eye field) to superior colliculus in the monkey. An autoradiographic study. *Brain Res.,* 117: 487 – 492.

Kuypers, H.G.J.M. and Lawrence, D.G. (1967) Cortical projections to the red nucleus and the brainstem in the rhesus monkey. *Brain Res.,* 4: 151 – 188.

Leichnetz, G.R., Spencer, R.F., Hardy, S.G.P. and Astruc, J. (1981) The prefrontal corticotectal projection in the monkey: an anterograde and retrograde horseradish peroxidase study. *Neuroscience,* 6: 1023 – 1041.

Lund, J.S., Lund, R.D., Hendrickson, A.E., Bunt, A.H. and Fuchs, A.F. (1975) The origin of efferent pathways from the primary visual cortex, area 17, of the macaque monkey as shown by retrograde transport of horseradish peroxidase. *J. Comp. Neurol.,* 164: 287 – 304.

Lynch, J.C., Graybiel, A.M. and Lobeck, L.J. (1985) The differential projection of two cytoarchitectonic subregions of the inferior parietal lobule of macaque upon the deep layers of the superior colliculus. *J. Comp. Neurol.,* 235: 241 – 254.

Mays, L.E. and Sparks, D.L. (1980) Dissociation of visual and saccade-related responses in superior colliculus neurons. *J. Neurophysiol.,* 43: 207 – 232.

Mesulam, M.-M. (1978) Tetramethylbenzidine for horseradish peroxidase neurohistochemistry: a non-carcinogenic blue reaction-product with superior sensitivity for visualizing neural afferents and efferents. *J. Histochem. Cytochem.,* 26: 106 – 117.

Mesulam, M.-M., Van Hoesen, G.W., Pandya, D.N. and Geschwind, N. (1977) Limbic and sensory connections of the inferior parietal lobule (area PG) in the rhesus monkey: a study with a new method for horseradish peroxidase histochemistry. *Brain Res.,* 136: 393 – 414.

Mohler, C.W. and Wurtz, R.H. (1976) Organization of monkey superior colliculus: Intermediate layer cells discharging before eye movements. *J. Neurophysiol.,* 39: 722 – 744.

Mountcastle, V.B., Lynch, J.C., Georgopoulos, A., Sakata, H. and Acuna, C. (1975) Posterior parietal association cortex of the monkey: command functions for operations within extrapersonal space. *J. Neurophysiol.,* 38: 871 – 908.

Ogasawara, K., McAffie, J.G. and Stein, B.E. (1984) Two visual corticotectal systems in cat. *J. Neurophysiol.,* 52: 1226 – 1245.

Pandya, D.N. and Kuypers, H.G.J.M. (1969) Cortico-cortical connections in the rhesus monkey. *Brain Res.,* 13: 13 – 36.

Robinson, D.A. and Fuchs, A.F. (1969) Eye movements evoked by stimulation of the frontal eye fields. *J. Neurophysiol.,* 32: 637 – 648.

Schell, G.R. and Strick, P.L. (1984) The origin of thalamic inputs to the arcuate premotor and supplementary motor areas. *J. Neurosci.*, 4: 539 – 560.

Schiller, P.H. and Koerner, F. (1971) Discharge characteristics of single units in the superior colliculus of the alert rhesus monkey. *J. Neurophysiol.*, 34: 920 – 936.

Schiller, P.H., Stryker, M.P., Cynader, M. and Berman, N. (1974) Response characteristics of single cells in the monkey superior colliculus following ablation or cooling of visual cortex. *J. Neurophysiol.*, 37: 181 – 194.

Schiller, P.H., True, S.D. and Conway, J.L. (1979) Paired stimulation of the frontal eye fields and the superior colliculus of the rhesus monkey. *Brain Res.*, 179: 162 – 164.

Schlag, J. and Schlag-Rey, M. (1985) Unit activity related to spontaneous saccades in frontal dorsomedial cortex of monkey. *Exp. Brain Res.*, 58: 208 – 211.

Schlag, J. and Schlag-Rey, M. (1987) Evidence for a supplementary eye field. *J. Neurophysiol.*, 57: 179 – 200.

Segal, R.L. and Beckstead, R.M. (1984) The lateral suprasylvian corticotectal projection in cats. *J. Comp. Neurol.*, 225: 259 – 275.

Segraves, M.A. and Goldberg, M.E. (1985) Functional properties of tectal projection neurons in the monkey frontal eye field. *Soc. Neurosci. Abstr.*, 11: 472.

Shibutani, H., Sakata, H. and Hyvärinen, J. (1984) Saccade and blinking evoked by microstimulation of the posterior parietal association cortex of the monkey. *Exp. Brain Res.*, 55: 1 – 8.

Spatz, W.B. and Tigges, J. (1973) Studies on the visual area MT in primates. II. Projection fibers to subcortical structures. *Brain Res.*, 61: 374 – 378.

Stanton, G.B., Bruce, C.J. and Goldberg, M.E. (1982) Organization of subcortical projections from saccadic eye movement sites in the macaque's frontal eye fields. *Soc. Neurosci. Abstr.*, 8: 293.

Tigges, J. and Tigges, M. (1981) Distribution of retinofugal and corticofugal axon terminals in the superior colliculus of squirrel monkey. *Invest. Ophthalmol. Visual Sci.*, 20: 149 – 158.

Tigges, J., Spatz, W.B. and Tigges, M. (1974) Efferent corticocortical fiber connections of area 18 in the squirrel monkey (*Saimiri*). *J. Comp. Neurol.*, 158: 219 – 236.

Tigges, J., Tigges, M., Anschel, S., Cross, N.A., Letbetter, W.D. and McBride, R.L. (1981) Areal and laminar distribution of neurons interconnecting the central visual cortical areas 17, 18, 19, and MT in squirrel monkey (*Saimiri*). *J. Comp. Neurol.*, 202: 539 – 560.

Ungerleider, L.G., Desimone, R., Galkin, T.W. and Mishkin, M. (1984) Subcortical projections of area MT in the macaque. *J. Comp. Neurol.*, 223: 368 – 385.

Ungerleider, L.G. and M. Mishkin (1982) Two cortical visual systems. In: Ingle et al. (Eds.), *Analysis of Visual Behaviour,* MIT Press, Cambridge, MA, pp. 549 – 586.

Updyke, B.V. (1974) Characteristics of unit responses in superior colliculus of the *Cebus* monkey. *J. Neurophysiol.*, 37: 896 – 909.

Updyke, B.V. (1977) Topographic organizations of the projections from cortical areas 17, 18 and 19 onto the thalamus, pretectum and superior colliculus in the cat. *J. Comp. Neurol.*, 173: 81 – 122.

Van Essen, D.C. (1985) Functional organization of primate visual cortex. In: A. Peters and E.G. Jones (Eds.), *Cerebral Cortex, Vol. 3,* pp. 259 – 329.

Weber, J.T. and Yin, T.C.T. (1984) Subcortical projections of the inferior parietal cortex (area 7) in the stump-tailed monkey. *J. Comp. Neurol.*, 224: 206 – 230.

Weller, R.E. (1988) Two cortical visual systems in Old World and New World primates. In: T.P. Hicks and G. Benedek (Eds.), *Progress in Brain Research, Vol. 75,* ch. 27, Elsevier Science Publishers, Amsterdam, pp. 293 – 306.

Weller, R.E. and Kaas, J.H. (1987) Subdivisions and connections of inferior temporal cortex in owl monkeys. *J. Comp. Neurol.*, 256: 137 – 172.

Weller, R.E., Steele, G. and Cusick, C.G. (1987) Cortical connections of a dorsal visual area in squirrel monkeys. *Soc. Neurosci. Abstr.*, 13, 626.

Wiesendanger, R. and Wiesendanger, M. (1985) The thalamic connections with medial area 6 (supplementary motor cortex) in the monkey (*Macaca fascicularis*). *Exp. Brain Res.*, 59: 91 – 104.

Wilson, M.E. and Toyne, M.J. (1970) Retino-tectal and cortico-tectal projections in *Macaca mulatta. Brain Res.*, 24: 395 – 406.

Wong-Riley, M.T.T. (1979) Changes in the visual system of monocularly sutured or enucleated cats demonstrable with cytochrome oxidase histochemistry. *Brain Res.*, 171: 11 – 28.

Wurtz, R.H. and Goldberg, M.E. (1972) Activity of superior colliculus in behaving monkey. III. Cells discharging before eye movements. *J. Neurophysiol.*, 35: 575 – 586.

T.P. Hicks and G. Benedek (Eds.)
Progress in Brain Research, Vol. 75
© 1988 Elsevier Science Publishers B.V. (Biomedical Division)

CHAPTER 2

Retinal and cortical inputs to cat superior colliculus: composition, convergence and laminar specificity

David M. Berson

Section of Neurobiology, Division of Biology and Medicine, Brown University, Providence, RI 02912, U.S.A.

The extreme diversity of tectofugal efferent projections implies a multiplicity of functional roles for the superior colliculus, including visual guidance of eye and head movements and transmission of visual signals to the extrastriate cortex. Many of these functions may be subserved by more or less distinct collicular subsystems: major colliculofugal pathways arise from largely separate sets of tectal output neurons, distinguishable in part by their characteristic laminar distributions. These output pathways are under afferent control exerted by a bewildering array of visual structures, the most prominent being the retina and visual cortex. Both the retino- and corticotectal projections exhibit substantial heterogeneity in their areal origins, morphologies and visual response properties. The key to understanding the functional significance of such heterogeneity is probably to be found in its relation to the efferent organization of the colliculus, because individual components of these afferent projections, like the major classes of efferent cells, exhibit distinctive laminar distributions. In principle, such an arrangement could permit each class of collicular output neuron to sample a unique subset of inputs from the afferent array, thereby assembling a characteristic output signal matched to the requirements of its target structure.

Whether this represents a valid model of collicular input-output relations has yet to be fully tested. What is required is a detailed accounting of the functional properties of visual afferents terminating in individual collicular sublayers, and of the response properties and output projections of collicular cells with which these afferents make synaptic contact. To date, the most comprehensive evidence of this sort is available in the cat, for which we have arguably the most complete understanding of ganglion-cell typology and visual cortical organization. In a landmark study, Hoffmann (1973) provided the first detailed view of the functional composition of retino- and corticotectal influences on cells of the cat's colliculus. From the latencies of collicular unit responses evoked electrically at several points in the optic pathway, he determined the conduction velocities, and therefrom the functional composition, of retinotectal afferents. He detected two major components of the direct retinotectal projection: a 'fast-direct' pathway originating in retinal Y cells, and a 'slow-direct' pathway arising from W cells. (He detected no input from X cells, a major contributor to the retinogeniculate projection.) The two components of the retinocollicular pathway appeared to drive separate populations of collicular cells differing in their laminar distribution: those driven by the 'W direct' pathway predominated throughout the superficial layers, while a smaller number excited by the 'Y direct' input occupied the deepest part of the superficial gray layer (SGS) and stratum opticum. Hoffmann identified a third afferent pathway which was mediated by the fast axons of Y cells, but which drove collicular cells at paradoxically long latencies, presumably reflecting a polysynaptic influence. He provided evidence that this 'Y indirect' pathway was relayed to the colliculus by the corticotectal projections of complex cells in area 17.

Hoffmann's pioneering observations on the superficial layers prompted a number of questions that have formed the primary focus of my research over the past few years. First, might a similar experimental approach be used to clarify the nature of visual control over the deep collicular layers? Second, in view of what we know now to be a very heterogeneous W cell population, can the functional composition of the W direct pathway be specified more precisely? Do all subclasses of W cells contribute to the projection, or only a few? Finally, what is the nature of retino- and corticotectal convergence? Does Y indirect corticotectal influence reach only cells driven by direct Y cell input or does it also affect W direct cells? In this chapter, I briefly review recent findings concerning these questions and their implications for collicular physiology.

Composition of visual input to deep collicular layers

The visual responsiveness of neurons in the superficial layers (stratum opticum and above) have traditionally been contrasted with the polysensory and preoculomotor behavior of cells of the deeper layers (intermediate gray and below). But many deeper-layer cells exhibit frank visual responses or visual gating of presaccadic discharges (for review see Sparks 1986). The origin of such visual influence has been unclear in the absence of compelling evidence for direct synaptic input to the deep layers from the retina, visual cortex or superficial collicular layers.

I found that under ketamine anesthesia most cells of the deeper collicular layers could be activated by electrical stimulation of retinofugal fibers (Berson and McIlwain 1982). This allowed

me to use conduction-velocity analysis to identify the retinal origin of such visual influence, just as Hoffmann had done for the superficial layers. The results suggested that deep-layer cells were influenced by both of the Y cell pathways that Hoffmann had identified superficially.

About a third of deep-layer cells appeared to receive direct excitatory input from retinal Y cells. Like Y direct cells of the superficial layers, these neurons responded at extremely short latencies to stimulation of retinofugal fibers and exhibited small latency differences (Fig. 1A – C). There is little doubt that at least some of this rapid retinal activation is mediated by monosynaptic inputs from retinal Y cell afferents. Some of these direct synaptic contacts may occur upon dendritic processes of deeper-layer cells arborizing in the deep SGS or stratum opticum, the main terminal zone of Y cell afferents (Hoffmann 1973; Itoh et al. 1981). Other contacts are probably made in the deeper layers themselves which are now known to receive at least weak direct retinal projections (Beckstead and Frankfurter 1983).

A far larger proportion of deep-layer cells (at least 75%) were driven indirectly by Y cell input (Fig. 1A – C). Like their superficial-layer counterparts, these cells exhibited very small latency differences and paradoxically long absolute latencies; many received convergent input from the Y direct pathway. In light of Hoffmann's evidence for cortical mediation of the Y in direct influence, these results suggested strongly that the visual cortex exerted a profound excitatory influence on the deep collicular layers. This hypothesis was supported by evidence that extensive ablation of the visual cortex, including areas 17, 18, 19, and the lateral suprasylvian (LS) areas, virtually eliminated Y indirect driving of deep-layer cells. In addition, intracortical stimulation in areas 17, 18, 19 and LS activated many cells of the deep layers, and at latencies suggesting at least some monosynaptic input. Both the direct and indirect Y cell pathways drove deep-layer cells with descending efferent axons (Fig. 1D, E), suggesting that these visual signals could play a role in the control of gaze.

W cell input to the superficial gray layer

The dominance of the cat's retinotectal projection by W cells has been amply confirmed (Hoffmann 1973; Cleland and Levick 1974a,b; Fukuda and Stone 1974; McIlwain 1978; Wässle and Illing 1980; Itoh et al. 1981; Ogawa and Takahashi 1981; Freeman and Singer 1983; Leventhal et al. 1985; Crabtree et al. 1986; Stanford 1987), but its significance for collicular visual function has been obscured by the extreme heterogeneity within the W cell class. There are at least seven functional subtypes of W cells, exhibiting wide variation in visual response properties (Cleland and Levick 1974a,b; Stone and Fukuda 1974a). Do these subtypes contribute equally to the W direct input to

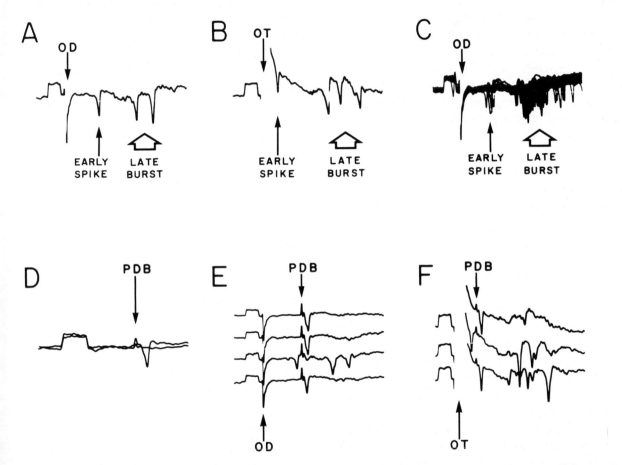

Fig. 1. Convergent direct and indirect Y cell inputs to an output cell of the intermediate gray layer of the cat's superior colliculus. (A) Shock to contralateral optic disk (OD) evokes short-latency action potential ('early spike') and longer latency burst. (B) Early spike and late burst evoked by shock to ipsilateral optic tract (OT). Extremely small shift in latency of these responses as compared with those in A (about 1 ms) reflect their mediation by rapidly conducting Y cell axons. Short latency of early spike suggests monosynaptic Y cell input to this cell ('Y direct' pathway); longer latency of late burst indicates polysynaptic ('Y indirect') activation. (C) Variable latency of early spike, as shown by multiple superimposed traces, confirms that the Y direct input is synaptically mediated. (D – F) Demonstration of descending efferent projections of same cell by antidromic activation from the predorsal bundle (PDB). (D) All-or-none nature of antidromic spike evoked by near-threshold shock of PDB. (E,F) Collision of antidromic spike with orthodromic spikes elicited from the optic disk (E) or optic tract (F). Square wave calibration pulses at beginning of each trace: +200 μV, 1 ms. Reproduced from Berson and McIlwain (1982) with permission.

the colliculus? The anatomy of the retinotectal projection provides a partial answer because the response properties of W cells tend to be correlated with their soma size and pattern of decussation at the optic chiasm (Fukuda and Stone 1974; Stone and Fukuda 1974b; Kirk et al. 1976; Rowe and Stone 1977; Stanford 1987). The main collicular target of W cell input is the 'upper SGS', a thin lamina occupying the upper $50-100$ μm of the superficial gray layer (Graybiel 1975; Harting and Guillery 1976; Behan 1982a; Freeman and Singer 1983). Retinal input to the upper SGS is almost exclusively crossed, and appears to arise from ganglion cells that are exceedingly small, even for presumed W cells (Graybiel 1975; Harting and Guillery 1976; McIlwain 1978; Wässle and Illing 1980; Itoh et al. 1981; Stanford 1987). Thus, preliminary indications are that a subset of W cell receptive-field types may supply most of the W direct input to the colliculus.

Because the receptive-field properties of W cells are also correlated with their axonal conduction velocities (Cleland and Levick 1974a,b; Stone and Fukuda 1974a; Stanford 1987), I reasoned that a detailed conduction-velocity analysis of retinotectal afferents might provide further clues to the functional composition of the W direct pathway. Ideally, such an analysis would employ direct recordings from W cell afferents to the colliculus. The small caliber of W cell terminal arbors makes this impractical, but one can do nearly as well by exploiting a unitary extracellular potential unique to the upper SGS that provides an index of the activity of single W cell afferents. McIlwain (1978), who discovered and termed it the juxtazonal potential (JZP), showed that it results when an action potential invades a single retinal afferent terminal arbor in the upper SGS, triggering synchronous EPSPs in postsynaptic collicular neurons.

I have used three methods to estimate the conduction velocities of W cell afferents mediating the JZPs (Berson 1987b). In each, weak shocks to the optic disk, chiasm or tract evoked single, isolated JZPs. When the same JZP could be evoked in

isolation from two sites, I was able to estimate the conduction velocity of the axon mediating it by dividing the JZP's latency difference into the distance between the stimulating electrodes (Fig. 2). For many JZPs, I used a collision method to determine the conduction velocity. A conditioning shock to the more central of two stimulus sites caused the JZP evoked from the peripheral site to fail in an all-or-none manner. The failure indicated that the conditioning shock had exceeded the spike threshold of the axon mediating the JZP, eliciting an antidromic action potential which collided with the orthodromic spike initiated at the peripheral site. Assessments of the critical interval for producing such a collision, of the axon's refractory period, and of the interelectrode separation, permitted estimation of the axon's conduction velocity. In a third approach, conduction velocities were

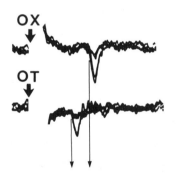

LATENCY DIFFERENCE: 2.4 ms

50 μV

2 ms

Fig. 2. Evidence for extremely slowly conducting W cell innervation of the upper SGS. Traces show electrically evoked responses of a single unitary juxtazonal potential (JZP) recorded in the upper superficial gray layer. Near-threshold stimulation of the optic chiasm (OX; upper trace) evoked the JZP about half the time in all-or-none fashion, and in two of the four superimposed records shown. Same JZP was evoked at a shorter latency from the optic tract (OT; lower trace). Dividing the difference in latency (2.4 ms) into the conduction distance between the stimulating electrodes (13.5 mm) yielded an estimated conduction velocity of 5.6 m/s for the retinal axon triggering this potential. Reproduced from Berson (1987b) with permission.

estimated by dividing the absolute latency of unitary JZPs, minus an estimate of synaptic delay, into the conduction distance from stimulus to recording site.

Regardless of the method used, retinal afferents triggering JZPs proved to have among the most slowly conducting axons of all W cells. The estimates for individual axons ranged from 1.9 to 6.8 m/s, with means of about 3 – 5 m/s, depending on the method. This may be compared with the conduction velocities of W cells overall, which range from roughly 1 to 20 m/s and average about 9 m/s (Cleland and Levick 1974a,b; Stone and Fukuda 1974a). These results suggest strongly that a subset of retinal W cells distinguished by slow axonal conduction velocities innervates the upper SGS and triggers JZPs. These W cells probably respond phasically to standing contrast in their receptive fields, because such 'phasic W cells' are far more slowly conducting on average than the 'tonic W cells' (Cleland and Levick 1974a,b; Stone and Fukuda 1974a; Rowe and Stone 1977; but see Stanford 1987). This inference is supported by evidence that the retinal input to the upper SGS originates predominantly in very small ganglion cells of the contralateral retina, including its temporal half (Stone and Keens 1980; Stone et al. 1980; Wässle and Illing 1980; Itoh et al. 1981; Stanford 1987), because phasic W cells are thought to have smaller somas and to decussate more completely at the optic chiasm than the tonic subtypes (Kirk et al. 1976; Rowe and Stone 1977; Stone and Keens 1980; Stanford 1987). The phasic subclass of W cells ('W2' subgroup of Rowe and Stone (1977)) is itself quite heterogeneous functionally, with respect to preferred sign of center contrast (ON-, OFF- or ON/OFF) and direction selectivity. Ongoing retinal recordings may help to identify which of these subtypes innervate the upper SGS.

Retinal afferents generating JZPs probably constitute only one component of W cell input to the colliculus. At least some W cells with relatively large somas, fast axons, ipsilateral projections and tonic responses to standing contrast apparently innervate the colliculus (Cleland and Levick 1974a,b;

Fukuda and Stone 1974; Stone and Keens 1980; Wässle and Illing 1980; Freeman and Singer 1983). Current source-density and anatomical studies suggest that faster, ipsilateral W cell input terminates predominantly below the upper SGS (Graybiel 1975; Harting and Guillery 1976; Behan 1982b; Freeman and Singer 1983). Substantial input from such cells to the upper SGS seems unlikely in view of the properties of the JZPs, but cannot be excluded.

Though the W direct pathway is thus probably not strictly homogeneous, I now have reason to believe it is dominated by the slowly conducting phasic W cells that innervate the upper SGS. Careful measurements of the activation latencies of collicular W direct cells have shown nearly all of

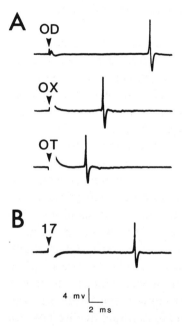

Fig. 3. Convergence of retinal W cell and corticotectal input to a neuron of the superficial gray layer. (A) Responses evoked by electrical stimulation of the contralateral optic disk (OD), optic chiasm (OX) and optic tract (OT). Stimuli were many times threshold and responses shown represent minimum latencies of activation. Differences between the latencies of these evoked responses yielded conduction-velocity estimates ranging from 3.4 to 5.2 m/s for the retinal afferents driving this unit. Such slow conduction velocities are typical of the very slowly conducting retinal W cells innervating the upper SGS and triggering the juxtazonal potentials.

them to be driven by extremely slowly conducting W cell axons (Fig. 3A). This is despite the fact that in making such measurements I have used stimuli many times threshold and minimum activation latencies, thus biasing the observations in favor of detecting faster inputs. (The intense stimuli proved necessary because response latency often dropped dramatically as the intensity of near-threshold stimuli was increased, apparently reflecting spatiotemporal convergence of multiple W cell afferents. This rendered the conduction velocity estimates very sensitive to the stimulus parameters used. Use of suprathreshold shocks yielded good agreement among the various estimates obtained for single cells from multiple latency-difference values.)

Laminar specificity of corticotectal input

Hoffmann's observations led him to propose that the polysynaptic Y cell input he detected reached the colliculus by way of complex cells in the striate cortex. Subsequent studies have repeatedly confirmed that the corticotectal output of area 17 (and 18) is driven by the Y cell stream (e.g., Singer et al. 1975; Schiller et al. 1979; Harvey 1980), but there are reasons to question whether the striate cortex alone is responsible for the Y indirect activation of collicular cells. For instance, corticotectal afferents from the striate cortex terminate predominantly in the upper half of the SGS (Kawamura et al. 1974; Updyke 1977; Mize 1983; Behan 1984), where collicular neurons exhibit W direct, not Y indirect input (Berson, in preparation). The failure to observe Y indirect input in this stratum is probably not attributable to masking by direct W cell input because Y indirect activation generally precedes direct W cell activation of collicular cells (Hoffmann 1973). Nor does it appear to be an anesthetic effect: regardless of whether ketamine or barbiturate anesthesia is used, I have never observed Y indirect activation of collicular cells in the upper 400 μm of the superficial layers. Paradoxically, cells driven by the Y indirect pathway are frequently encountered in the stratum opticum and in-

termediate gray layer (Berson and McIlwain 1982), laminae with little direct input from the striate cortex. Such discrepancies have prompted me to reexamine the origin of the Y indirect pathway and the nature of corticotectal influence on the upper SGS.

The striate cortex gives rise to but one of the many parallel corticotectal projections from the areas of the parieto-occipital cortex. These projections terminate within progressively deeper tiers of the colliculus as one moves out from the striate cortex (e.g., Kawamura et al. 1974), and in this sense the extrastriate cortex seemed to me a more likely source than the striate cortex of Y indirect influence on the stratum opticum and deeper collicular layers. Making the case for such a role hinged in part on identifying corticotectal cells in the extrastriate areas that, like those in areas 17 and 18, were driven by Y cell signals. In this respect, the posteromedial lateral suprasylvian area (PMLS) seemed a particularly good candidate, since it was known to receive afferent projections directly from geniculate laminae containing Y cells, as well as from areas 17 and 18 (see Berson (1985) for references). By analyzing afferent conduction velocities, I found that most cells in PMLS, including corticotectal cells, were driven indirectly by geniculate Y cells. The conduction times through this pathway from geniculate Y cells through PMLS to the colliculus were consistent with the view that it contributed to the polysynaptic Y cell activation of collicular cells (Berson and McIlwain 1983; Berson 1985). This idea is also supported by evidence that the lateral suprasylvian region projects heavily to the deep SGS, stratum opticum and intermediate gray (Segal and Beckstead 1983), where Y indirect driving is common. Moreover, inactivation of the lateral suprasylvian region alters or abolishes the visual responsiveness of many deep layer cells while inactivation of the striate cortex seems to affect only the superficial layers (Ogasawara et al. 1984). Taken together, these data suggest that much of the Y indirect influence on the superior colliculus, especially its deeper layers, may be derived from the lateral suprasylvian region or other extrastriate areas rather than from the striate cortex.

But if this is so, which collicular cells receive input from area 17? The failure of collicular W direct cells to exhibit Y indirect influence might be interpreted to mean that such cells lack input from the visual cortex. This idea is lent some credence by the partial complementarity in the laminar and topographic distributions of afferents from the retina and striate cortex (Updyke 1977; Mize 1983). On the other hand, the idea of a strict segregation is difficult to credit: corticotectal in-

puts from areas 17, 18 and 19 terminate most heavily in laminae where W direct cells predominate (Kawamura et al. 1974; Updyke 1977; Behan 1984) and are reported to drive most cells of the superficial gray (McIlwain 1977). To test directly for convergence of corticotectal and retinal W cell input to single collicular cells, I have examined the responses of identified W direct cells to intracortical stimulation of area 17 (Berson 1987a). The great majority of W direct cells are driven readily from the striate cortex (Fig. 3B). Whether this activation reflects direct inputs from

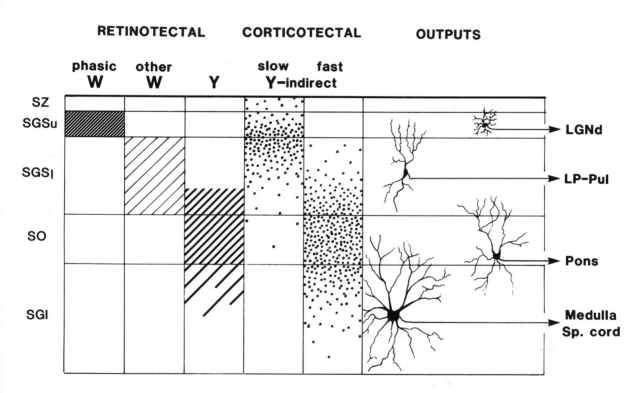

Fig. 4. Schematic diagram summarizing proposed laminar organization of some inputs and outputs of the cat's superior colliculus, as outlined in text. Major components of retinotectal projection include crossed inputs to the upper SGS (SGSu) from very slowly conducting, presumably phasic W cells; and bilateral inputs to the deep SGS, stratum opticum (SO) and stratum griseum intermediale (SGI) from retinal Y cells. More rapidly conducting W cells and a few X cells probably contribute to the projection, perhaps terminating in the lower SGS (SGSl). At least two functional components contribute to the corticotectal projection. A long-latency ('slow') pathway may originate partly in the striate cortex. A shorter-latency ('fast') pathway probably originates largely in the extrastriate cortex, including LS. Both presumably convey polysynaptic Y cell signals, but only the fast pathway mediates the overt Y indirect activation described by Hoffmann (1973). Cells in the upper half of the SGS are driven by convergent input from phasic W cells and the slow corticotectal path; some probably project to the lateral posterior-pulvinar complex (LP-Pul) and dorsal lateral geniculate nucleus (LGNd). Cells in the SO and SGI are driven by convergent input from the direct Y cell and fast Y indirect corticotectal paths; these presumably include tectopontine and tectobulbospinal neurons. SZ = stratum zonale.

cells in area 17 itself or an indirect pathway involving extrastriate corticotectal cells, the input almost certainly carries signals from the Y cell stream of the geniculocortical system. This may explain why experimental manipulations that affect the integrity of Y cell pathways alter the receptive field properties of W direct cells (Crabtree et al. 1986). But why, then, do W direct cells lack demonstrable Y indirect input in Hoffmann's paradigm? One possibility is that different sets of cortical neurons drive W direct cells and cells exhibiting frank Y indirect activation. The corticotectal output of area 17 is itself heterogeneous (Kawamura and Konno 1979; Weyand et al. 1986) and may differ functionally from that of the extrastriate areas. The geniculocorticotectal loop affecting W direct cells could be less responsive to electrical stimulation of primary retinal fibers than that mediating Y indirect activation; or it might involve longer conduction times so that its influence is masked by direct W cell activation. This latter possibility is supported by evidence that W direct cells are driven from the cortex at longer latencies than are cells with demonstrable Y indirect input (Fig. 3B; Berson 1987a).

Overview

The available data offer a number of refinements to the classical view of collicular afferent circuitry (Fig. 4). The direct retinocollicular projection consists primarily of Y and W cell components, as Hoffmann showed, but the W cell input is probably more specialized than appreciated previously. Most of the W cell input probably originates predominantly in one, or at most a few, subtypes of phasic W cell. These have very small somas, very slowly conducting axons, lie almost entirely in the contralateral retina and project to the upper 50–100 μm of the SGS. There appears to be a second, functionally distinct W cell component which terminates somewhat deeper in the SGS. Its functional identity is unclear, but it appears to have a substantial ipsilateral component and to be somewhat more rapidly conducting than the main

W direct pathway. Finally, there appears to be a weak X cell input of unknown laminar distribution (Sawai et al. 1985). The direct Y cell and slowly conducting W cell inputs appear to drive distinct sets of collicular neurons. Y cell axons ramify in the deep SGS, stratum opticum and intermediate gray, and drive cells within or just below these layers. Very slow W cell inputs drive most of the cells in the SGS, particularly its upper half. Collicular neurons driven by X cell or faster W cell input have not been unequivocally identified.

Descending cortical projections appear to exert profound excitatory influence over most collicular cells, regardless of their laminar position or source of retinal innervation. All such corticotectal influences probably convey polysynaptic Y cell signals, but only one component is overtly expressed in collicular cells as the Y indirect pathway identified by Hoffmann (1973). This component affects cells primarily in the deep SGS, stratum opticum and deeper laminae, where it converges with input from the Y direct pathway. It is mediated by a relatively fast corticotectal pathway that probably originates primarily in the extrastriate cortex, including the lateral suprasylvian areas. A slower corticotectal pathway, probably originating partly in the striate cortex, activates W direct cells in the upper half of the SGS.

An important goal for future work will be to specify how the output signals of individual collicular cell types are shaped by the admixtures of afferent information they receive. From what is currently known of the laminar origin of collicular efferents, it seems likely that tectal output signals to the visual thalamus will reflect the influence of the phasic W cell and slow corticotectal inputs described above. By contrast, descending collicular influences on the gaze control centers of the brainstem and spinal cord seem more likely to be shaped by direct Y cell and faster corticotectal inputs.

Acknowledgments

I am grateful to James T. McIlwain for advice and

support. Experiments described here were supported from one or more of the following sources: NIH grants EY05425 and EY06108 to the author; NIH grant EY02505 and a Grass Foundation Trustee Grant to J.T. McIlwain; and a Biomedical Research Support Grant PHS RR05664-18 to Brown University.

References

Beckstead, R.M. and Frankfurter, A. (1983) A direct projection from the retina to the intermediate gray layer of the superior colliculus demonstrated by anterograde transport of horseradish peroxidase in monkey, cat and rat. *Exp. Brain Res.*, 52: 261 – 268.

Behan, M. (1982a) Identification and distribution of retinocollicular terminals in the cat: an electronmicroscopic autoradiographic study. *J. Comp. Neurol.*, 199: 1 – 15.

Behan, M. (1982b) A quantitative analysis of the ipsilateral retinocollicular projection in the cat: an EM degeneration and EM autoradiographic study. *J. Comp. Neurol.*, 206: 253 – 258.

Behan, M. (1984) An EM-autoradiographic analysis of the projection from cortical areas 17, 18, and 19 to the superior colliculus in the cat. *J. Comp. Neurol.*, 225: 591 – 604.

Berson, D.M. (1982) Retinal Y-cell activation of deep-layer cells in superior colliculus of the cat. *J. Neurophysiol.*, 47: 700 – 714.

Berson, D.M. (1983) Visual cortical inputs to deep layers of cat's superior colliculus. *J. Neurophysiol.*, 50: 1143 – 1155.

Berson, D.M. (1985) Cat lateral suprasylvian cortex: Y-cell inputs and corticotectal projection. *J. Neurophysiol.*, 53: 544 – 556.

Berson, D.M. (1987a) Convergence of cortical and retinal W-cell input to cells of cat superior colliculus. *Soc. Neurosci. Abstr.*, 13, 1435.

Berson, D.M. (1987b) Retinal W-cell input to the upper superficial gray layer of the cat's superior colliculus: a conduction velocity analysis. *J. Neurophysiol.*, 58: 1035 – 1051.

Cleland, B.G. and Levick, W.R. (1974a) Brisk and sluggish concentrically organized ganglion cells in the cat's retina. *J. Physiol.*, 240: 421 – 456.

Cleland, B.G. and Levick, W.R. (1974b) Properties of rarely encountered types of ganglion cells in the cat's retina and an overall classification. *J. Physiol.*, 240: 457 – 492.

Crabtree, J.W., Spear, P.D., McCall, M.A., Jones, K.R. and Kornguth, S.E. (1986) Contributions of Y- and W-cell pathways to response properties of cat superior colliculus neurons: comparison of antibody- and deprivation-induced alterations. *J. Neurophysiol.*, 56: 1147 – 1156.

Freeman, B. and Singer, W. (1983) Direct and indirect visual inputs to superficial layers of cat superior colliculus: a current source-density analysis of electrically evoked potentials. *J. Neurophysiol.*, 49: 1075 – 1091.

Fukuda, Y. and Stone, J. (1974) Retinal distribution and central projections of Y-, X-, and W-cells of the cat's retina. *J. Neurophysiol.*, 37: 749 – 772.

Graybiel, A.M. (1975) Anatomical organization of retinotectal afferents in the cat: an autoradiographic study. *Brain Res.*, 96: 1 – 23.

Harting, J.K. and Guillery, R.W. (1976) Organization of retinocollicular pathways in the cat. *J. Comp. Neurol.*, 166: 133 – 144.

Harvey, A.R. (1980) A physiological analysis of subcortical and commissural projections of areas 17 and 18 of the cat. *J. Physiol.*, 302: 507 – 534.

Hoffmann, K.-P. (1973) Conduction velocity in pathways from retina to superior colliculus in the cat: a correlation with receptive-field properties. *J. Neurophysiol.*, 36: 409 – 424.

Itoh, K., Conley, M. and Diamond, I.T. (1981) Different distributions of large and small ganglion cells in the cat after HRP injections of single layers of the lateral geniculate body and the superior colliculus. *Brain Res.*, 207: 147 – 152.

Kawamura, K. and Konno, T. (1979) Various types of corticotectal neurons of cats as demonstrated by means of retrograde axonal transport of horseradish peroxidase. *Exp. Brain Res.*, 35: 161 – 175.

Kawamura, S., Sprague, J.M. and Niimi, K. (1974) Corticofugal projections from the visual cortices to the thalamus, pretectum and superior colliculus in the cat. *J. Comp. Neurol.*, 158: 339 – 362.

Kirk, D.L., Levick, W.R. and Cleland, B.G. (1976) The crossed or uncrossed destination of axons of sluggish-concentric and non-concentric cat retinal ganglion cells, with an overall synthesis of the visual field representation. *Vision Res.*, 16: 233 – 236.

Leventhal, A.G., Rodieck, R.W. and Dreher, B. (1985) Central projections of cat retinal ganglion cells. *J. Comp. Neurol.*, 237: 216 – 226.

McIlwain, J.T. (1977) Topographic organization and convergence in corticotectal projections from areas 17, 18, and 19 in the cat. *J. Neurophysiol.*, 40: 189 – 198.

McIlwain, J.T. (1978) Cat superior colliculus: Extracellular potentials related to W-cell synaptic actions. *J. Neurophysiol.*, 41: 1343 – 1358.

Mize, R.R. (1983) Patterns of convergence and divergence of retinal and cortical synaptic terminals in the cat superior colliculus. *Exp. Brain Res.*, 51: 88 – 96.

Ogasawara, K., McHaffie, J.G. and Stein, B.E. (1984) Two visual corticotectal systems in cat. *J. Neurophysiol.*, 52: 1226 – 1245.

Ogawa, T. and Takahashi, Y. (1981) Retinotectal connectivities within the superficial layers of the cat's superior colliculus. *Brain Res.*, 217: 1 – 11.

Rowe, M.H. and Stone, J. (1977) Naming of neurons:

classification and naming of cat retinal ganglion cells. *Brain Behav. Evol.,* 14: 185 – 216.

Sawai, H., Fukuda, Y. and Wakakuwa, K. (1985) Axonal projections of X-cells to the superior colliculus and to the nucleus of the optic tract in cats. *Brain Res.,* 341: 1 – 6.

Schiller, P.H., Malpeli, J.G. and Schein, S.J. (1979) Composition of geniculostriate input to superior colliculus of the rhesus monkey. *J. Neurophysiol.,* 42: 1124 – 1133.

Segal, R.L. and Beckstead, R.M. (1984) The lateral suprasylvian corticotectal projection in cats. *J. Comp. Neurol.,* 225: 259 – 275.

Singer, W., Tretter, F. and Cynader, M. (1975) Organization of cat striate cortex: a correlation of receptive-field properties with afferent and efferent connections. *J. Neurophysiol.,* 38: 1080 – 1098.

Sparks, D.L. (1986) Translation of sensory signals into commands for control of saccadic eye movements: role of primate superior colliculus. *Physiol. Rev.,* 66: 118 – 171.

Stanford, L.R. (1987) W-cells in the cat retina: correlated morphological and physiological evidence for two distinct classes. *J. Neurophysiol.,* 57: 218 – 244.

Sterling, P. (1973) Quantitative mapping with the electron microscope: retinal terminals in the superior colliculus. *Brain Res.,* 54: 347 – 354.

Stone, J. and Fukuda, Y. (1974a) Properties of cat retinal ganglion cells: a comparison of W-cells with X- and Y-cells. *J. Neurophysiol.,* 37: 722 – 748.

Stone, J. and Fukuda, Y. (1974b) The nasotemporal division of the cat's retina examined in terms of the Y-, X- and W-cells. *J. Comp. Neurol.,* 155: 377 – 394.

Stone, J. and Keens, J. (1980) Distribution of small and medium-sized ganglion cells in the cat's retina. *J. Comp. Neurol.,* 192: 235 – 246.

Stone, J., Leventhal, A.G., Watson, C.R.R., Keens, J. and Clarke, R. (1980) Gradients between nasal and temporal areas of the cat retina in the properties of retinal ganglion cells. *J. Comp. Neurol.,* 192: 219 – 233.

Updyke, B.V. (1977) Topographic organization of the projections from cortical areas 17, 18, and 19 onto the thalamus, pretectum, and superior colliculus in the cat. *J. Comp. Neurol.,* 173: 81 – 122.

Wässle, H. and Illing, R.-B. (1980) The retinal projection to the superior colliculus in the cat: a quantitative study with HRP. *J. Comp. Neurol.,* 190: 333 – 356.

Weyand, T.G., Malpeli, J.G., Lee, C. and Schwark, H.D. (1986) Cat area 17. IV. Two types of corticotectal cells defined by controlling geniculate inputs. *J. Neurophysiol.,* 56: 1102 – 1108.

T.P. Hicks and G. Benedek (Eds.)
Progress in Brain Research, Vol. 75
© 1988 Elsevier Science Publishers B.V. (Biomedical Division)

CHAPTER 3

Organisation of efferent projections from superior colliculus to brainstem in rat: evidence for functional output channels

Paul Dean, Peter Redgrave and Ian J. Mitchell

Department of Psychology, University of Sheffield, Sheffield S10 2TN, U.K.

Introduction

Because the superior colliculus receives direct visual input, and projects directly to premotor areas of the brainstem and spinal cord, it has been used as a preparation in which to study certain kinds of visuomotor transformation, i.e. to understand how visual input signals can be processed to produce appropriate motor output (for recent reviews see, e.g., Chalupa 1984; Schiller 1985; Sparks 1986). As these reviews make clear, the visual input to the superior colliculus has been investigated extensively with anatomical, electrophysiological, and behavioural techniques. Collicular outputs, however, have received less attention, so that important questions concerning the information that they carry have yet to be answered. Since understanding the nature of collicular output signals is a necessary part of understanding sensorimotor transforms within the superior colliculus, we have begun investigating the functional anatomy of collicular projections to the brainstem.

This work has been carried out on rats, an animal in which a very high proportion (probably > 90%) of retinal ganglion cells have collicular projections (Linden and Perry 1983; Dreher et al. 1985). In contrast, the dorsal lateral geniculate nucleus in rat receives a substantially smaller pro-

jection, variously estimated to arise from 20 to 50% of retinal ganglion cells (Linden and Perry 1983; Dreher et al. 1985; Martin 1986). This anatomical arrangement may underly the well-known behavioural observations that damage to the superior colliculus in rat (and similar animals such as hamsters) produces a very severe visual neglect (for recent review, see Dean and Redgrave 1984a,b,c). These effects of collicular damage in rat appear to be much more evident than those observed in, for example, rhesus monkeys (see, e.g., Schiller 1985), animals in which the retinal projection to the thalamus is about 9 times more extensive than that to the superior colliculus (Perry and Cowey 1984). Insofar as the superior colliculus in rats is less 'overshadowed' by the geniculostriate system than it is in primates, the rat may be a good preparation for investigating certain aspects of collicular function.

The original work on the neglect produced by damage to the superior colliculus in rodents was carried out by Schneider (summarised in Schneider 1969). His well-known conclusion was that the function of the superior colliculus was to produce orienting movements of the eyes and head to stimuli appearing outside the central visual field: the orienting movements would then bring the stimulus into the central field for analysis and identification by the geniculostriate system. The collicular and cortical visual projections can thus be thought of as constituting part of 'two visual systems', with the superior colliculus being specialised to produce a particular kind of response, namely orienting movements of the eyes and head.

This model offers a powerful guide for research on the functions of the efferent projections of the superior colliculus to the brainstem. However, our initial findings on the anatomy of these projections, described in the next section, raised some concern about whether the model was complete.

Organisation of descending projections from superior colliculus in rat

Previous investigations of the descending projections of the superior colliculus either had taken place before the arrival of modern tract-tracing techniques or had concentrated on the projection to a particular terminal area (for references, see Redgrave et al. 1987b). We therefore studied the overall organisation of these pathways using the orthograde transport of wheatgerm agglutinin conjugated with horseradish peroxidase (Redgrave et al. 1987b). As it turned out, this organisation appears very similar to that described in a number of other mammals, including cat and monkey: it is shown in schematic form in Fig. 1. There are two major descending pathways. One travels caudally and laterally to innervate target areas mainly in lateral midbrain and pons. The second projection travels ventrally and medially, crosses the midline in the dorsal tegmental decussation, then turns caudally to run in the predorsal bundle. From there it innervates a succession of targets mainly in medial pons and medulla, and eventually reaches the cervical spinal cord. It is sometimes called the tectospinal tract, although on account of its prominent projections to the medial brainstem reticular formation, a better term might be the tecto-reticulospinal (TRS) projection (cf. Grantyn and Berthoz 1985).

A puzzling feature of these projections, if their function is to mediate orienting movements of the head and eyes, is their extent. Why are there *two*

main projections? Why does each contact so many terminal areas? At first sight there seems to be a mismatch between the complexity of collicular efferents and the apparent simplicity of the response they are presumed to control.

A second puzzling feature of these projections is revealed by studies of their cells of origin within the superior colliculus. We used a retrograde double-labelling technique with the fluorescent tracers True Blue and Diamidino Yellow to examine the cells of origin of the crossed and uncrossed descending pathways (Redgrave et al.

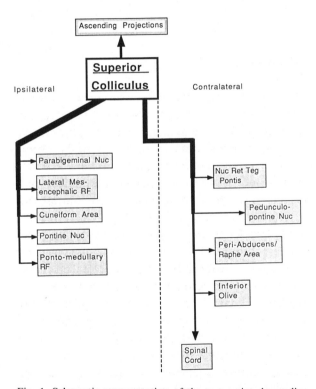

Fig. 1. Schematic representation of the two major descending projections of superior colliculus in rat, as shown by orthograde transport of WGA-HRP (Redgrave et al. 1987b). The ipsilateral projection, shown on the left of the dotted line representing midline, travels caudally, ventrally and laterally from the superior colliculus to innervate structures mainly in midbrain and pons (Nuc = nucleus; RF = reticular formation). The contralateral projection travels ventrally and medially to cross midline in the dorsal tegmental decussation, then turns caudally within the predorsal bundle to innervate structures throughout the brain stem, eventually reaching the cervical spinal cord (Nuc. Ret. Teg. Pontis = nucleus reticularis tegmenti pontis).

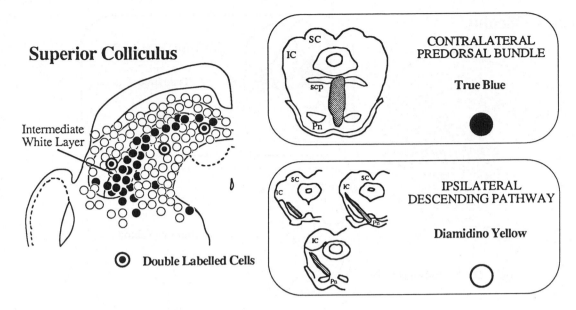

Fig. 2. Semi-schematic representation of retrograde labelling within left superior colliculus (coronal view) after injections of the fluorescent tracers True Blue into the right predorsal bundle, and Diamidino Yellow into the left brainstem. Adapted from Redgrave et al. (1986).

1986). Large injections of True Blue were made into the fibres of the predorsal bundle, together with even larger injections aimed at the midbrain and pontine terminal areas of the uncrossed projection. This procedure gave thousands of single-labelled cells in the superior colliculus (Fig. 2), but very few double-labelled cells. In fact, the cells of origin of the two pathways were segregated spatially from one another, with the majority of the cells that projected into the predorsal bundle lying in the lateral half of the intermediate white layer, where they were surrounded by cells in the deep and intermediate grey layers projecting into the uncrossed descending pathway.

Further studies have indicated that a similar organisation is also present within each of the two major descending collicular projections.

(i) Injections of fluorescent tracers into two of the major targets of the uncrossed descending pathway, namely basolateral pons and the cuneiform nucleus, again produce many single-labelled but very few double-labelled cells (Redgrave et al. 1987a: Fig. 3).

(ii) Preliminary data indicate that few double-labelled cells are found when the injection sites are in two targets of the crossed descending projection, namely the periabducens area, and the rostral spinal cord with adjacent caudal medulla (cf. Fig. 1).

These findings suggest that the brainstem projections in rat are organised at least in part as a collection of relatively independent output channels, each with distinct targets and cells of origin. Previous results from experiments using orthograde transport, or retrograde transport of single label have indicated that a similar arrangement is present in other animals, including garter snake, squirrel and cat (e.g., Edwards 1980; Holcombe and Hall 1981a,b; Harting and Huerta 1984; Dacey and Ulinski 1986), a range that suggests that anatomically distinct output channels to the brainstem may be a fundamental feature of vertebrate tectal anatomy. If so, it becomes very important to understand their functional significance.

One possibility is that individual output chan-

Superior Colliculus

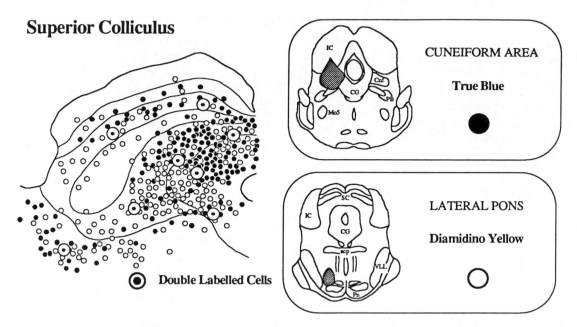

Fig. 3. Representative coronal section through superior colliculus, illustrating the retrograde labelling seen after injections of the fluorescent tracers True Blue into the cuneiform nucleus and surrounding area, and Diamidino Yellow into the basolateral pons. Labelled cells are located mainly in the deep layers ventral to the intermediate white layer (Fig. 2). Adapted from Redgrave et al. (1987a).

nels mediate functionally distinct responses. Although this would seem to be the obvious reason for having independent output channels, it is not clear how it would fit with the idea that the superior colliculus mediates only orienting responses. In the next section, therefore, we consider evidence that the superior colliculus is involved in a wider range of responses to visual stimuli than orienting movements of the eyes and head.

Functions of superior colliculus: evidence from ablation and stimulation studies

We have argued in detail elsewhere (Dean and Redgrave 1984a) that the effects of removing the superior colliculus, at any rate in rats and hamsters, are not confined to orienting movements. At least three other classes of response are affected.

(i) Normal animals stop what they are doing (e.g., running to a target, sucking a tube for milk) when an appropriate novel visual stimulus is presented. This interruption of current behaviour

can be abolished completely by collicular damage (e.g., Goodale and Murison 1975; Overton et al. 1985).

(ii) In some circumstances, unexpected visual stimuli cause rats and hamsters to freeze or flee — appropriate responses for small animals with many predators. These visually evoked defensive responses may also be impaired or abolished by lesions of the superior colliculus (e.g. Goodale and Murison 1975; Merker 1980).

(iii) Novel visual stimuli are capable of producing a variety of autonomic responses in rats as in people. These responses include desynchronisation of the cortical EEG and changes in heart-rate and blood pressure and their function is probably to prepare the organism for subsequent action. The effects of collicular damage have been examined so far only for one of the autonomic responses, namely desynchronisation of the cortical EEG by intense flashes of light. Once again, removal of the superior colliculus almost abolished light-induced arousal of the cortical EEG (Dean et al. 1984).

The effects of stimulating the superior colliculus in rats are consistent with these findings. We have conducted an extensive series of mapping studies using both chemical and electrical stimulation, and have found that sites within the superior colliculus can give not only movements of the head and body resembling orienting responses (Sahibzada et al. 1986; Dean et al. 1987a; cf. McHaffie and Stein 1982), but also each of the classes of response affected by collicular ablation. Specifically, we have obtained interruption of ongoing exploratory behaviour (Dean et al. 1988a): prolonged freezing (Redgrave et al. 1981; Dean et al. 1987a,b); movements resembling avoidance and flight (Redgrave et al. 1981; Sahibzada et al. 1986; Dean et al. 1988b): desynchronisation of the cortical EEG (Redgrave and Dean 1985); and changes in blood pressure and heart rate (Keay et al. 1986, 1987).

These two sets of behavioural data indicate that the rat superior colliculus is capable of mediating a large number of the responses appropriate to unexpected visual stimuli (Fig. 4; cf. Dean and Redgrave 1984b,c), and provide a possible functional role for the anatomically distinct output channels described in the previous section. The next question, therefore, is whether there is any evidence that different output channels in fact mediate different responses.

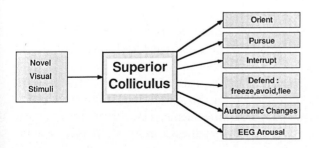

Fig. 4. Summary diagram of data from ablation and stimulation experiments, which suggests that the superior colliculus can mediate a wide range of responses, both somatomotor and autonomic, appropriate to novel visual stimuli.

Evidence for functional output channels

We have investigated the roles of two brainstem projections in the head and body movements mediated by the rat superior colliculus. The projections are (i) the crossed tectoreticulospinal (TRS) projection (Figs. 1 and 2), and (ii) that part of the uncrossed descending projection that terminates in the cuneiform nucleus, immediately ventral to the inferior colliculus (Figs. 1 and 3). Three kinds of behavioural experiment were carried out: (i) stimulation in the vicinity of a pathway's collicular cells of origin; (ii) stimulation of the pathway itself or its terminal area; and (iii) collicular stimulation after the projection had been interrupted. We hoped that these three kinds of experiment would constitute a set of convergent operations, inasmuch as the uncertainties of inference associated with any one of them could be reduced by results from the other two. We describe their application first to the crossed descending pathway, and secondly to the cuneiform nucleus.

Studies of the crossed tectoreticulospinal system

Stimulation within superior colliculus

As outlined above, electrical or chemical stimulation of the superior colliculus gives a variety of head and body movements. Some of these are directed contralaterally; given the organisation of spatial maps within the colliculus (reviewed in, e.g., Chalupa 1984; Schiller 1985), such contralateral movements resemble orienting or approach responses. Other movements resemble defensive responses, including retreat from a contralateral stimulus, freezing, or violent escape (Redgrave et al. 1981; Sahibzada et al. 1986; Dean et al. 1988b).

Because the cells of origin of the crossed descending pathway are concentrated mainly within the lateral half of the intermediate white layer (Fig. 2), it is possible to use the results of systematic mapping studies to ask whether particular movements are likely to be mediated by that pathway. The relevant information is whether those movements are observed after stimulation at sites in or close to lateral intermediate white layer.

Data from a number of studies suggest that these sites produce little if any defensive responding, but rather contralaterally directed movements of the eyes, head and body (McHaffie and Stein 1982; Kilpatrick et al. 1982; Sahibzada et al. 1986; Dean et al. 1988a,b). In addition, there is some evidence that only a particular type of contralateral head movement may be mediated by cells in the lateral part of the intermediate white layer. Stimulation of this region with the cell excitant glutamate produces head movements with a downward component, often accompanied by contralateral circling movements of the body (Dean et al. 1988a). The animal seems to be *pursuing* a stimulus that continues to move away from the midline, a resemblance often heightened by the appearance of sniffing or (if the stimulant is a GABA-blocker or antagonist) biting movements (Redgrave et al. 1981; Kilpatrick et al. 1982) appropriate to the pursuit of prey. In contrast, the contralateral head movements produced by stimulation of other tectal sites often have an upward component, and are not accompanied by circling.

Stimulation of the predorsal bundle

Electrical stimulation of the predorsal bundle produces ipsilateral head movements and circling (consistent with the collicular projection having a crossed midline). The circling is sufficiently reliable that it has been used as the dependent measure in experiments to investigate current spread during electrical stimulation of nervous tissue (Miliaresis and Philippe 1984; Yeomans et al. 1984). Electrophysiological evidence suggests that part of the substrate for this circling is formed by axons running from the contralateral superior colliculus (Tehovnik and Yeomans 1986).

Effects of section of the dorsal tegmental decussation

We have examined the effects on head and body movements elicited either by direct electrical stimulation of the superior colliculus, or by visual and tactile stimuli, of interrupting the contralateral TRS projection as it crosses the midline in the dorsal tegmental decussation (Dean et al. 1986). The lesions were verified by approximately placed injections of retrograde tracer within the predorsal bundle to show that cells in the contralateral intermediate white layer were no longer labelled. The results for electrically elicited responses were as follows.

(i) Thresholds for movements resembling avoidance or escape were little affected.

(ii) Contralateral circling movements were almost abolished.

(iii) Contralateral head movements were not abolished: indeed, the movements obtained at low currents seemed not to be affected at all unless the lesions caused substantial incidental damage. There was some suggestion that the very short latency head movements obtained with higher currents were impaired.

(iv) In addition, the initial orienting head movement to a visual or tactile stimulus was apparently unaffected. However, subsequent exploration of that stimulus was curtailed and inaccurate.

These results are in reasonable agreement with the stimulation data from intact animals. Taken together, they suggest that the crossed TRS pathway plays little if any role in defence-like head and body movements, but does mediate a particular subset of contralaterally-directed head and body movements (see below).

Studies of the tectocuneiform projection

Stimulation within the superior colliculus

The cells of origin of the tectal projection to the cuneiform nucleus are less clearly segregated than the cells of origin of the TRS pathway (Figs. 2 and 3). It may be for this reason that stimulation in the medial part of the deep layers, where they are most concentrated, produces a number of different responses.

(i) Contralateral head movements can be obtained from this area, with both electrical (Sahibzada et al. 1986) and chemical stimulation (Dean et al.

1988a). These are associated with circling and downward head movements when electricity is used: glutamate, however, gives sustained postures or discontinuous movements, both with an upward component. We have not resolved these differences, but one obvious possibility is that the electrical effects are mediated by fibres of passage.

(ii) It has also proved possible to obtain defence-like responses from the medial deep layers. These are rather varied, whichever form of stimulation used, and include prolonged freezing, ipsilateral movements of the body and locomotion, and finally very rapid running and jumping (Sahibzada et al. 1986; Dean et al. 1988b).

Stimulation within the cuneiform nucleus

In contrast to the somewhat confusing results of the previous section, stimulation within the cuneiform area itself produced clear effects. Injections of glutamate initially gave freezing; then, if the injections were repeated, very fast running resembling escape was observed (Mitchell et al. 1987). There appeared to be no clear directional component, i.e. no systematic contralateral head movement, and no systematic sideways cringing or shying. It is as if a particular subset of the animal's defensive repertoire was selectively activated.

Lesions of cuneiform nucleus

Preliminary studies of large bilateral lesions of the cuneiform nucleus that also damaged surrounding structures such as the inferior colliculus suggested that they had no effect on orienting or approach responses whether elicited by natural stimuli or by electrical or chemical stimulation of the superior colliculus. In contrast, escape-like responses to collicular injection of the GABA-antagonist bicuculline appeared to be abolished.

The results of these preliminary lesion studies are thus consistent with the data obtained from stimulating the cuneiform nucleus in suggesting that the tectocuneiform projection is involved in some aspect of defensive behaviour, but is unlikely to be involved in tectally-mediated orientation or approach.

Evidence for functional output channels – conclusions

Equivalent manipulations of the crossed TRS and of the mainly uncrossed tectocuneiform pathways have sharply contrasting effects on behaviour (Fig. 5). Stimulating the TRS pathway produces contralateral circling, whereas stimulating the cuneiform nucleus gives freezing or strong running.

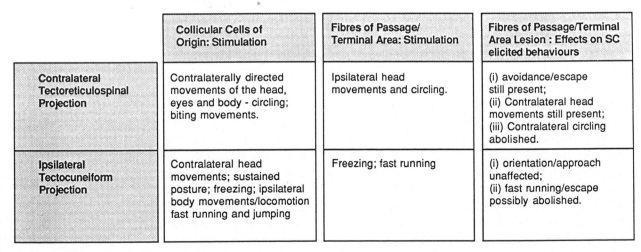

	Collicular Cells of Origin: Stimulation	Fibres of Passage/ Terminal Area: Stimulation	Fibres of Passage/Terminal Area Lesion : Effects on SC elicited behaviours
Contralateral Tectoreticulospinal Projection	Contralaterally directed movements of the head, eyes and body - circling; biting movements.	Ipsilateral head movements and circling.	(i) avoidance/escape still present; (ii) Contralateral head movements still present; (iii) Contralateral circling abolished.
Ipsilateral Tectocuneiform Projection	Contralateral head movements; sustained posture; freezing; ipsilateral body movements/locomotion fast running and jumping	Freezing; fast running	(i) orientation/approach unaffected; (ii) fast running/escape possibly abolished.

Fig. 5. Summary of behavioural data obtained by stimulating or interrupting (i) the contralateral tectoreticulospinal projections, and (ii) the (predominantly) ipsilateral tectocuneiform projection.

Damaging the TRS projection interferes with a quite different set of tectally-elicited movements than does ablation of the cuneiform nucleus. These results are consistent with the two collicular projections having distinct functions.

At present those functions cannot be specified precisely, though the data raise some intriguing possibilities. The observation that the TRS projection is involved in some kinds of head movement but not others invites a conjecture, as far as we are aware not made previously, that the superior colliculus mediates more than one functional class of contralaterally directed movement. What might these be? A priori considerations suggest that two different kinds of control information are needed for a general 'orienting' system (Dean et al. 1986). (a) To cope with very transient stimuli, which disappear before the movement can be completed or even initiated, the system needs to remember the position of the stimulus. Since no sensory feedback is available in this situation, the response has been referred to as open-loop orienting. (b) In contrast, variably moving stimuli can only be accurately oriented to and pursued by use of sensory feedback. The behavioural data raise the possibility that the crossed descending pathway may be more concerned with the second kind of control than the first. A system concerned with sensorily-guided following or pursuit might be expected to give continuous movements (e.g., circling) when stimulated rather than particular postures. The effects of its interruption would be felt on pursuit and exploration rather than on initial orienting. We have argued (Dean et al. 1986) that this view is consistent with electrophysiological data on predorsal bundle cells in cat (e.g., Berthoz et al. 1986).

But whether this particular conjecture concerning the precise function of the TRS projection proves to be correct or not, the currently available data indicate that this function must be very different from that of the tectocuneiform projection. The data therefore support the intuitively appealing idea that projections from the superior colliculus to the brainstem that are anatomically distinct, are functionally distinct also. In the final section, we briefly discuss the implications of this idea for future investigations of collicular function.

Functional output channels – implications

The existence of functionally distinct output channels from the superior colliculus was postulated by Casagrande et al. (1972), on the basis of anatomical and behavioural experiments on tree shrews. They suggested that the superficial and deeper layers of the superior colliculus performed different functions, and had different efferent projections. It has subsequently become apparent that the deeper layers too are anatomically heterogeneous (Edwards 1980; Holcombe and Hall 1981a,b; Harting and Huerta 1984), and the behavioural data presented here raise the possibility that this heterogeneity also has its functional counterpart.

The most direct implications of this idea are clearly for future research on functions of collicular output pathways themselves. It appears that the superior colliculus may be able to mediate many responses appropriate to suddenly changing visual stimuli, and it becomes important to know which efferent channel mediates which response.

There may also, however, be implications for collicular research not immediately concerned with the functions of output pathways, for example, investigations of the electrophysiological properties of cells in the intermediate and deep layers.

(a) It has become apparent that the properties of these cells with respect to eye movements are very varied (for review see, e.g., Sparks 1986). Does this variation arise because the cells of origin of different pathways are being sampled? Recent data on the properties of identified TRS cells in cat support this possibility: the firing patterns of these cells suggested that they are concerned with eye movements that pursued moving visual targets, rather than with eye movements to precise positions in space (Berthoz et al. 1986). These results, which are consistent with the behavioural data described above, imply that some other collicular output cells are concerned with saccades to particular positions, and that these will therefore have different electrophysiological properties from TRS cells in relation to eye movements.

(b) If individual output pathways are functionally distinct, it is possible that their cells of origin within the superior colliculus have distinct inputs. For example, stimuli that initiate approach are likely to differ from those that initiate defensive movements: in the case of the rat, preliminary evidence suggests that visual stimuli in the upper visual field are more likely to elicit defensive movements whereas stimuli in the lower field are more likely to elicit approach (Sahibzada et al. 1986). Recent evidence has suggested that a major feature of afferent input to the intermediate and deeper layers of the superior colliculus is its inhomogeneity with terminal zones appearing in particular layers or in patches within a layer (e.g., Harting and Huerta 1984; Illing and Graybiel 1986). At least in one instance a close spatial relationship has been demonstrated between an afferent projection (the nigrotectal pathway) and an output channel (the crossed TRS projection) (May and Hall 1984). It may therefore be the case that electrophysiological investigations of the inputs to identified collicular output neurons will reveal major differences between different projections.

Finally, the existence of functionally distinct output channels has implications for the investigation of sensorimotor transformations within the superior colliculus. If the superior colliculus is in fact carrying out a number of *different* transformations, it becomes important to identify the one under study. For example, the transformation necessary to generate movements appropriate for pursuit of a moving stimulus may differ from that required for a movement to fixate a particular position (cf. Dean et al. 1986; Grantyn et al. 1986). Characterising visuomotor transformations, a major reason for studying the superior colliculus in the first place is thus likely to be made a much easier task by first understanding "the organization of the superior colliculus as a mosaic of discrete functionally specialized domains" (Illing and Graybiel 1986, p.391).

Acknowledgement

This study was supported by S.E.R.C. grant GR/C 46963.

References

Berthoz, A., Grantyn, A. and Droulez, J. (1986) Some collicular efferent neurons code saccadic eye velocity. *Neurosci. Lett.,* 72: 298 – 294.

Casagrande, V.A., Harting, J.K., Hall, W.C., Diamond, I.T. and Martin G.F. (1972) Superior colliculus of the tree shrew: a structural and functional subdivision into superficial and deep layers. *Science,* 177: 444 – 447.

Chalupa, L.M. (1984) Visual physiology of the mammalian superior colliculus. In: H. Vanegas (Ed.), *Comparative Neurology of the Optic Tectum,* Plenum Press, New York, pp. 775 – 818.

Dacey, D.M. and Ulinski, P.S. (1986) Optic tectum of the eastern garter snake, *Thamnophis sirtalis.* II. Morphology of efferent cells. *J. Comp. Neurol.,* 245: 198 – 237.

Dean, P. and Redgrave, P. (1984a) The superior colliculus and visual neglect in rat and hamster. I. Behavioural evidence. *Brain Res. Rev.,* 8: 129 – 141.

Dean, P. and Redgrave, P. (1984b) The superior colliculus and visual neglect in rat and hamster. II. Possible mechanisms. *Brain Res. Rev.,* 8: 143 – 153.

Dean, P. and Redgrave, P. (1984c) Superior colliculus and visual neglect in rat and hamster. III. Functional implications. *Brain Res. Rev.,* 8: 155 – 163.

Dean, P., Redgrave, P. and Molton, L. (1984) Visual desynchronization of cortical EEG impaired by lesions of superior colliculus in rats. *J. Neurophysiol.,* 52: 625 – 637.

Dean, P., Redgrave, P., Sahibzada, N. and Tsuji, K. (1986) Head and body movements produced by electrical stimulation of superior colliculus in rats: Effects of interruption of crossed tectoreticulospinal pathway. *Neuroscience,* 19: 367 – 380.

Dean, P., Mitchell, I.J. and Redgrave, P. (1988a) Contralateral head movements produced by microinjection of glutamate into superior colliculus of rats: evidence for mediation by multiple output pathways. *Neuroscience,* 24: 491 – 500.

Dean, P., Mitchell, I.J. and Redgrave, P. (1988b) Responses resembling defensive behaviour produced by microinjection of glutamate into superior colliculus of rats. *Neuroscience,* 24: 501 – 510.

Dreher, R., Sefton, A.J., Ni, S.Y.K. and Nisbett, G. (1985) The morphology, number, distribution and central projections of class I retinal ganglion cells in albino and hooded rats. *Brain Behav. Evol.,* 26: 10 – 48.

Edwards, S.B. (1980) The deep cells of the superior colliculus: Their reticular characteristics and structural organisation. In:

36

J.A. Hobson and M.A.R. Brazier (Eds.), *The Reticular Formation Revisited,* Raven Press, New York, pp. 193 – 209.

Goodale, M.A. and Murison, R.C.C. (1975) The effects of lesions of the superior colliculus on locomotor orientation and the orienting reflex in the rat. *Brain Res.,* 88: 243 – 261.

Grantyn, A. and Berthoz, A. (1985) Burst activity of identified tecto-reticulo-spinal neurons in the alert cat. *Exp. Brain Res.,* 57: 417 – 421.

Harting, J.K. and Huerta, M.F. (1984) The mammalian superior colliculus: studies of its morphology and connections. In: H. Vanegas (Ed.), *The Comparative Neurology of the Optic Tectum,* Plenum Press, New York, pp. 687 – 773.

Holcombe, V. and Hall, W.C. (1981a) Laminar origin of ipsilateral tectopontine pathways. *Neuroscience,* 6: 255 – 260.

Holcombe, V. and Hall, W.C. (1981b) The laminar origin and distribution of the crossed tectoreticular pathways. *J. Neurosci.,* 1: 1103 – 1112.

Illing, R.-B. and Graybiel, A.M. (1986) Complementary and non-matching afferent compartments in the cat's superior colliculus: innervation of the acetylcholinesterase-poor domain of the intermediate gray layer. *Neuroscience,* 18: 373 – 394.

Keay, K.A., Redgrave, P. and Dean, P. (1986) Changes in blood pressure and respiration elicited by electrical and chemical stimulation of the superior colliculus in rats. *Neurosci. Lett.,* Suppl., 26: S328.

Keay, K.A., Redgrave, P. and Dean, P. (1987) Cardiovascular changes elicited by microinjection of *N*-methyl-D-aspartate (NMDA) into the superior colliculus of the hooded Lister rat. *Neurosci. Lett.,* Suppl. 29: S127.

Kilpatrick, I.C., Collingridge, G.L. and Starr, M.S. (1982) Evidence for the participation of nigrotectal gamma-aminobutyrate containing neurones in striatal and nigral derived circling in the rat. *Neuroscience,* 7: 207 – 222.

Linden, R. and Perry, V.H. (1983) Massive retinotectal projection in rats. *Brain Res.,* 272: 145 – 149.

Martin, P.R. (1986) The projection of different retinal ganglion cell classes to the dorsal lateral geniculate nucleus in the hooded rat. *Exp. Brain Res.,* 62: 77 – 88.

May, P.J. and Hall, W.C. (1984) Relationships between the nigrotectal pathway and the cells of origin of the predorsal bundle. *J. Comp. Neurol.,* 226: 357 – 376.

McHaffie, J.G. and Stein, R.E. (1982) Eye movements evoked by electrical stimulation in the superior colliculus of rats and hamsters. *Brain Res.,* 247: 243 – 254.

Merker, B. (1980) *The sentinel hypothesis: A role for the mammalian superior colliculus.* Unpublished doctoral thesis, Massachusetts Institute of Technology.

Miliaresis, F. and Philippe, L. (1984) The pontine substrate of circling behavior. *Brain Res.,* 293: 143 – 152.

Mitchell, I.J., Redgrave, P. and Dean, P. (1987) Potentiation of glutamate-elicited defensive responses from tecto-recipient zone of cuneiform area in rat. *Neurosci. Lett.,* Suppl. 29: S127.

Overton, P., Dean, P. and Redgrave, P. (1985) Detection of visual stimuli in far periphery by rats: possible role of superior colliculus. *Exp. Brain Res.,* 59: 559 – 569.

Perry, V.H. and Cowey, A. (1984) Retinal ganglion cells that project to the superior colliculus and pretectum in the macaque monkey. *Neuroscience,* 12: 1125 – 1137.

Redgrave, P. and Dean, P. (1985) Tonic desynchronisation of cortical EEG by electrical stimulation of superior colliculus and surrounding structures in urethane-anaesthetised rats. *Neuroscience,* 16: 659 – 671.

Redgrave, P., Dean, P., Souki, W. and Lewis, G. (1981) Gnawing and changes in reactivity produced by microinjections of picrotoxin into the superior colliculus of rats. *Psychopharmacology,* 75: 198 – 203.

Redgrave, P., Odekunle, A. and Dean, P. (1986) Tectal cells of origin of predorsal bundle in rats: Location and segregation from ipsilateral descending pathway. *Exp. Brain Res.,* 63: 279 – 293.

Redgrave, P., Mitchell, I. and Dean, P. (1987a) Further evidence for segregated output channels from superior colliculus in rat: ipsilateral tecto-pontine and tecto-cuneiform projections have different cells of origin. *Brain Res.,* 413: 170 – 174.

Redgrave, P., Mitchell, I. and Dean, P. (1987b) Descending projections from the superior colliculus in rat: a study using orthograde transport of wheatgerm-agglutinin conjugated horseradish peroxidase. *Exp. Brain Res.,* 68: 147 – 167.

Sahibzada, N., Dean, P. and Redgrave, P. (1986) Movements resembling orientation or avoidance elicited by electrical stimulation of the superior colliculus in rats. *J. Neurosci.,* 6: 723 – 733.

Schiller, P.H. (1985) The superior colliculus and visual function. In: I. Darien-Smith (Ed.), *Handbook of Physiology – The Nervous System, Vol. 3,* American Physiological Society, Bethesda, MD, pp. 457 – 505.

Schneider, G.E. (1969) Two visual systems. *Science,* 163: 895 – 902.

Sparks, D.L. (1986) Translation of sensory signals into commands for control of saccadic eye movements: role of primate superior colliculus. *Annu. Rev. Neurosci.,* 66: 118 – 171.

Tehovnik, E.J. and Yeomans, J.S. (1986) Two converging brainstem pathways mediating circling behavior. *Brain Res.,* 385: 329 – 342.

Yeomans, J.S., Pearce, R., Wen, D. and Hawkins, R.D. (1984) Mapping midbrain sites for circling using current-frequency trade-off data. *Physiol. Behav.,* 32: 287 – 294.

T.P. Hicks and G. Benedek (Eds.)
Progress in Brain Research, Vol. 75
© 1988 Elsevier Science Publishers B.V. (Biomedical Division)

CHAPTER 4

Superior colliculus-mediated visual behaviors in cat and the concept of two corticotectal systems

Barry E. Stein

Department of Physiology, Medical College of Virginia, Virginia Commonwealth University, Richmond, VA 23298, U.S.A.

The present chapter is the outgrowth of a series of experiments my colleagues and I began in cat in an attempt to understand how cortex and midbrain (specifically, the superior colliculus) interact in the production of visual behaviors. A number of years ago we (and others) examined how primary visual cortex affects the most visually 'dominant' area of the superior colliculus (SC), its superficial laminae. This proved to be an excellent model for determining how the brain builds receptive fields from converging afferents. But the superficial laminae have little to do with the most striking visual role of the superior colliculus: attentive and orientation behavior. Just as visual cortex encompasses a multiplicity of distinct visual areas, the label SC covers at least two functionally separate regions, and, oddly enough, the visual role for which the SC is best known involves an area more poorly endowed with visual cells than the superficial laminae, yet whose visual inputs have more obvious behavioral consequences. These deeper layers are, in turn, controlled by a visual area far removed from 'primary' visual cortex.

The results of these studies are simple enough to describe in a few sentences. An extrastriate cortical area has now been identified as controlling the deep laminae SC cells that connect to those areas of the brainstem and spinal cord through which overt responses are initiated. Compromising any station along this circuit seriously impairs visual attention and orientation capability.

Despite my statement that these experiments can be summarized briefly, the reader has undoubtedly noticed the alarming number of subsequent pages that seem to belie this claim. Unfortunately, putting this information in a context in which it can be evaluated properly requires substantial text. Nevertheless, if absolutely necessary, it is possible to skip the introductory sections and begin on p. 39.

Overview of the SC

Studies of the role of the superior colliculus (SC) in vision have a long history. Among the earliest are those of Adamuk (1872) demonstrating a role of the SC in generating eye movements. Yet for much of this history the SC was mentioned in passing. However, during the mid 1960s a great deal of attention was directed toward the visual role of the SC. This was a consequence of Sprague and Meikle's (1965) study showing that its ablation produced a profound contralateral visual neglect despite an intact geniculostriate system. This was a rather startling finding at the time, and because removal of the SC and ablation of visual cortex appeared to produce qualitatively different visual dysfunctions, it was postulated, or intimated, that there were actually "two visual systems" (Sprague 1966; Diamond and Hall 1969; Schneider 1969). We now know that these 'systems' are interrelated components, in part, because removal of visual cortex changes the physiological properties of SC cells. Nevertheless, they do have different contributions to specific aspects of visual behavior: the SC is involved primarily in attention and orientation, whereas the visual cortex plays its major (though not exclusive) role in analyzing detail.

The heightened interest in the SC grew, even when the original 'two visual system' hypothesis no longer was tenable. A wealth of anatomical and physiological information about this structure now has been generated, much of which also is summarized in a number of review articles (e.g., Kruger 1970; McIlwain 1972; Palmer et al. 1972; Schiller 1972; Sprague 1972; Gordon 1975; Schneider 1975; Sparks and Pollack 1977; Goldberg and Robinson 1978; Stein 1978; Coulter et al. 1979; Wurtz and Albano 1980; Huerta and Harting 1982; Chalupa 1984; Stein 1984).

Sensory and motor organization

While the SC consists of at least seven reasonably well-defined laminae (Kanaseki and Sprague 1974), for most purposes it is separated into only two divisions: superficial (layers I – III) and deep (layers IV – VII). These divisions reflect differences between them in morphology, afferent – efferent connections, physiology, and behavioral involvements (see Edwards 1980; Stein and Gordon 1981; Stein 1984). Nevertheless, both superficial and deep laminae contain visual cells and exhibit the same general map-like organization: cells with nasal receptive fields are located rostrally in the superior colliculus, whereas those with temporal receptive fields are located caudally. Similarly, superior visual space is represented medially in the SC, and inferior visual space is represented laterally. It is through the output, or efferent, cells that the sensory roles of the SC can be transformed into overt responses.

The deep laminae send their outputs to a variety of extraoculomotor-related structures (Graham 1977; Edwards and Henkel 1978), and these 'motor' cells are in topographic register with the visuotopy. Consequently, a focal electrical stimulus produces an eye movement that centers the area centralis on the same point in space represented at the stimulation site in the visual map (Syka and Radil-Weiss 1971; Straschill and Rieger 1973; Roucoux and Crommelinck 1976; Stein et al. 1976; Harris 1980). Presumably, during 'normal' behavior a visual stimulus produces a localized region of sensory activity, which in turn is converted into an output signal that moves the eyes.

Receptive field properties

By understanding the receptive field characteristics of these cells, we not only characterize how they deal with stimulus parameters but we learn which stimuli have access to the sensorimotor circuitry of the SC.

Because visual cells are encountered most readily in superficial laminae, these were the cells most often studied in cat SC (e.g., Marchiafava and Pepeu 1966; Straschill and Taghavy 1967; McIlwain and Buser 1968; Sprague et al. 1968; Sterling and Wickelgren 1969; Berman and Cynader 1972; Stein and Arigbede 1972; Dreher and Hoffmann 1973; Harutiunian-Kozak et al. 1973; Pinter and Harris 1982), and there is good agreement that the most obvious characteristics of these cells are that they: (1) prefer moving to stationary flashed stimuli; (2) prefer stimuli moved in specific directions across the receptive field (directionally selective) within a specific velocity range; (3) receive inputs from both eyes (binocular); (4) exhibit receptive fields that are not systematically divided into separate 'on' and 'off' regions; (5) have larger receptive fields than generally found in the geniculostriate system; (6) have suppressive flanks bordering the excitatory receptive field; (7) are excited optimally by stimuli far smaller than the borders of their receptive fields; (8) exhibit transient responses even to maintained stimuli.

Many of the receptive field properties of these visual cells were found to be dependent on the inputs received from primary visual cortex. This dependency was apparent when removal of striate cortex eliminated from these SC cells their binocularity, directional selectivity, and preferences for moving rather than stationary flashed stimuli (Wickelgren and Sterling 1969; Rosenquist and Palmer 1971; Berman and Cynader 1975; Stein and Magalhães-Castro 1975; Mize and Murphy 1976). These studies also demonstrated that the SC cell was an excellent model for evaluating the manner in which the brain constructs complex properties by the convergence of two (retinotectal and corticotectal) afferent pathways, but they provided little insight into the circuitry involved most directly with visual attention and orientation.

Although less attention has been directed toward visual cells in the deep laminae (IV – VII), it is these cells that are critical for the SC to perform its role in visually guided behavior (Casagrande et al. 1972; Stein and Arigbede 1972; Abrahams and Rose 1975; Stein 1978; Meredith and Stein 1983a,b). Superficial layer cells seem to be more like those in the geniculostriate system in that they are involved in spatial analysis (Casagrande et al. 1972). It is curious to note that deep laminae visual cells possess many of the same receptive field properties exhibited by superficial laminae cells (see Table 1), yet their afferents are distinctly different. In contrast to the very heavy direct retinal projection to superficial layers, it was not until quite recently that the deep laminae were thought to receive any direct retinal input (Harting and Guillery 1976; Edwards 1980; Berson and McIlwain 1982; but also see Sterling 1973; Mize 1983). Furthermore, the corticotectal inputs to deep layers from the primary visual cortex are sparse and diffuse (Garey et al. 1968; Kawamura 1974; Mize 1983). Therefore, although it was possible that the similarities in the receptive-field properties of deep and superficial laminae cells could be derived from the same sources, the paucity of deep layer retinotectal and primary visual corticotectal inputs made it seem unlikely.

Corticotectal projections to the deep layers have now been shown to originate in the extrastriate cortex, especially the posterior regions of the suprasylvian cortex (PSSC; Segal et al. 1982;

Baleydier et al. 1983; Berson 1983; Segal and Beckstead 1984). So as a first step we sought to compare the corticotectal influences of the striate cortex and the PSSC on SC cells. Since these corticotectal projections are not segregated completely in the SC (i.e., both cortices project to superficial and deep laminae), superficial and deep laminae cells were studied before, during and after the temporary deactivation of each cortical region.

Two corticotectal systems

Cortical deactivation

Cortex was reversibly depressed using a cooling probe that could be positioned as necessary and which is shown in Fig. 1. Although the laminar locations of the SC cells affected by cooling the two areas studied (area 17 – 18 and PSSC) proved to be quite different (see below), the general depressive changes observed did not differ accord-

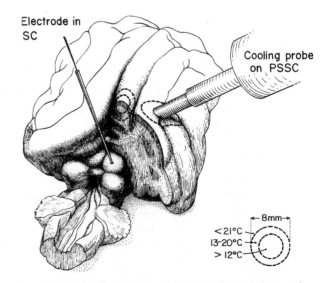

Fig. 1. Diagram showing recording microelectrode in superior colliculus (SC) while cortex is being cooled. Area of cortex to be cooled was restricted by using a cooling probe with a 5-mm tip diameter and placing it on dura directly overlying area 17 – 18 or posterior suprasylvian cortex (PSSC). Cortical temperature was progressively higher with increasing distance from probe tip; this is indicated by concentric circles on surface of each cortical area studied, and is described in detail through depth of brain in Fig. 3. (From Ogasawara et al. 1984.)

ing to the area deactivated. The changes in activity were exhibited as either a substantial decrease in the number of impulses evoked or in the elimination of responses to a previously optimal stimulus. These changes were reversed by rewarming cortex with warm saline.

Receptive-field properties: cortical cooling

A variety of receptive-field properties were examined and ocularity and directional selectivity distinguished most clearly between SC cells affected or not affected by cortical cooling. The majority of directionally selective or binocular cells

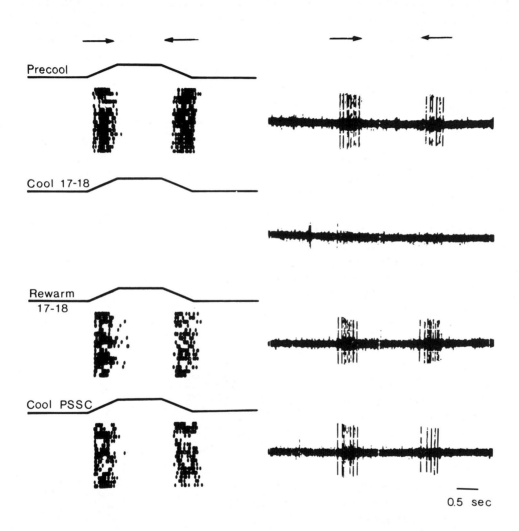

0.5 sec

Fig. 2. Responses of superficial laminae SC cells were depressed by cooling area 17–18, but often were unaffected by cooling PSSC. Cell represented here is typical of cells in superficial portion of stratum griseum superficiale. It responded vigorously to stimuli moved across its receptive field as illustrated in top row by raster display and oscillograms (precool). Ramps above raster display represent electronic signal controlling stimulus movement (left to right is nasal to temporal). Upward ramp produced movement in one direction, downward ramp produced movement in opposite direction; arrows indicate direction of movement. No movement occurs during plateau. Deactivation of area 17–18 (cool 17–18) eliminated responses to these stimuli, but responses were re-instated after 8 min of rewarming (rewarm 17–18). Cooling PSSC (cool PSSC) had no apparent effect on responsiveness of this cell. Each dot in rasters represents 1 neuronal impulse, and raster traces are ordered from bottom (1st stimulus presentation) to top (last stimulus presentation). These conventions also are followed in Fig. 3. (From Ogasawara et al. 1984.)

TABLE 1

	Stationary stimulus	Moving stimulus	Both	Directionally selective	Directionally non-selective	Binocular	Monocular
Superficial ($n = 75$)	2 (3)	26 (34)	47 (63)	43 (57)	32 (43)	61 (81)	14 (19)
Deep ($n = 62$)	2 (3)	32 (52)	28 (45)	42 (68)	20 (32)	49 (79)	13 (21)

Numbers in parentheses are percents of total.

were depressed by cooling. When both these properties were evident in the same cell, that cell was always depressed by cortical cooling. In contrast, very few monocular, non-directionally selective cells were affected. The single best predictor of a cooling-induced change in activity proved to be the presence of binocularity and of 110 binocular cells (some directionally selective, some not), 98% ($n = 108$) were depressed; of these, 27% became completely unresponsive.

Effects of cooling area 17 – 18 and PSSC on visually active SC cells

The overwhelming majority of binocular superficial laminae cells (95%, 58/61) were influenced by cooling area 17 – 18, but many of them (59%, 36/61) were affected by cooling the PSSC as well. Yet, the nature of the cooling-induced changes was strikingly different. The most obvious difference was the magnitude of the changes observed.

Cooling PSSC produced only a slight reduction in the excitability of these cells, but cooling area 17 – 18 profoundly depressed them, often rendering them totally unresponsive to stimuli that previously evoked vigorous activity. Figure 2 shows an example of response elimination to an optimal stimulus after cooling area 17 – 18. The difference of greatest functional importance, however, was that deactivating area 17 – 18 altered the receptive-field properties of these cells, but deactivating the PSSC did not.

Receptive-field properties of superficial laminae SC cells depend on area 17 – 18

In many SC cells ($n = 36$), responses were depressed but not eliminated by cooling area 17 – 18. In studying these cells, it became apparent that removing the influence of area 17 – 18 produced dramatic changes in the characteristic receptive field properties of SC cells. The most obvious of these was the removal of directional selectivity and binocularity. Similarly, a decrement in the spatial analyzing properties of the cells (i.e., spatial summation, spatial inhibition, and suppressive surround) was often apparent, and the range of effective stimulus velocities changed. On the other hand, cooling the PSSC never produced changes in superficial laminae receptive-field properties. Because there are reciprocal connections between area 17 – 18 and the PSSC (Heath and Jones 1971; Kawamura 1973a,b; Naito 1980), there was the possibility that the effect of cooling the PSSC on superficial laminae SC cells was mediated by area 17 – 18. This did not appear to be the case. After ablating area 17 – 18 cooling the PSSC still depressed the excitability in 6 of the 10 cells studied.

Deep laminae SC cells are affected by PSSC but not by area 17 – 18

In every deep laminae visual cell affected by cooling, the effective site was the PSSC. Cooling the PSSC not only depressed the excitability of

42

these cells, but altered their complex receptive-field properties as well. No such changes were observed when area 17 − 18 was cooled (see Table 2).

The changes in receptive-field properties of deep laminae cells produced by cooling the PSSC paralleled the changes described earlier in superficial laminae cells during deactivation of area 17 − 18. Figure 3 illustrates the dramatic changes in the excitability of a directionally selective cell produced by cooling the PSSC; the responses evoked by a moving visual stimulus were eliminated during the cooling of the PSSC, but were unaffected by cooling area 17 − 18.

The presence of either binocularity or directional selectivity was a reliable predictor that the activity of a given deep laminae cell would be depressed when the PSSC was cooled. Binocularity was the single best predictor, accurate in 98% of the cells studied; the presence of directional selectivity was an accurate indicator in 85% of the cells studied. When both properties occurred in the same cell, the likelihood that it would be influenced by cooling the PSSC became 100%.

The spatial properties of deep laminae cells were also disrupted by cooling the PSSC, in the same way that these properties in superficial laminae cells were affected by cooling 17 − 18.

These experiments demonstrated that the same receptive-field properties of superficial and deep laminae SC cells are dependent on the cortex, but that the relevant cortical areas are different (see Table 2). Apparently, there are two, largely independent, corticotectal systems; the only exception to a complete separation is the ability of the PSSC to affect the general activity level of some superficial laminae SC cells. This influence was independent of area 17 − 18 and was expressed even in animals from which area 17 − 18 had been removed.

Some implications of two visual corticotectal systems

Functionally separated corticotectal influences on superficial and deep SC laminae is consistent with a number of other distinctions. Superficial and deep laminae cells exhibit morphological differences (Sterling 1971; Norita 1980), are involved in different behavioral functions (Casagrande et al. 1972; Meredith and Stein 1983), receive different inputs (Sprague 1975; Edwards et al. 1979), and project to different targets (Graham 1977). This superficial-deep layer segregation prompted Edwards (1980) to suggest that they are independent structures. Thus, it is surprising that despite these differences, the cells in both divisions of the SC exhibit many of the same receptive-field characteristics, which apparently suit equally well their very different functional roles (Sprague 1966; Casagrande et al. 1972). This seems even more surprising given the widespread belief that different behavioral functions require different receptive-field properties. Yet these data indicate that the same bits of information are needed by superficial laminae cells to perform their role in pattern or detail analysis and by deep laminae cells to perform their role in visually guided behavior. Perhaps the behavioral role of these different divisions of the SC may be more an expression of their different efferent connections than of the manner in which their visual receptive fields are organized.

Behavioral consequences of two visual corticotectal systems

At this point it should be evident that (1) it is the cells of the deep laminae that are most directly involved in visual attentive and orientation behaviors and (2) these cells are controlled by, and owe their

TABLE 2

Cells affected by cooling

	Area 17 − 18	PSSC	Area 17 − 18 + PSSC	Un-affected
Superficial (n = 75)	22	4	36	13
Deep (n = 62)	0	49	0	13

complex receptive field properties to, PSSC. The implication of these findings was that removal of 17 – 18, which affects only superficial laminae, would have no obvious effect on visual attentive and orientation behavior, but removing PSSC should.

Just as Sprague and colleagues had shown that the SC was involved in visual attentive and orientation behavior, Sprague also showed that cortex plays an important role in those behaviors because it controls the SC.

It had been known for some time that a large posterior neocortical lesion produces a persistent contralateral visual neglect ('cortical blindness'). However, Sprague's (1966a,b) experiments in cats revealed that this cortical blindness, produced by removal of all known visual cortex in one hemisphere, was in large part reversible by removing the opposite superior colliculus. Thus, a lesion-induced deficit could be ameliorated by a second lesion. The most obvious conclusion was that there is a delicate balance among the central nervous

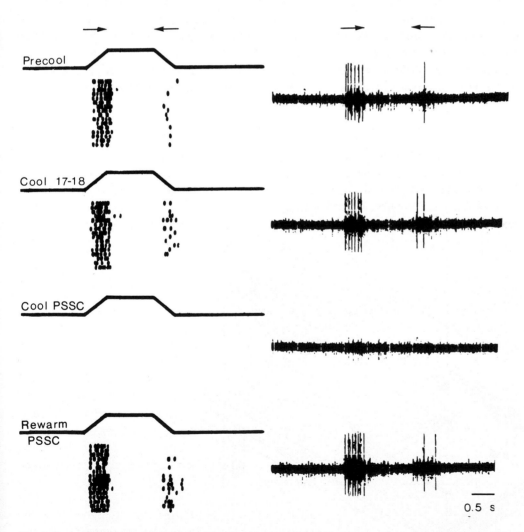

Fig. 3. Responses of deep laminae directionally selective visual SC cells were depressed by cooling PSSC, but not by cooling area 17 – 18. Responses of the deep laminae cell shown here were eliminated after 6 min of cooling PSSC. However, cooling area 17 – 18 for same period had no apparent effect on cell's responsiveness. (From Ogasawara et al. 1984.)

system structures subserving visual attention and visually-guided behaviors. This balance was thought to consist of (a) descending excitatory influences from each visual cortex to its ipsilateral superior colliculus and (b) counterbalancing inhibitory inputs via the connection between the colliculi: the intercollicular commissure. The elimination of contralateral visual attention after a cortical lesion is due to the functional loss of visual cortex itself which allows the ipsilateral superior colliculus to be dominated by intercollicular inhibition. The basic scheme as suggested by Sprague continues to be supported by physiological studies demonstrating that corticotectal influences are predominantly excitatory (see Stein (1984) for a recent review), and intercollicular projections are largely inhibitory (Goodale 1973; Saraiva et al.

1978), and behavioral studies showing that cutting the intercollicular commissure restores vision in animals 'blinded' by bilateral cortical lesions (Sherman 1974).

Since deep laminae cells depend on PSSC for their normal excitability and receptive field properties, it seemed likely that damage to this area alone could, in large part, account for the visual neglect induced by posterior neodecortication. This was the basis for our next set of experiments. In these, cats were trained in a perimetry device as shown in Fig. 4. The animal was trained to fix its gaze at the 0° mark while a piece of food (bait) was held in the opening. As the animal was released, a pingpong ball on the end of a metal rod was introduced at some point within the testing device. If the animal approached the ball, a correct response, it was

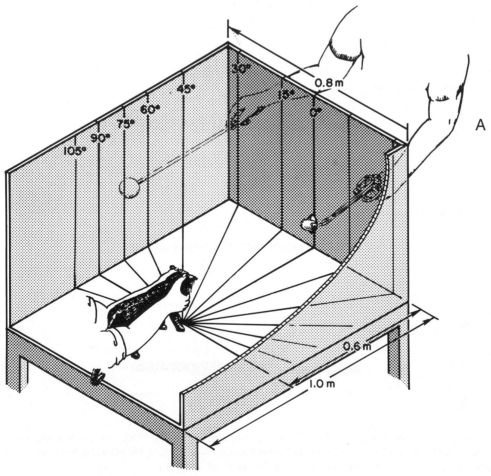

Fig. 4A.

rewarded with food. If the animal ignored the ball and continued toward the fixation point (0°), it was still given food there, but this was considered an 'incorrect' response. These tests were labeled the 'Baited Method'. In some cases no food was present at 0° ('unbaited method') or release of the animal was delayed 1 or 2 s after the pingpong ball was introduced ('delayed-release'). One additional test involved a stationary animal. While it fixated at 0°, food in a forceps was introduced from above the animal's head and within a foot of its eyes. A

correct response was a prompt orientation toward the food. Animals were tested binocularly or monocularly (one eye was occluded with an opaque contact lens after applying an ophthalmic anesthetic) before and then again after a cortical lesion. In 12/20 animals, another set of trials was run after the contralateral SC was lesioned. In this way, each animal served as its own control.

Lesions of various sizes were placed in the cortex and involved portions of the crown of the suprasylvian gyrus and/or parts of PMLS, PLLS, VLS and

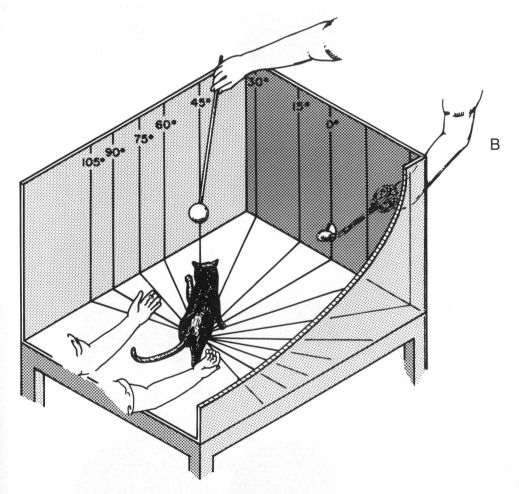

Fig. 4. (A) The baited testing method. Each animal was first trained to fix its gaze on the food (bait) at the eye-level opening in the forward wall (0° mark). When released, the animal was trained to move directly forward to the bait without altering fixation. (From Hardy and Stein 1986.) (B) During testing, a pingpong ball on a thin rod was randomly introduced at one of 14 visual angles at the same time that the animal was released. Normal animals approached the pingpong ball on nearly 100% of the trials. (From Hardy and Stein 1986.)

46

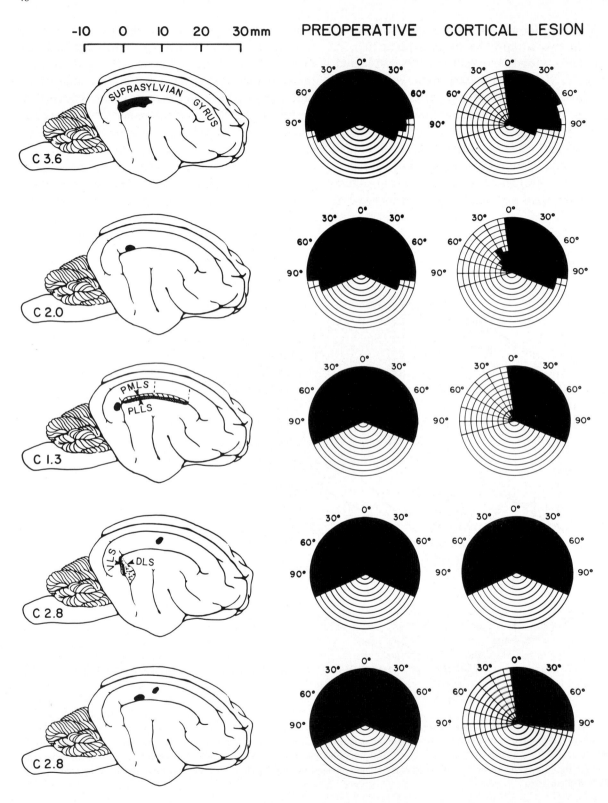

DLS, where multiple visual representations have been described (Palmer et al. 1978) (see Fig. 5). None of these lesions produced obvious visual defects in free-field situations. The animals readily avoided obstacles, were able to jump onto a table, and had normal pupillary responses to light. However, gross abnormalities could be demonstrated experimentally in the perimetry apparatus.

Surprisingly, neither the severity of the visual field defects that were demonstrated nor their representation in the visual field changed substantially as a consequence of lesion position when the baited method was used. Lesions in any portion of PSSC reduced the probability that the animal would orient to a contralateral stimulus. Cats No. 3.6, 2.0 and 1.3 had lesions restricted primarily to PLLS, PMLS, or VLS, respectively, yet showed similar visual neglect throughout the contralateral hemifield when tested by the baited method (Fig. 5). When released, they ignored a contralateral pingpong ball (but oriented to an ipsilateral one) and moved briskly forward to the fixation point.

All posterior neocortical lesions did not produce visually-guided deficits. The lesion shown in cat 2.8 (Fig. 5) that was placed on the crown of the anterior middle suprasylvian gyrus (outside the topographic visual representations described by Palmer et al. (1978) and beyond the principal corticotectal zone of PSSC (Ogasawara et al. 1984; Segal and Beckstead 1984)) of cat 2.8 (Fig. 5) produced no change in visually-guided behavior. However, a second lesion placed caudal to the first so that it was within PMLS produced one of the most severe contralateral visual deficits observed: the animal did not respond to any stimuli in the contralateral hemifield (Fig. 5). Similarly, an auditory cortex lesion in one animal produced no visually-guided deficits in any of the tests.

Of the tests used, the baited method proved to be the most sensitive. When the same animals were examined post-operatively by using other methods to assess their visual capabilities, different visual perimetries were recorded. The severe deficits observed using the baited method were somewhat less severe with the delayed release method and were no longer evident with the stationary method.

These data indicate that the PSSC lesions did not induce 'blindness' in the contralateral field. The term 'visual neglect' was previously used as a description of the visual defects produced by posterior neodecortication (see Sprague and Meikle 1965) and seems particularly apt for describing the visual defects seen here. This neglect was most obvious using the testing paradigm in which the animal was required to respond immediately by breaking fixation on an object of interest and to move its entire body toward the new stimulus.

To determine if the lesion-induced visual neglect could be ameliorated by removing 'inhibition' via the intercollicular commissure, the contralateral SC was aspirated in 12 cortically lesioned animals. Their deficits were immediately eliminated or significantly ameliorated (Fig. 6). Frequently, they oriented to stimuli in the previously blind hemifield more rapidly than normal, perhaps because

◄ Fig. 5. Small lesions at various loci along the principal corticotectal region of the posterior aspect of the suprasylvian cortex produce profound contralateral visual neglect. Neither the severity of the deficit nor its representation in the visual field varied substantially with the position of the lesion within the middle and posterior suprasylvian sulcus. The suprasylvian gyrus is labelled in the upper schematic, PMLS (posteromedial lateral suprasylvian) and PLLS (posterolateral lateral suprasylvian) in the third from the top, and VLS (ventrolateral suprasylvian) and DLS (dorsolateral suprasylvian) in the fourth from the top. Cats 3.6, 2.0, 1.3 and 2.8 (lower) had normal preoperative visually-guided behavior, but after lesions (shown in black on the schematics of the brain) restricted to various subregions of the posterior suprasylvian cortex (i.e., PLLS, PMLS, VLS and PMLS, respectively), the animals showed similar patterns of contralateral visual neglect. Note that a lesion rostral and medial in animal 2.8 (second from bottom) produced no detectable visual defect, but a second (more caudal and lateral) lesion in the same animal did produce a characteristic visual defect. Similar lesions elsewhere in cortex (e.g., auditory cortex, not shown) produced no discernible defect on this visual task. The percentage of correct orientations at each visual angle is plotted in black on each polar coordinate graph of the visual field. (From Hardy and Stein 1986.)

48

BINOCULAR

MONOCULAR

(left eye)   (right eye)

PREOPERATIVE

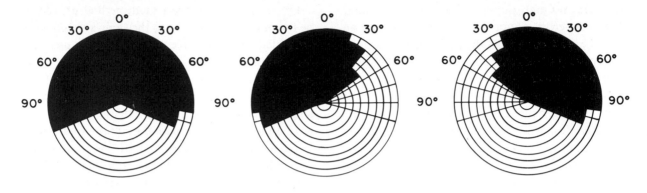

RIGHT CORTICAL LESION

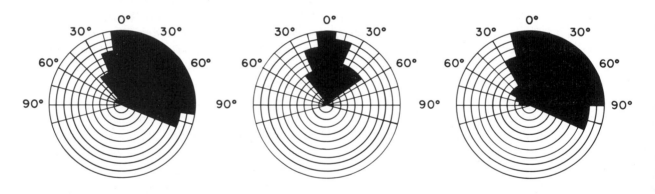

RIGHT CORTICAL AND LEFT SC LESIONS

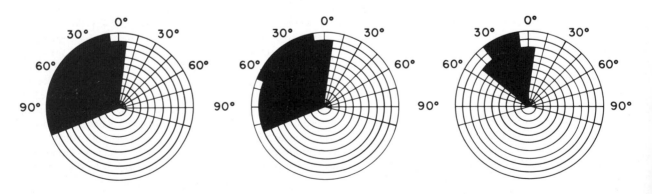

of the 'new' visual defect induced contralateral to the aspirated SC. Reinstatement of visually-guided behavior could not be produced by a control lesion of the inferior colliculus, indicating that this effect was not a general consequence of damage to the contralateral midbrain.

Because of the approach used in removing the SC, we sometimes undercut the SC and did comparatively little damage to the superficial laminae. Yet these lesions reversed the visual neglect as ef-

fectively as did complete removal of the structure. The best example of an undercut SC is shown in Fig. 7. In this example, only the lateral borders of the superficial laminae were damaged, and the major course of the cut is in the subjacent tegmentum.

Conclusions

The data indicate that normal, visually-guided behavior depends on functional corticotectal visual areas of PSSC. Even small lesions here produce a neglect in the entire contralateral visual field. Although complete posterior neodecortication produces a more debilitating homonymous hemianopia (Sprague 1966a), these defects were quite dramatic considering the small size of the lesions. They were most apparent in a task that required the animal to: (a) interrupt fixation on an object of interest (e.g., food) when another stimulus was introduced into the contralateral visual hemifield, (b) move its entire body in order to capture that stimulus, and (c) begin forward movement immediately upon the presentation of that stimulus. Eliminating these task requirements often led to progressively better performance. When they were all eliminated, so that the animal had only to orient its head toward a stimulus, no defect was apparent.

It is important to note that there are many limitations of the tasks used to document visual anomalies and an unfortunate inadequacy of broad operational terms to describe them. 'Visual neglect' distinguishes blindness from a failure to respond to visual stimuli, but does not specify in which conditions this failure will become evident. In the studies described here, cortically-lesioned cats reliably 'neglected' stimuli when they were

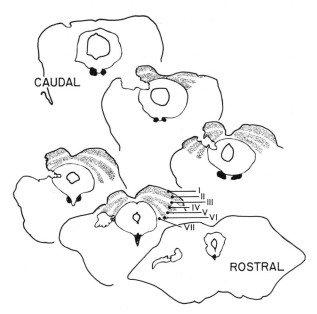

Fig. 7. Undercutting the superior colliculus contralateral to a cortical lesion reversed visual neglect even though superficial laminae remained functional (visual activity was recorded in the superficial laminae). The lesion shown on the tracing of coronal sections through the superior colliculus undercut the structure while leaving most of the superficial laminae and much of the deep laminae intact. However, the lesion reinstated visually-guided behavior that previously had been disrupted by a suprasylvian cortex lesion in the opposite hemisphere. (From Hardy and Stein 1986.)

Fig. 6. Visual neglect induced by suprasylvian cortex lesions is reversed by damaging the opposite SC. The data from 12 animals are combined here. Each animal exhibited normal preoperative binocular and monocular visual fields (top). A lesion in right posterior suprasylvian cortex produced a profound contralateral visual neglect (middle) in each animal (baited method) that was later reversed by a lesion of the left SC. The visual fields pre- and postoperatively are shown as the average number of correct responses at each visual angle for all animals combined, and accurately reflect the data obtained in each animal. Note that while visual orientation returned in the left visual field following the left SC lesion, this lesion always eliminated visually-guided behavior in its contralateral (right) visual field. (From Hardy and Stein, 1986.)

tested in some situations, but reliably responded to them in others. The shift from complete neglect to complete attentiveness, given the minimal changes in the task, emphasizes how important it is to choose the appropriate task to expose specific perceptual, attentive or sensorimotor integrative defects. The defects produced by larger lesions may be more readily detectable because they degrade sensory function more broadly.

One unexpected result was the absence of topographies in the lesion-induced defects and in the restoration of visually-guided behavior via SC lesions. With even the smallest lesions in cortex, orientation defects were evident across the entire contralateral visual field. Although there were many variations in lesion location in the 20 cats studied, and a corticotectal topography is known to exist here (Segal and Beckstead 1984), no animal retained 'islands' of normal visually-guided behavior (although the defect became more pronounced far peripherally). Our inability to demonstrate a clear topography in the defects may reflect several representations of the contralateral visual field within small regions of PSSC. On the other hand, perhaps the topographies within PSSC may be somewhat less discrete than previously thought (Zumbroich et al. 1986) so that even small lesions can damage areas that represent large areas of visual space.

Similarly, incomplete lesions of the opposite SC readily restored vision throughout the previously blind hemifield. Several of the SC lesions left superficial laminae largely intact, and even some of the deeper laminae. Yet these lesions were no less effective at restoring contralateral visual behavior than were more complete lesions. This finding is now less perplexing due to recent experiments showing that intercollicular inhibition is mediated in large part by fibers originating from outside the SC (e.g., substantia nigra – Graybiel 1978; Edwards et al. 1979; Karabelas and Moschovakis 1985; Wallace and Rosenquist 1986), but traveling within the intercollicular commissure (Sprague et al. 1986). Even lesions that undercut the superior colliculus would sever these fibers en route to the commissure and would therefore be effective in restoring contralateral visually-guided behaviors. Consequently, any attempts to account for the normal influences of the intercollicular commissure on the superior colliculus must take into account those fibers originating from the contralateral superior colliculus cells and those fibers coming from extrinsic sources.

These experiments illustrate the delicate balance that must be maintained among structures at various levels of the neuraxis to support seemingly simple visual behaviors. Removing even a small region of extraprimary visual cortex, from which deep laminae superior colliculus cells receive input, disrupts this balance. The consequence of this disruption is a striking decrement in the effectiveness of contralateral visual stimuli. This deficit is clearly apparent even though the integrity of the principal visual cortical areas (17, 18 and 19) and their projection targets have not been compromised.

References

Abrahams, V.C. and Rose, P.K. (1975) Projections of extraocular, neck muscle, and retinal afferents to superior colliculus in the cat: their connections to cells of origin of tectospinal tract. *J. Neurophysiol.*, 38: 10–18.

Adamuk, E. (1872) Über angeborene und erworbene Association von F.C. Donders, Albrecht V. Graefes. *Arch. Ophthalmol.*, 18: 153–164.

Baleydier, C., Kahungu, M. and Mauguière, F. (1983) A crossed corticotectal projection from the lateral suprasylvian area in the cat. *J. Comp. Neurol.*, 24: 344–351.

Berman, N. and Cynader, M. (1972) Comparison of receptive-field organization of the superior colliculus in Siamese and normal cats. *J. Physiol.*, 244: 363–389.

Berman, N. and Cynader, M. (1975) Receptive fields in cat superior colliculus after visual cortex lesions. *J. Physiol.*, 245: 261–270.

Berson, D.M. (1983) Y-cell input to the lateral suprasylvian area: a substrate for Y-indirect influence on the deep superior colliculus. *Soc. Neurosci. Abstr.*, 9: 37.

Berson, D.M. and McIlwain, J.T. (1982) Retinal Y-cell activation of deep-layer cells in superior colliculus of the cat. *J. Neurophysiol.*, 47: 700–714.

Casagrande, V.A. Harting, J.K., Hall, W.C. and Diamond, I.T. (1972) Superior colliculus of the tree shrew: a structural and functional subdivision into superficial and deep layers. *Science,* 177: 444–447.

Chalupa, L.M. (1984) Visual physiology of the mammalian superior colliculus. In: H. Vanegas (Ed.), *Comparative Neurology of the Optic Tectum,* Plenum, New York, pp. 775–818.

Coulter, J.D., Bowker, R.M., Wise, S.P., Murray, E.A., Castiglioni, A.J. and Westlund, K.N. (1979) Cortical, tectal and medullary descending pathways to the cervical spinal cord. *Prog. Brain Res.,* 50: 263–279.

Diamond, I.T. and Hall, W.C. (1969) Evolution of neocortex. *Science,* 164: 251–262.

Dreher, B. and Hoffmann, K.-P. (1973) Properties of excitatory and inhibitory regions in the receptive fields of single units in the cat's superior colliculus. *Exp. Brain Res.,* 16: 333–353.

Edwards, S.B. (1980) The deep cell layers of the superior colliculus. Their reticular characteristics and structural organization. In: A. Hobson and M. Brazier (Eds), *The Reticular Formation Revisited,* Raven Press, New York, p. 193.

Edwards, S.B., Ginsburgh, C.L., Henkel, C.K. and Stein, B.E. (1979) Sources of subcortical projections to the superior colliculus in the cat. *J. Comp. Neurol.,* 198: 309–330.

Garey, L.J., Jones, E.G. and Powell, T.P.S. (1968) Interrelationships of striate and extrastriate cortex with the primary relay sites of the visual pathway. *J. Neurol. Neurosurg. Psychiat.,* 31: 135–157.

Goldberg, M.E. and Robinson, D.L. (1978) Visual system: superior colliculus. In: R.B. Masterton (Ed.), *Handbook of Behavioral Neurobiology,* Plenum Press, New York, pp. 119–164.

Goodale, M. (1973) Corticotectal and intertectal modulation of visual responses in the rat's superior colliculus. *Exp. Brain Res.,* 17: 75–86.

Gordon, B.G. (1975) Superior colliculus: structure, physiology and possible functions. *MTP Int. Rev. Sci.,* 3: 185–230.

Graham, J. (1977) An autoradiographic study of the efferent connections of the superior colliculus in the cat. *J. Comp. Neurol.,* 173: 629–654.

Graybiel, A.M. (1979) Organization of the nigrotectal connection: an experimental tracer study in the cat. *Brain Res.,* 143: 339–348.

Hardy, S.C. and Stein, B.E. (1986) Small lesions in suprasylvian cortex produce contralateral visual neglect and a lowered incidence of deep laminae visual cells in the superior colliculus. *Soc. Neurosci. Abstr.,* 12: 1368.

Harris, L.R. (1980) The superior colliculus and movements of the head and eyes in cats. *J. Physiol.,* 300: 367–391.

Harting, J.K. and Guillery, R.W. (1976) Organization of retinocollicular pathways in the cat. *J. Comp. Neurol.,* 166: 133–144.

Harutiunian-Kozak, B., Dec, K. and Wrobel, A. (1973) The organization of visual receptive fields of neurons in the cat colliculus superior. *Acta Neurobiol. Expl. (Warsaw),* 33: 563–573.

Heath, C.J. and Jones, E.G. (1971) The anatomical organization of the suprasylvian gyrus of the cat. *Ergeb. Anat. Entwicklungsgesch.,* 45: 1–64.

Huerta, M.F. and Harting, J.K. (1982) Tectal control of spinal cord activity: Neuroanatomical demonstration of pathways connecting the superior colliculus with the cervical spinal cord grey. *Prog. Brain Res.,* 51: 293–328.

Karabelas, A.B. and Moschovakis, A.K. (1985) Nigral inhibitory termination on efferent neurons of the superior colliculus: An intracellular horseradish peroxidase study in the cat. *J. Comp. Neurol.,* 239: 309–329.

Kawamura, K. (1973a) Corticocortical fiber connections of the cat cerebrum. II. The parietal region. *Brain Res.,* 51: 23–40.

Kawamura, K. (1973b) Corticocortical fiber connections of the cat cerebrum. III. The occipital region. *Brain Res.,* 51: 41–60.

Kawamura, K., Konno, T. and Chiba, M. (1978) Cells of origin of corticopontine and corticotectal fibers in the medial and lateral banks of the middle suprasylvian sulcus in the cat. An experimental study with the horseradish peroxidase method. *Neurosci. Lett.,* 9: 129–135.

Kawamura, S., Sprague, J.M. and Niimi, K. (1974) Corticofugal projections from the visual cortices to the thalamus, pretectum and superior colliculus in the cat. *J. Comp. Neurol.,* 158: 339–362.

Kruger, L. (1970) The topography of the visual projection to the mesencephalon: a comparative survey. *Brain Behav. Evol.,* 3: 169–177.

Marchiafava, P.L. and Pepeu, G.C. (1966) Electrophysiological study of tectal responses to optic nerve volley. *Arch. Ital. Biol.,* 104: 406–420.

McIlwain, J.T. (1972) Central vision: visual cortex and superior colliculus. *Annu. Rev. Physiol.,* 34: 291–314.

McIlwain, J.T. and Buser, P. (1968) Receptive fields of single cells in cat's superior colliculus. *Exp. Brain Res.,* 5: 314–325.

Meredith, M.A. and Stein, B.E. (1983a) Descending efferents of the superior colliculus relay integrated multimodal information. *Soc. Neurosci. Abstr.,* 9: 817.

Meredith, M.A. and Stein, B.E. (1983b) Interactions among converging sensory inputs in the superior colliculus. *Science,* 221: 389–391.

Mize, R.R. (1983) Patterns of convergence and divergence of retinal and cortical synaptic terminals in the cat superior colliculus. *Exp. Brain Res.,* 51: 88–96.

Mize, R.R. and Murphy, E.H. (1976) Alterations in receptive field properties of superior colliculus cells produced by visual cortex ablation in infant and adult cats. *J. Comp. Neurol.,* 168: 393–424.

Naito, J. (1980) Corticocortical connections of the cat sensory areas studied by means of retrograde axonal transport of horseradish peroxidase. *Arch. Hist. Jap.,* 43: 99 – 114.

Norita, M. (1980) Neurons and synaptic patterns in the deep layers of the superior colliculus of the cat: a Golgi and electron microscopic study. *J. Comp. Neurol.,* 190: 29 – 48.

Ogasawara, K., McHaffie, J.G. and Stein, B.E. (1984) Two visual corticotectal systems in cat. *J. Neurophysiol.,* 52: 1226 – 1245.

Palmer, L.A., Rosenquist, A.C. and Sprague, J.M. (1972) Corticotectal systems in the cat: Their structure and function. In: T. Frigyesi, E. Rinvik and M.D. Yahr (Eds.), *Corticothalamic Projections and Sensorimotor Activities,* Raven Press, New York, pp. 491 – 523.

Palmer, L.A., Rosenquist, A.C. and Tusa, R.J. (1978) The retinotopic organization of lateral suprasylvian visual areas in the cat. *J. Comp. Neurol.,* 177: 237 – 256.

Pinter, R.B. and Harris, L.R. (1981) Temporal and spatial response characteristics of the cat superior colliculus. *Brain Res.,* 207: 73 – 94.

Rosenquist, A.C. and Palmer, L.A. (1971) Visual receptive field properties of cells of the superior colliculus after cortical lesions in the cat. *Exp. Neurol.,* 33: 629 – 652.

Roucoux, A. and Crommelinck, M. (1976) Eye movements evoked by superior colliculus stimulation in the alert cat. *Brain Res.,* 106: 349 – 363.

Saraiva, P., Magalhaes-Castro, B., Magalhaes-Castro, H. and Torres, S.R. (1978) Electrophysiological aspects of the superior colliculus of the opossum. Cortico-tectal and tectotectal influences. In: C.E. Rocha-Miranda and R. Lent (Eds.), *Opossum Neurobiology,* Academia Brasileira de Ciências, Rio de Janeiro, pp. 151 – 165.

Schiller, P.H. (1972) The role of the monkey superior colliculus in eye movement and vision. *Invest. Ophthalmol.,* 11: 451 – 460.

Schneider, G.E. (1969) Two visual systems: brain mechanisms for localization and discrimination are dissociated by tectal and cortical lesions. *Science,* 163: 895 – 902.

Schneider, G.E. (1975) Two visuomotor systems in the Syrian hamster. *Neurosci. Res. Prog. Bull.,* 13: 255 – 258.

Segal, R.L. and Beckstead, R.M. (1984) The lateral suprasylvian corticotectal projection in cats. *J. Comp. Neurol.,* 225: 259 – 275.

Segal, R.L., Edwards, S.B. and Beckstead, R.M. (1982) Identification of visual cortical areas that project to the superficial or deep layers of the superior colliculus in cats. *Soc. Neurosci. Abstr.,* 8: 672.

Sherman, S.M. (1974) Visual fields of cats with cortical and tectal lesions. *Science,* 185: 355 – 357.

Sparks, D.L. and Pollack, J.G. (1977) The neural control of saccadic eye movements: the role of the superior colliculus. In: B.A. Brooks and F.J. Bajandas (Eds.), *Eye Movements,* Plenum Press, New York, pp. 179 – 219.

Sprague, J.M. (1966a) Interaction of cortex and the superior colliculus in mediation of visually guided behavior in the cat.

Science, 153: 1544 – 1546.

Sprague, J.M. (1966b) Visual, acoustic, and somesthetic deficits in the cat after cortical and midbrain lesions. In: D.D. Purpura and M. Yahr (Eds.), *The Thalamus,* Columbia, New York, pp. 319 – 417.

Sprague, J.M. (1972) The superior colliculus and pretectum in visual behavior. *Invest. Ophthalmol.,* 11: 473 – 482.

Sprague, J.M. (1975) Mammalian tectum: intrinsic organization, afferent inputs, and integrative mechanisms. In: D. Ingle and J.M. Sprague (Eds.), *Sensorimotor Functions of the Midbrain Tectum, Vol. 13,* MIT Press, Cambridge, pp. 204 – 214.

Sprague, J.M. and Meikle, T.H., Jr. (1965) The role of the superior colliculus in visually guided behavior. *Exp. Neurol.,* 11: 115 – 146.

Sprague, J.M., Marchiafava, P.L. and Rizzolatti, G. (1968) Unit responses to visual stimuli in the superior colliculus of the unanesthetized midpontine cat. *Arch. Ital. Biol.,* 106: 169 – 193.

Sprague, J.M., Wallace, S.F. and Rosenquist, A.C. (1986) Sprague effect mediated by removal of non tecto-tectal fibers in the commissure of the superior colliculus. *Soc. Neurosci. Abstr.,* 12: 1032.

Stein, B.E. (1978) Development and organization of multimodal representation in cat superior colliculus. *Fed. Proc.,* 37: 2240 – 2245.

Stein, B.E. (1984) Development of the superior colliculus. *Annu. Rev. Neurosci.,* 7: 95 – 125.

Stein, B.E. and Arigbede, M.O. (1972) A parametric study of movement detection properties of neurons in the cat's superior colliculus. *Brain Res.,* 45: 437 – 454.

Stein, B.E. and Gordon, B.G. (1981) Maturation of the superior colliculus. In: R.N. Aslin, J.R. Alberts and M.R. Petersen (Eds.), *The Development of Perception: Psychobiological Perspectives, Vol. 2,* Academic Press, New York, pp. 157.

Stein, B.E. and Magalhaes-Castro, B. (1975) Effects of neonatal cortical lesions upon the cat superior colliculus. *Brain Res.,* 83: 480 – 485.

Stein, B.E., Goldberg, S.J. and Clamann, H.P. (1976) The control of eye movements by the superior colliculus in the alert cat. *Brain Res.,* 118: 469 – 474.

Sterling, P. (1971) Receptive fields and synaptic organization of the superficial gray layer of the cat superior colliculus. *Vision Res. Suppl.,* 3: 309 – 328.

Sterling, P. (1973) Quantitative mapping with the electron microscope: retinal terminals in the superior colliculus. *Brain Res.,* 54: 347 – 354.

Sterling, P. and Wickelgren, B.G. (1969) Visual receptive fields in the superior colliculus of the cat. *J. Neurophysiol.,* 32: 1 – 15.

Straschill, M. and Rieger, P. (1973) Eye movements evoked by focal stimulation of the cat's superior colliculus. *Brain Res.,*

59: 211 – 227.

Straschill, M. and Taghavy, H. (1967) Neuronale Reaktionen im Tectum Opticum der Katze auf bewegte und stationäre Lichtreize. *Exp. Brain Res.*, 3: 353 – 367.

Syka, S. and Radil-Weiss, T. (1971) Electrical stimulation of the tectum in freely moving cats. *Brain Res.*, 28: 567 – 572.

Wallace, S.F. and Rosenquist, A.C. (1986) The role of the substantia nigra (pars reticularis) in the mediation of the Sprague effect. *Soc. Neurosci. Abstr.*, 12: 1032.

Wickelgren, B.G. and Sterling, P. (1969) Influence of visual cortex on receptive fields in the superior colliculus of the cat. *J. Neurophysiol.*, 32: 16 – 23.

Wurtz, R.H. and Albano, J.E. (1980) Visual-motor function of the primate superior colliculus. *Annu. Rev. Neurosci.*, 3: 189 – 226.

Zumbroich, T.J., von Grünau, M., Poulin, C. and Blakemore, C. (1986) Differences of visual field representations in the medial and lateral banks of the suprasylvian cortex (PMLS/PLLS) of the cat. *Exp. Brain Res.*, 64: 77 – 93.

T.P. Hicks and G. Benedek (Eds.)
Progress in Brain Research, Vol. 75
© 1988 Elsevier Science Publishers B.V. (Biomedical Division)

CHAPTER 5

Electrophysiological and behavioral experiments on the primate pulvinar

D.B. Bender

Department of Physiology, University at Buffalo, State University of New York, Buffalo, NY 14226, U.S.A.

Our ignorance of pulvinar function is almost total, despite the many anatomical, physiological, and behavioral studies directed at this structure. These studies do show, however, that a major part of the pulvinar is concerned with vision. Two of its three main subdivisions, the inferior and lateral nuclei, are visually responsive and contain at least two retinotopic maps of the contralateral hemifield (Bender 1981, 1982). Both nuclei have reciprocal connections with widespread areas of visual cortex, including striate, prestriate, and inferior temporal cortex (Benevento and Rezak 1976; Ogren and Hendrickson 1976; Benevento and Davis 1977; Ungerleider et al. 1983, 1984). We still, however, have no clear idea of how either subdivision might contribute to visual function.

Most ideas about pulvinar function have been based on the functions of those structures with which it is connected. Thus, the extensive connections with prestriate and inferior temporal cortex have suggested a role in visual learning or memory. This idea has received virtually no experimental support; pulvinar lesions do not impair performance on a wide variety of tasks which are affected by lesions of prestriate or of inferotemporal cortex (Chow 1954; Mishkin 1972; Ungerleider et al. 1977; Ungerleider and Pribram 1977).

A different view of pulvinar function, based on projections it receives from the superior colliculus, is that it serves as a thalamic link forwarding visual information from midbrain to extrastriate cortex.

In tree shrew, squirrel, and other non-primates, both anatomical and behavioral evidence suggest that this 'second visual system' makes an important contribution to visual function that is complementary to the geniculostriate pathway and that can function independently of it (e.g., see Diamond 1976). In monkeys, there have been few direct tests of this notion. The anatomical basis for a second visual system is now well documented: the superficial layers of the superior colliculus project to the inferior pulvinar, and this projection is retinotopically organized and is in register with the inferior pulvinar's visuotopic map (Benevento and Fallon 1975; Partlow et al. 1977; Harting et al. 1980). What contribution this tectopulvinar system makes to visual function, however, is unknown.

In trying to understand the role of the tectopulvinar system, we have used both physiological and behavioral approaches. In the next section, we describe the results of microelectrode recordings from the pulvinar's tectorecipient zone. The findings suggest that the colliculus contributes rather little to neuronal response properties in the pulvinar, in contrast to what one would expect if the pulvinar served a major role as a 'relay' nucleus. We then describe a series of behavioral experiments comparing the effects of tectal and pulvinar lesions. These results likewise suggest a surprising degree of functional independence between tectum and pulvinar.

Studies with single neurons

In monkeys, the tectorecipient zone of the pulvinar also receives topographically organized projections from both striate and prestriate cortex. Interestingly, receptive field properties of inferior pulvinar neurons suggest that it is cortex, not colliculus, which provides the crucial visual input (Bender 1982). Most pulvinar cells are sensitive to stimulus orientation or direction of movement, as are cells in visual cortex. Almost all collicular cells, by contrast, are non-oriented. Furthermore, the non-oriented cells found in the pulvinar differ from non-oriented colliculus cells in that many give sustained responses to flashed stimuli, whereas most colliculus cells give transient responses (Cynader and Berman 1972; Goldberg and Wurtz 1972). Only about 15% of pulvinar neurons are both non-oriented and transient, and thus likely to be driven directly from the colliculus. In order to verify the suggestion that cortical input plays the major role in organizing pulvinar receptive fields, pulvinar neurons were studied following lesions of either striate cortex or the superior colliculus (Bender 1983).

Effects of striate cortex lesions

We made subtotal striate cortex lesions, involving just the representation of the central 15 degrees. Since the inferior pulvinar has a clear retinotopic organization, these restricted cortical removals should affect only those pulvinar cells within the representation of the field defect that resulted from the lesion.

The lesions had a dramatic effect: they eliminated all responsiveness to visual stimuli within the field defect for about three weeks. On a typical electrode penetration through the inferior pulvinar (see Fig. 1), the first cells encountered were visually responsive and had receptive fields near the vertical meridian, just as in intact animals. As the electrode entered the representation of the field defect, a series of unresponsive cells was recorded. The cells were spontaneously active, and easily isolated, but did not respond to any visual stimuli.

Still deeper in the penetration, cells were again visually responsive, with receptive fields in the upper visual quadrant, peripheral to the field defect. This complete lack of responsiveness for cells within the representation of the field defect was in sharp contrast to recordings in normal animals, in which more than 85% of inferior pulvinar neurons can be visually driven.

At survival times longer than 3 weeks, there was a modest recovery of visual responsiveness. About 15% of the cells within the 'scotoma' could be activated by visual stimuli. These cells had response properties strikingly similar to those of colliculus cells: they lacked selectivity for stimulus orienta-

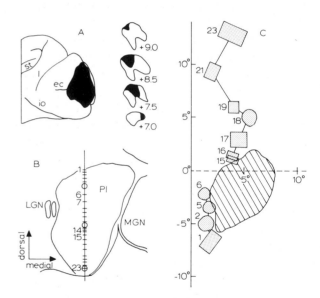

Fig. 1. Receptive fields recorded from the inferior pulvinar of an animal which received a striate cortex lesion 12 days prior to recording. (A) Lateral view of hemisphere showing reconstruction of the lesion (black). Cross-sections to the right show resulting retrograde degeneration (black) in the LGN. (B) Reconstruction of the electrode penetration (vertical line) and recording sites (horizontal bars); small circles indicate electrolytic marking lesions. (C) Receptive fields corresponding to recording sites in (B). A sequence of unresponsive cells was found between sites 6 and 15. The field defect (cross-hatched region) resulting from the cortical lesion was determined by microelectrode mapping of the LGN. ec, external calcarine sulcus; io, inferior occipital sulcus; l, lunate sulcus; st, superior temporal sulcus; LGN, lateral geniculate nucleus; MGN, medial geniculate nucleus; PI, inferior pulvinar. (Adapted from Bender 1983.)

tion or direction of movement, receptive field size was comparable to that in the colliculus, and virtually all gave short-latency, transient, on-off responses to light flashes. These properties suggest that the recovery of responsiveness might well have been mediated by the tectopulvinar projection.

Effects of superior colliculus lesions

Cortical input is thus clearly necessary for activation of pulvinar cells, but might colliculus input make an essential contribution to receptive field properties when cortex is intact? To test this possibility, we made large, bilateral colliculus lesions, which destroyed both superficial and deep layers throughout almost all of the colliculus. This virtually total loss of tectal input had only minimal effects on pulvinar receptive fields. All receptive field types were present after the lesions, and in roughly the same proportions as in intact animals (see Fig. 2). The lesions did have one small effect: the proportion of non-oriented cells that gave transient, on-off, short-latency responses was reduced from the 15% found in normal animals to less than 5%. Hence these non-oriented cells, which bear a

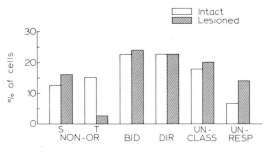

Fig. 2. Effects of superior colliculus lesions on the distribution of receptive field classes in the inferior pulvinar. The results are based on 192 neurons in 4 lesioned animals and 252 neurons in 18 intact animals. Receptive fields were classified into 3 main groups. Non-oriented (NON-OR) cells responded equally well to all orientations of a light bar and gave either sustained (S) or transient (T) responses. Bidirectional (BID) cells preferred one orientation and responded well to back and forth stimulus movement. Directional cells (DIR) preferred one direction of movement over the opposite. UNCLASS, visually responsive cells with undetermined orientation and direction selectivity; UNRESP, visually unresponsive cells. (Adapted from Bender 1983.)

strong resemblance to collicular cells, may indeed be dependent on the tectopulvinar pathway.

Together, the results following striate cortex and superior colliculus lesions indicate that most inferior pulvinar neurons are dominated by input from visual cortex. Orientation-selective, direction-selective, and even many non-oriented cells are permanently lost after cortical but not collicular lesions. The tectopulvinar projection must therefore contribute little to the organization of classical receptive field properties in the intact animal. This pathway might, nonetheless, mediate some of the visual capacity that remains after striate cortex damage, since a few cells did have receptive fields inside the field defect at long survival times. While these cells could not report stimulus orientation or direction of movement, they could indicate stimulus onset and location to about the same degree of precision as do tectal cells. We do not yet know, however, whether these cells project to cortex and whether or not their receptive fields do, in fact, derive from tectal input.

While these results seem incompatible with the view of the pulvinar as a thalamic relay nucleus, it is important to bear in mind the limitations of these experiments. We used the immobilized and anesthetized animal; it is conceivable that in the awake behaving animal, pulvinar cells might be strongly affected by behavioral factors, such as attention, mediated by tectal input. Furthermore, we examined the effects of lesions only on classical receptive field properties. There may be more complex properties that do depend on collicular input. For example, we have recently found that most cells in the tectal layers that project to the pulvinar are remarkably sensitive to movement of a stimulus relative to movement of a textured background (Bender and Davidson 1986). Such local-global comparisons may be present in the pulvinar, and could derive from the tectopulvinar projection. Finally, other parts of the pulvinar, such as the lateral margin of the lateral pulvinar, receive tectal input but have not yet been examined following tectal lesions.

These studies provide one perspective on the tectopulvinar system. In the following section, I describe experiments directed at understanding the contribution of the tectopulvinar system to visually guided behavior.

Behavioral studies

Few behavioral deficits have been seen following destruction of the pulvinar. Only two studies report clear impairments. Chalupa et al. (1976) found that inferior pulvinar lesions impair tachistoscopic pattern discrimination learning, and suggested that the pulvinar is involved in the control of attention. Ungerleider and Christensen (1979) found that pulvinar lesions prolong fixations during spontaneous viewing of a complex scene, and suggested a possible role for the pulvinar in the control of eye movements. Although we have tried to replicate these studies, our main concern has been to compare the behavioral effects of pulvinar and superior colliculus lesions. We assumed that if the colliculus and pulvinar work together in some aspect of visual function then lesions of the tectorecipient zone of the pulvinar and lesions of the colliculus should produce similar impairments. We used several different tasks, each sensitive to colliculus damage, but dependent to different degrees on eye – hand coordination, shifts of attention, and oculomotor performance. Unfortunately, the results failed to support our assumption: although collicular lesions impaired performance in each task, pulvinar lesions did not. The results did suggest, however, that projections from cortex to the colliculus, via the corticotectal tract, play an important role in some, but not all, of these behaviors.

There were two problems which we had to solve in making the pulvinar lesions for these studies. The first was the difficulty of making lesions that were complete, confined to the pulvinar, and consistent across animals. The solution was to record first with microelectrodes from the thalamus and locate the caudal pole of the lateral geniculate nucleus. Having found this landmark, it was possible to choose lesion sites which damaged the LGN only minimally, destroyed virtually all of the inferior and lateral pulvinar, and did so consistently. Second was the problem that radiofrequency (RF) lesions inevitably damage fibers of passage (Bender and Baizer 1984). This was particularly critical since two major fiber systems, corticotectal and retinotectal fibers, pass through the pulvinar on their way to the colliculus. Fortunately, it was possible to solve this problem by making lesions with injections of kainic acid. Such lesions destroy essentially all pulvinar cells without damaging fibers of passage.

Localization and color discrimination with displaced cues

In our first test of the idea that pulvinar and colliculus function together in visually guided behavior, we used two tasks which clearly required eye – hand coordination; in both, the animals were obliged to touch the discriminanda.

The first task tested the ability to detect and localize brief light flashes (Butter et al. 1978; Leiby et al. 1982). The animal faced a horizontal array of response panels on which the stimuli were presented when the animal pressed a start key. On half the trials, a 50 ms flash appeared on one of the panels, and the animal was required to push that panel for reward. The remaining trials were catch trials: no flash was presented and the animal had to press a 'no light' key for reward. Monkeys were trained on this task, given either superior collicular lesions or RF pulvinar lesions, and then retested.

The collicular lesions produced persistent deficits for stimuli presented more than 40 degrees into the periphery (see Fig. 3). The animals mislocalized the flash (pressed a panel neighboring the target panel) on some trials, and failed to detect it (pressed the 'no light' key) on others. Performance was normal when the flashes were presented in the central 30 degrees, and also when the flash duration was increased to 1 s. The pulvinar lesions gave somewhat unexpected results, and first drew our attention to the importance of the corticotectal tract. These lesions pro-

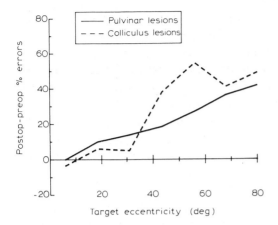

Fig. 3. Effect of pulvinar and colliculus lesions on the localization task. Light flashes were presented to the right and left of a central fixation point; ordinate values represent the difference between preoperative and postoperative percent total errors (localization errors plus detection errors) for flashes at a given eccentricity, averaged over right and left sides. Solid curve is the average of 3 pulvinar-lesioned animals with damaged corticotectal tract; dashed line is the average for 3 colliculus-lesioned animals (Sherm et al., in Butter et al. 1978).

cues were located at the edge of the plaque farthest from the animal, interposing a 3-inch separation between cue and response site. Butter (1974) had shown that colliculus lesions impair learning in this second stage, the animals apparently failing to shift their gaze between the response site and the displaced cues (Kurtz et al. 1982). Since we were concerned about the possible confounding effects of damage to corticotectal fibers, we tested two groups of animals. One received RF pulvinar lesions, destroying both the pulvinar and corticotectal fibers; the other received kainic acid (KA) lesions which destroyed pulvinar cells, but spared corticotectal fibers.

Neither pulvinar-lesioned group was impaired in the first stage of testing, confirming earlier findings that pulvinar lesions do not impair color discrimination learning. In the stimulus – response separation stage, however, the animals with RF lesions were impaired relative to normal controls. They required more trials to relearn the discrimina-

duced deficits similar to the colliculus deficit, but only when there was damage to corticotectal fibers. Three animals had destruction of the pulvinar's tectorecipient zone, but they also had marked shrinkage of the brachium of the superior colliculus, indicating severe loss of corticotectal fibers. These animals made localization errors as well as detection errors when peripheral flashes were presented (see Fig. 3). Four additional animals also had pulvinar damage, but in each case the brachium appeared normal and the animals were unimpaired.

In the second task, pulvinar-lesioned animals were trained in a Wisconsin General Test Apparatus on two-choice color discriminations in which the cues were spatially separated from the response sites (Nagel-Leiby et al. 1984). The animals learned the discrimination with the cues initially placed at the base of the stimulus plaques, the part that is habitually touched by the animal as it pushes it away to retrieve a reward. They were then tested in a second stage in which the color

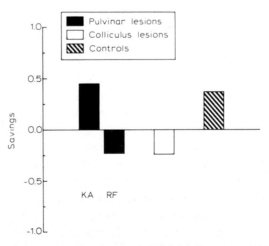

Fig. 4. Savings scores for color discriminations with a stimulus-response (S-R) separation. Savings were calculated from the formula $(x - y)/(x + y)$, where x and y are trials to criterion in the 1st (no S-R separation) and 2nd (S-R separation) learning stages, respectively; bars represent performance averaged over two different color discriminations. Controls include unoperated and subcortical lesion groups in Nagel-Leiby et al. (1984). KA, 3 animals with kainic acid lesions; RF, 3 animals with radiofrequency lesions.

tion than they had to learn it in the first stage, whereas control animals showed substantial savings (see Fig. 4). By contrast, the animals with KA lesions showed no impairment.

Both studies, then, fail to support the idea that the pulvinar and superior colliculus share some aspect of visual function. Although the colliculus is necessary for stimulus localization, and for learning in the face of a stimulus – response separation, the ascending projection from colliculus to pulvinar is not. At the same time, the results indicate that damage to the corticotectal tract can be as devastating as direct damage to the colliculus. It is thus important to consider such damage in interpreting earlier studies using lesions of the pulvinar. While it is far from clear what role the projections from cortex to colliculus play, they may be particularly critical for eye – hand coordination, as this was required in both of our tasks. Furthermore, this factor was not prominent in the two tasks described below, and in these tasks performance was not impaired by corticotectal tract damage.

Visual search and tachistoscopic discrimination

Since several studies had suggested that the pulvinar plays a role in control of attention (Gould et al. 1974; Chalupa et al. 1976; Petersen et al. 1984), we next used two tasks which clearly seemed to depend on attention. The first was a visual search task in which the animals searched for a small target pattern within an array of irrelevant patterns (Bender and Butter 1987). Normal animals perform the search by shifting their gaze, and attention, serially through the display, a fact reflected in search times and errors that increase linearly with the number of irrelevant patterns (Azzato and Butter 1984). The second task was almost identical to the tachistoscopic pattern discrimination that Chalupa et al. (1976) had used; rather than measure rate of learning, however, we measured the minimum necessary exposure for discriminating the patterns.

In both tasks, animals viewed two large response panels on which the stimuli were presented. They started a trial by pushing an observing-response key which, in turn, presented the stimuli. For the visual search task, the target pattern, together with various numbers of irrelevant patterns, appeared on one of the panels, and an equal number of irrelevant stimuli appeared on the other. For the tachistoscopic task, the stimuli appeared as flashes whose duration was gradually reduced until the animals reached asymptotic performance at about 80% correct responses. Animals were trained on the visual search task, received either colliculus or pulvinar lesions and were then retested. Finally, they were tested on the tachistoscopic task. For these experiments, we started with massive RF pulvinar lesions which destroyed both inferior and lateral pulvinar, part of the medial pulvinar, and much of the corticotectal tract. We had planned to use a third group with KA lesions, had a deficit been found.

In the visual search task, the colliculus lesions

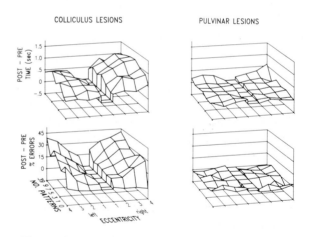

Fig. 5. Visual search performance for 3 animals with RF pulvinar lesions and 3 animals with colliculus lesions. Differences between preoperative and postoperative times and errors were averaged across animals within each group. Animals began each trial with gaze and hand directed at an observing response (OR) key located between the two display panels. The target was presented on either the left or right panel, within one of 4 approximately equal-area eccentricity ranges (11 – 35, 35 – 46, 46 – 54, 54 – 57 degrees with respect to the OR key), together with 0, 1, 3, 5, 7, 9, or 39 irrelevant stimuli; an equal number of stimuli, all irrelevant, appeared on the opposite panel. See Bender and Butter (1987) for details.

resulted in longer search times and increased errors (see Fig. 5). Search times and errors increased more steeply with target eccentricity, and with number of irrelevant patterns, following surgery than before. This probably reflects an impaired ability to shift gaze, and presumably attention, from one site to the next in the display. In contrast, the pulvinar lesions did not alter search performance. As shown in Fig. 5, neither search time nor errors increased after surgery.

The results of tachistoscopic discrimination testing were similar. As seen in Fig. 6, colliculus lesions increased the threshold exposure durations by almost 20-fold, on average, over those of control animals. By contrast, thresholds for the animals with pulvinar lesions did not differ from those of controls.

Once again, both studies fail to support the idea that the pulvinar shares visual functions with the superior colliculus. Furthermore, they make it difficult to accept the idea that the pulvinar plays a major and indispensible role in the control of attention. Certainly the pulvinar is not essential for

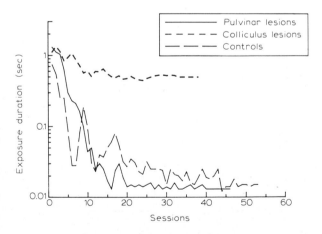

Fig. 6. Median exposure durations during estimation of thresholds for tachistoscopic pattern discrimination. During each 210-trial session, the exposure duration was decreased by 10 ms for 3 consecutive correct responses, and was increased by 10 ms for every error. The exposure durations were averaged over the session for each animal; the ordinate for each group is the median of the average durations for the 3 animals in the group. See Bender and Butter (1987) for details.

the shifts of attention that must occur during visual search, and it must not play a very fundamental role in the attentional requirements of tachistoscopic performance. We do not yet know which of the many minor methodological differences between this study and that of Chalupa et al. (1976) might account for their finding of a tachistoscopic performance deficit.

While colliculus lesions altered visual search performance, it is worth emphasizing that loss of both retinal and cortical afferents to the colliculus, as a result of the pulvinar lesions, had no effect whatever on visual search. Some other afferent system, possibly the nigrotectal pathway (Wurtz and Hikosaka 1986), must underlie the contribution of the colliculus to this behavior.

Saccadic eye movements

There were several reasons for thinking that the pulvinar might be involved in oculomotor performance. The tectal laminae that project to the pulvinar contain cells which discharge in relation to eye movements (Schiller and Koerner 1971; Wurtz and Mohler 1976; Harting et al. 1980); some pulvinar cells discharge in association with eye movements (Petersen et al. 1985), and alterations in eye movements have been seen following pulvinar lesions in both man and monkey. Ungerleider and Christensen (1979) reported that monkeys with pulvinar lesions were 'visually captured'. During scanning of a complex scene, fixations were twice as long as in normal monkeys. A similar lengthening of fixations has been described in two human patients with pulvinar damage, although additional damage to parietal cortex make these cases hard to interpret (Zihl and von Cramon 1979; Ogren et al. 1984).

We looked at eye movements made in response to three different types of target movements (Bender and Baizer 1986). We used a single-step movement in which a target jumped from a fixation point to a point 12, 24 or 36 degrees to the right or left, at the same time that the fixation point turned off. To test for 'visual capture', we used two additional conditions. On 'overlap' trials, the fixation point remained lit while an identical target jumped to the right or left. If the lesioned animals were 'visually captured', latencies of saccades to the target jump should be prolonged relative to those on single-step trials. We also used a double-step condition, the 'pulse-undershoot' paradigm of Becker and Jurgens (1979), in which the target jumped from the straight-ahead position to 24 degrees to the right or left, and then after a brief delay, jumped halfway back to the 12 degree position. Normal animals respond to this motion with an initial saccade whose amplitude varies from 24 to 12 degrees, depending on the time between the second target jump and saccade onset. This decrease of amplitude with time is the 'amplitude transition function', or ATF, of Becker and Jurgens (1979). If animals with pulvinar lesions are slow to change fixation because of an inability to process new target information, there should be a change in the ATF. Animals were trained on the three different types of target movements, received KA lesions, and then were retested.

Despite the fact that the lesions were large, destroying virtually all of the visual pulvinar, they had almost no effect on saccadic latency for any type of target movement. On single-step trials, only latencies to the most peripheral target (36 degrees eccentricity) were affected, and for these the change was a slight (20 – 50 ms) decrease in latency (see Fig. 7A). On overlap trials, where one might have expected an increase in latency, there was again only a slight postoperative decrease in latency, averaging 20 msec, at the most eccentric target positions (Fig. 7B). Finally, the saccadic responses on double-step trials were essentially unaffected, with the amplitude transition functions showing no consistent change (see Fig. 8).

Although these massive pulvinar lesions had little effect on saccades evoked by target movements, it was still conceivable that spontaneous eye movements might have been affected by the lesions, particularly in view of Ungerleider and Christensen's findings, but also since spontaneous saccades are more severely affected by collicular lesions than are saccades evoked by a target movement (Schiller

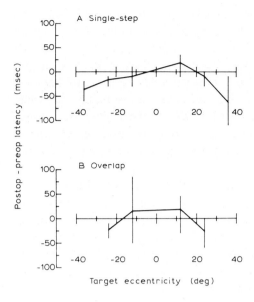

Fig. 7. Difference between preoperative and postoperative median saccadic latencies following kainic acid lesions of the pulvinar. Differences are averaged across 3 animals; vertical bars represent the range of the differences. (A) Single-step trials, on which the fixation point turned off synchronously with the target jump. (B) Overlap trials, on which the fixation point remained on during and after the target jump.

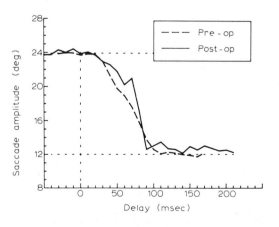

Fig. 8. Amplitude transition functions for one animal with a kainic acid pulvinar lesion. The target jumped 24 degrees to the right of the fixation point, and then 12 degrees back after an interval of 30 – 180 ms. The ordinate is the average amplitude of the first saccade evoked by the target movement as a function of the time (Delay) between the start of that saccade and the second target jump.

et al. 1980). Thus we tried to replicate Ungerleider and Christensen's experiment. We used subjects from the above-mentioned saccade study, and followed Ungerleider and Christensen's experimental procedure, simply measuring the average duration of fixations while the animals gazed at a complex scene. As shown in Fig. 9, we found that animals with KA pulvinar lesions did not make significantly longer fixations than did unoperated control animals.

These findings once again emphasize the functional independence of tectum and pulvinar. Collicular lesions increase latency of saccades to visual targets and increase fixation length during spontaneous viewing, yet pulvinar lesions alter neither. The animals with pulvinar lesions also showed no signs of 'visual capture'. On overlap trials, they shifted gaze to a peripheral target, despite the presence of a competing central target, as readily as they had prior to the operation. Likewise, they were just as able to reprogram saccades in response to the sudden changes of target position that occurred on double-step trials. Even using the same procedures that Ungerleider and Christensen used, we could find no hint of prolonged fixations. Most

likely, then, 'visual capture' does not result from damage to pulvinar neurons, but rather from corticotectal tract damage. Such damage was inevitable in Ungerleider and Christensen's study since all of their lesions encroached on the brachium of the colliculus.

Summary

The notion of a 'second visual system', in which the pulvinar conveys visual information from midbrain to cortex, has been a persistent and popular one. In the monkey, however, there is at present virtually no evidence to support this view of pulvinar function. Indeed, the present studies underline how little the colliculus seems to contribute to pulvinar function. Pulvinar receptive field properties are all but independent of colliculus input. Behavioral studies indicate a comparable independence. We have looked at a number of different aspects of visually guided behavior, including eye – hand coordination, visual attention, and oculomotor control, and found that the pulvinar is not critical for any of these. In sharp contrast, the colliculus is crucial for all; its contribution must be mediated by descending projections into the brainstem, rather than through ascending projections to the pulvinar. The critical afferent pathway to the colliculus, however, does seem to vary with the task. Corticotectal afferents are important when manual responses are directed at stimuli, or during unpracticed spontaneous inspection of a scene, but not during well-practiced search.

Beginning with Chow's original study in the early 1950s, there have been more than a dozen attempts to find behavioral impairments following pulvinar lesions. It is perplexing that so few deficits have been found. Now it appears that even those deficits cannot be reproduced when using a slightly different procedure or lesions that spare fibers of passage. The problem cannot be incompleteness of the lesions, as was once thought, since many of these studies involve complete destruction of the visual part of the pulvinar; nor

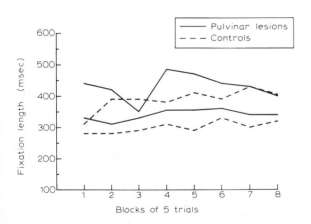

Fig. 9. Median length of fixations during spontaneous viewing of a complex scene for 2 animals with kainic acid lesions and 2 unoperated controls. The animals viewed the scene for 5-s trials, with a 30-s intertrial interval, 40 trials per day, for 2 consecutive days. Fixations were pooled in blocks of 5 successive trials, and corresponding blocks from the 2 sessions were then pooled.

can it be a lack of sensitivity of the behavioral tasks, since in every case performance is impaired by lesions of structures anatomically connected to the pulvinar. It may be that whatever function the pulvinar contributes by virtue of its thalamocortical relations, that function can be substituted adequately for, by direct cortico-cortical connections, thus making the lesion method useless. Alternatively, it may simply be that the right task has not been tried. In any case, it remains a considerable challenge to unravel the pulvinar's role in vision.

Acknowledgments

Many of the behavioral experiments were done in collaboration with Dr. C.M. Butter and his associates at the University of Michigan, Ann Arbor, MI. The eye movement studies were done in collaboration with Dr. J.S. Baizer at SUNY, Buffalo, NY. I am grateful to Beverly Caffery, Amy Stenger, and Diana Bozian for histological and technical assistance, and to Linda Smith for secretarial help. Supported by grant EY02254 from the National Eye Institute.

References

Azzato, M.C. and Butter, C.M. (1984) Visual search in cynomolgus monkeys: Stimulus parameters affecting two stages of visual search. *Percept. Psychophys.,* 36: 169 – 176.

Becker, W. and Jurgens, R. (1979) An analysis of the saccadic system by means of double step stimuli. *Vision Res.,* 19: 967 – 983.

Bender, D.B. (1981) Retinotopic organization of macaque pulvinar. *J. Neurophysiol.,* 46: 672 – 693.

Bender, D.B. (1982) Receptive-field properties of neurons in the macaque inferior pulvinar. *J. Neurophysiol.,* 48: 1 – 17.

Bender, D.B. (1983) Visual activation of neurons in the primate pulvinar depends on cortex but not colliculus. *Brain Res.,* 297: 258 – 261.

Bender, D.B. and Baizer, J.S. (1984) Anterograde degeneration in the superior colliculus following kainic acid and radiofrequency lesions of the macaque pulvinar. *J. Comp. Neurol.,* 228: 284 – 298.

Bender, D.B. and Baizer, J.S. (1986) Effects of kainic acid lesions of the pulvinar on saccadic eye movements in monkeys. *Soc. Neurosci. Abstr.,* 12: 1039.

Bender, D.B. and Butter, C.M. (1987) Comparison of the effects of superior colliculus and pulvinar lesions on visual search and tachistoscopic pattern discrimination in monkeys. *Exp. Brain Res.,* 69: 140 – 154.

Bender, D.B. and Davidson, R.M. (1986) Global visual processing in the monkey superior colliculus. *Brain Res.,* 381: 372 – 375.

Benevento, L.A. and Davis, B. (1977) Topographical projections of the prestriate cortex to the pulvinar nuclei in the macaque monkey: an autoradiographic study. *Exp. Brain Res.,* 30: 405 – 424.

Benevento, L.A. and Fallon, J.H. (1975) The ascending projections of the superior colliculus in the rhesus monkey (*Macaca mulatta*). *J. Comp. Neurol.,* 160: 339 – 362.

Benevento, L.A. and Rezak, M. (1976) The cortical projections of the inferior pulvinar and adjacent lateral pulvinar in the rhesus monkey (*Macaca mulatta*): An autoradiographic study. *Brain Res.,* 108: 1 – 24.

Butter, C.M. (1974) Effect of superior colliculus, striate and prestriate lesions on visual sampling in rhesus monkeys. *J. Comp. Physiol. Psychol.,* 87: 905 – 917.

Butter, C.M., Weinstein, C., Bender, D. and Gross, C.G. (1978) Localization and detection of visual stimuli following superior colliculus lesions in rhesus monkeys. *Brain Res.,* 156: 33 – 49.

Chalupa, L.M., Coyle, R.S. and Lindsley, D.B. (1976) Effect of pulvinar lesions on visual pattern discrimination in monkeys. *J. Neurophysiol.,* 39: 354 – 369.

Chow, K.-L. (1954) Lack of behavioral effects following destruction of some thalamic association nuclei in monkey. *Am. Med. Assoc. Arch. Neurol. Psychiat.,* 71: 762 – 771.

Cynader, M. and Berman, N. (1972) Receptive-field organization of monkey superior colliculus. *J. Neurophysiol.,* 35: 187 – 201.

Diamond, I.T. (1976) Organization of the visual cortex: comparative anatomical and behavioral studies. *Fed. Proc.,* 35: 60 – 67.

Goldberg, M.E. and Wurtz, R.H. (1972) Activity of superior colliculus in behaving monkey. I. Visual receptive fields of single neurons. *J. Neurophysiol.,* 35: 542 – 559.

Gould, J.E., Chalupa, L.M. and Lindsley, D.B. (1974) Modifications of pulvinar and geniculocortical evoked potentials during visual discrimination learning in monkeys. *Electroenceph. clin. Neurophysiol.,* 36: 639 – 649.

Harting, J.K., Huerta, M.F., Frankfurter, A.J., Strominger, N.L. and Royce, G.J. (1980) Ascending pathways from the monkey superior colliculus: An autoradiographic analysis. *J. Comp. Neurol.,* 192: 853 – 882.

Kurtz, D., Leiby, C.C. and Butter, C.M. (1982) Further analysis of S-R separation effects on visual discrimination performance of normal rhesus monkeys and monkeys with superior colliculus lesions. *J. Comp. Physiol. Psychol.,* 96: 35 – 46.

Leiby, III, C.C., Bender, D.B. and Butter, C.M. (1982)

Localization and detection of visual stimuli in monkeys with pulvinar lesions. *Exp. Brain Res.,* 48: 449 – 454.

Mishkin, M. (1972) Cortical visual areas and their interactions. In: A.G. Karczmar and J.C. Eccles (Eds.), *Brain and Human Behavior,* Springer, New York, pp. 187 – 208.

Nagel-Leiby, S., Bender, D.B. and Butter, C.M. (1984) Effects of kainic acid and radiofrequency lesions of the pulvinar on visual discrimination in the monkey. *Brain Res.,* 300: 295 – 303.

Ogren, M.P. and Hendrickson, A.E. (1976) Pathways between striate cortex and subcortical regions in *Macaca mulatta* and *Saimiri sciureus:* evidence for a reciprocal pulvinar connection. *Exp. Neurol.,* 53: 780 – 800.

Ogren, M.P., Mateer, C.A. and Wyler, A.R. (1984) Alterations in visually related eye movements following left pulvinar damage in man. *Neuropsychologia,* 22: 187 – 196.

Partlow, G.D., Colonnier, M. and Szabo, J. (1977) Thalamic projections of the superior colliculus in the rhesus monkey, *Macaca mulatta:* a light and electron microscopic study. *J. Comp. Neurol.,* 171: 285 – 318.

Petersen, S.E., Morris, J.D. and Robinson, D.L. (1984) Modulation of attentional behavior by injection of GABA-related drugs into the pulvinar of the macaque. *Soc. Neurosci. Abstr.,* 10: 475.

Petersen, S.E., Robinson, D.L. and Keys, W. (1985) Pulvinar nuclei of the behaving rhesus monkey: visual responses and their modulation. *J. Neurophysiol.,* 54: 867 – 886.

Schiller, P.H. and Koerner, F. (1971) Discharge characteristics of single units in superior colliculus of the alert rhesus monkey. *J. Neurophysiol.,* 34: 920 – 936.

Schiller, P.H., True, S.D. and Conway, J.L. (1980) Deficits in eye movements following frontal eye-field and superior colliculus ablations. *J. Neurophysiol.,* 44: 1175 – 1189.

Ungerleider, L.G. and Christensen, C.A. (1979) Pulvinar lesions in monkeys produce abnormal scanning of a complex visual array. *Neuropsychologia,* 17: 493 – 501.

Ungerleider, L.G. and Pribram, K.H. (1977) Inferotemporal versus combined pulvinar-prestriate lesions in the rhesus monkey: effects on color, object and pattern discrimination. *Neuropsychologia,* 15: 481 – 498.

Ungerleider, L.G., Ganz, L. and Pribram, K.H. (1977) Size constancy in rhesus monkeys: effects of pulvinar, prestriate and inferotemporal lesions. *Exp. Brain Res.,* 27: 251 – 269.

Ungerleider, L.G., Galkin, T.W. and Mishkin, M. (1983) Visuotopic organization of projections from striate cortex to inferior and lateral pulvinar in rhesus monkey. *J. Comp. Neurol.,* 217: 137 – 157.

Ungerleider, L.G., Desimone, R., Galkin, T.W. and Mishkin, M. (1984) Subcortical projections of area MT in the macaque. *J. Comp. Neurol.,* 223: 368 – 386.

Wurtz, R.H. and Hikosaka, O. (1986) Role of the basal ganglia in the initiation of saccadic eye movements. *Prog. Brain Res.,* 64: 175 – 190.

Wurtz, R.H. and Mohler, C.W. (1976) Organization of monkey superior colliculus: enhanced visual response of superficial layer cells. *J. Neurophysiol.,* 39: 745 – 765.

Zihl, J. and von Cramon, D. (1979) The contribution of the 'second' visual system to directed visual attention in man. *Brain,* 102: 835 – 856.

T.P. Hicks and G. Benedek (Eds.)
Progress in Brain Research, Vol. 75
© 1988 Elsevier Science Publishers B.V. (Biomedical Division)

CHAPTER 6

The consequences of the superior colliculus output on lateral geniculate and pulvinar responses

Stéphane Molotchnikoff, Christian Casanova and Alain Cérat

Department of Biological Sciences, University of Montreal, Montreal, Canada

Introduction

In the past two decades, it has been acknowledged that, in mammals, the retinofugal neuronal messages destined for the cortex are carried along two parallel channels. They pass through either the superior colliculus (SC) or more directly through thalamic relays. These two paths represent the anatomical substrates for a duality in visual functions. In broad terms, the geniculo-cortical network is associated with discrimination of discrete visual nuances, whether they are colored or not, while the colliculo-cortical system is linked to ambient vision and eye movements (Trevarthen 1968; Schneider 1969; Jeannerod 1974). There is a point of confluence in these two paths as the SC sends fibers to the thalamus; the latter then becomes a crossroads where colliculo-cortical and retino-cortical routes meet.

A first group of collicular cells, located in the superficial layer, sends axons to the dorsal lateral geniculate nucleus (LGN). These ascending fibers have been identified in a variety of mammals examined (Casagrande et al. 1972; Benevento and Fallon 1975; Robson and Hall 1976; Graham and Bergman 1981; Graham 1977; Harting et al. 1980;

Kawamura et al. 1980; Torrealba et al. 1981; Holstege and Collewijn 1982; Huerta and Harting 1983). The latter authors have shown that collicular axons terminate mostly in the interlaminar zone and S layers in primates. In cats, the densest collicular input is found in layers that contain the smallest geniculate neurons, that is, the C laminae. Collicular axons establish two types of synapses (Torrealba et al. 1981). In rodents such as rats, hamsters (Huerta and Harting 1983) and rabbits (Giolli and Pope 1971; Holstege and Collewijn 1982; Molotchnikoff and Lachapelle 1980) the colliculo-geniculate projections distribute themselves more diffusely.

A second major colliculofugal, ascending efferent route is made up of fibers that are destined for the lateral posterior-pulvinar complex (LP-P). In the remaining part of this text, it will be referred to as the pulvinar or LP-P. Indeed, these groups of thalamic cells receive their visual input mostly from the SC or the cortex, as the former lack a direct retinal input. Tectal cells that project to the LP-P are positioned slightly more ventrally than neurons that contact the LGN. Furthermore, there seems to be a dorsoventral segregation of tecto-LP-P cells, as the superficial units project to the anterior section while the deep cells contact the posterior pulvinar (Casanova 1986).

In view of these well-documented tecto-thalamic paths, it is legitimate to ask: what is the role of these fibers? This question is particularly impor-

Correspondence to: Dr. S. Molotchnikoff, Département des Sciences Biologiques, Université de Montréal, CP 6128, Succ. A, Montréal, P.Q., Canada, H3C 3J7.

tant as both tecto-pulvinar- and tecto-geniculate-recipient cells send their axons to supragranular layers of area 17 (Huerta and Harting 1984). Consequently, through these thalamic relay stations, the SC is potentially capable of influencing cortical responses. It is then reasonable to assume that this collicular impact upon cortical physiology is accomplished in relation with its role in visually guided eye reflexes (Chalupa 1984). At the present time there exist numerous observations that indicate that the collicular cells discharge in relation to short and long latency saccades (Sparks and Mays 1983; Sparks and Porter 1983; Schiller et al. 1987). In complement, electrical stimulation of the colliculus produces eye and/or head movements (Guitton et al. 1980). Conversely, the ablation of the colliculi results in a neglect of new targets (Goodale and Murison 1975) and slower or inaccurate saccades (Schiller et al. 1987). Hence, these tecto-thalamic paths must be intimately associated with the neuronal processing which integrates eye movements and visual perception (Wurtz and Albano 1980).

The aim of the experiments reported here was to determine the effects of collicular inactivation on LGN and LP-P responses. In addition, since the colliculus is linked to eye reflexes following the appearance of novel, disturbing targets, it is our assumption that the interactions between several stimuli in the visual field are neuronally integrated at the collicular level. Indeed, the results of Rizzolati et al. (1973) seem to lend credence to this assumption. The output of this processing is conveyed toward the collicular projection sites, including the thalamus. It then follows that, if the colliculus is rendered dysfunctional, the integration between two stimuli can no longer occur.

General methodology

Experiments were carried out on anesthetized and paralyzed rabbits prepared for acute single unit recordings. The detailed animal preparation procedure has been described elsewhere (Molotchni-koff et al. 1986a, b). Briefly, the neuronal activity of geniculate or pulvinar units was recorded with glass, NaCl-filled micropipettes. In retinotopic register with the geniculate cell, a second micropipette was lowered into the superior colliculus. This pipette was filled with lidocaine hydrochloride (2%), which blocks Na^+ channels. A pressure pump ejected 50 to 100 nl of the drug, which arrests all neuronal electrical activity. Consequently, all efferent collicular action potentials were interrupted while the drug was applied. A custom adaptation of the head stage of the ejecting pipette allowed the recording of collicular responses. The disappearance of these responses confirmed that the drug had been delivered, and conversely, the reappearance indicated that the drug had washed out and that the colliculus had recovered from the depression.

Hence, LGN and LP-P responses were measured prior to, during and after collicular inactivation.

In order to further understand the functions of the colliculo-thalamic system, two light sources were presented in the visual field. The first was a light emitting diode (LED) which was positioned within the visual receptive field of the geniculate cell. It was defined as the test stimulus. The second stimulus was a white, moving or stationary slit positioned in the periphery. This conditioning or 'disturbing' stimulus, when presented in solitary fashion, failed to influence the spontaneous activity of the tested geniculate cell. However, if paired with the LED, the conditioning stimulus modified significantly (>20% change) the evoked discharges to the first test stimulus. In this way, interactions between two discrete light sources could be revealed. An additional goal of this series of experiments was to verify if the interactions between two light stimuli in the visual field are processed by the colliculus. If this is the case, then collicular depression should suppress these interactions and the test response would be unchanged.

It must be emphasized that in all of these experiments, tests and controls were run randomly in order to reduce the effects of habituation.

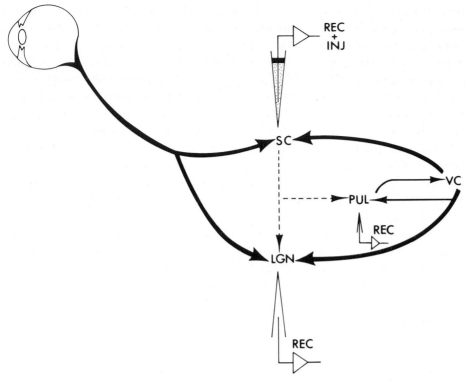

Fig. 1. Schematic drawing of the pathway involved in the present study. SC, superior colliculus; LGN, lateral geniculate nucleus; PUL, lateral posterior-pulvinar complex or LP-P; VC, visual cortex; REC + INJ, recording and lidocaine hydrochloride injection micropipette; REC, recording micropipette.

Results

Effect of collicular inactivation on LGN and LP-P responses

Figure 2 illustrates typical examples of collicular influences on LGN and LP-P cells. In response to the LED positioned in its receptive field, the geniculate neuron discharged with a phasic 'on' response, which rapidly declined well prior to the off-step of the LED. The 'off' stimulus did not excite the cell (trace 1). Interrupting the collicular input produced a significant facilitation of the geniculate excitation. The cell appears to have adopted a more sustained firing rate (trace 2). Indeed, the cell maintained a high rate of firing for the duration of the light pulse. The rate of action potentials decreased very gradually to the prestimulation level. A survey of data indicates that the injection of lidocaine hydrochloride increases geniculate ex-

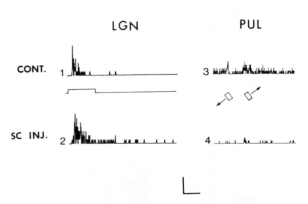

Fig. 2. Influence of collicular inactivation on lateral geniculate (LGN) and pulvinar (PUL) responses. Controls (Cont.) in traces 1 and 3: depressing the colliculus (SC. INJ.) produces an increase in the light response of the LGN. Trace 2: the same treatment produces a virtual arrest of neuronal excitation in the pulvinar. Trace 4: calibration, horizontal 300 ms, vertical 5 spikes. Poststimulus time histograms obtained following the summation of 20 stimuli presentations. LGN cell stimulated with an LED flashing on and off positioned in its receptive field. Pulvinar cell stimulated by sweeping a light square in its receptive field.

citability in 19% of cells ($n = 99$) whereas 25% of the neurons react with a decline of their responses. It is interesting to observe that the collicular blockade influences mostly the secondary discharges, while the initial responses, those which occurred with shortest latencies, remained undisturbed (Molotchnikoff et al., 1986a, b).

The majority of pulvinar cells reacted to collicular blockade with a decrease in their discharges. One typical example is shown in Fig. 2 (traces 3 and 4). The neuron responded to the back and forth sweeping of a white square ($10° \times 10°$) in its receptive field (trace 3, Fig. 2). The microinjection of lidocaine resulted in a virtual arrest of all neuronal electrical activity (trace 4, Fig. 2). This observation suggests that the pulvinar excitation strongly depends upon collicular afferents.

Comparison between the geniculate and the pulvinar

A comparative survey of these series of experiments disclosed interesting observations regarding colliculo-thalamic relations. The histogram in Fig. 3 displays the proportion of cells that augmented, diminished or were insensitive to collicular blockade. It appears that collicular cells ex-

ert a balanced dual impact on the geniculate, since about the same proportion of cells either significantly augmented (19%) or diminished (25%) their responses. Fifty-six percent of neurons failed to react to collicular blockade. In all of these studies we considered it a significant modification if the changes were of a magnitude greater than 20% relative to control responses. By contrast, most pulvinar cells (41%) had their responses reduced; only 19% showed a facilitation. Moreover, a facilitation superior to 60% occurred only in one cell (Casanova 1986). It is emphasized that a greater population of cells are affected in the pulvinar than in the LGN after interruption of collicular input. Finally, in the pulvinar, all segments of the evoked discharges, that is, the initial as well as the late responses, were affected. These observations are in agreement with the notion that visual inputs arise either from the superior colliculus or the cortex.

The role of colliculo-thalamic paths

In the Introduction, it was stated that the SC facilitates the orientation of gaze toward novel stimuli, suddenly introduced into the visual field. This hypothesis implicitly suggests that the neuronal interactions between several visual targets present in the visual field are processed, at least partially, at collicular levels. The outcome of this processing is 'read' by cells that are contacted by tectofugal axons. Obviously, geniculate and LP-P neurons are amongst those neurons. To test this hypothesis, two circumscribed stimuli were presented in the visual field, as described in the Methods. Figure 4 displays a typical example. In this case the conditioning or 'disturbing' stimulus was a moving slit travelling in the naso-temporal direction. This stimulus remained without effect on the spontaneous activity of the geniculate neuron (trace 1, Fig. 4). By contrast, the unit was excited by the LED positioned in its receptive field, as both 'on' and 'off' discharges were evoked (trace 2, Fig. 4). The 'off' response contains a robust secondary burst (bold arrow, trace 2).

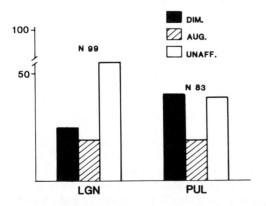

Fig. 3. Relative proportions and comparative influences of collicular inactivation on the LGN and PUL cells. Dark bars: cells which reacted with decreased (DIM) responses to collicular blockade; striped bars: cells which reacted with a facilitation (AUG); white bars: unaffected cells (UNAFF).

Although the conditioning or 'disturbing' stimulus was without influence on this geniculate neuron when presented in isolation, it exerted a profound effect when combined with the LED. As shown in trace 3, it was clear that the presence of the disturbing stimulus produced a profound change of the 'off' response: namely, the secondary burst was abolished (open arrow, trace 3, Fig. 4). It is essential to emphasize that test and control runs were presented in random sequences.

In the second step, the superior colliculus was injected with lidocaine hydrochloride (Fig. 4 INJ.: traces 4, 5 and 6). The collicular inactivation provoked an increased excitability of the geniculate unit. The cell became tonically active while the LED was on (trace 5). Interestingly and typically (Molotchnikoff et al. 1986b), the 'off' response

seemed to have lost the secondary bursts contained in its discharge. It was apparent that the addition of the remote stimulus failed to modify the firing pattern of responses to the test light. Indeed, both responses were quite comparable (traces 5 and 6). Hence, the interaction that occurred between two stimuli when the SC was intact, seemed to have disappeared. Thus, it appears that the disruption of a retinotopic ensemble of collicular neurons suppresses the interaction between two light sources present in the visual field.

Discussion

The major conclusion that stems from these investigations is the capability of the superior colliculus to influence the lateral geniculate nucleus and the lateral posterior-pulvinar complex. Since these structures convey their information to the cortex, it follows that the colliculi are participating in the visual properties of cortical cells. The colliculo-geniculate influences are dual in their nature, since excitatory and inhibitory responses are recorded with about the same frequency. This duality probably lies in the fact that two types of synaptic profiles are ascribed to colliculofugal axons. Such data were reported for cats (Torrealba et al. 1981). Somewhat differently, the tecto-LP-P influence is more homogeneous, as most cells decrease their responses with collicular decline. In addition, the excitation of geniculate cells is rarely fully abolished with collicular depression. By contrast, in many LP-P cells all excitation ceases after the same treatment. It may be that this reflects the fact that the geniculate receives its major visual inputs from the retina, while LP-P cells are visually driven either through the SC or the cortex. Furthermore, previous analysis from our laboratory has indicated that the colliculo-thalamic path is organized retinotopically.

It seems appropriate at this point to propose a functional role for the tecto-thalamic paths. The comparison of receptive field properties of the LGN and LP-P cells may provide some clues about this role. Two prominent characteristics seem to

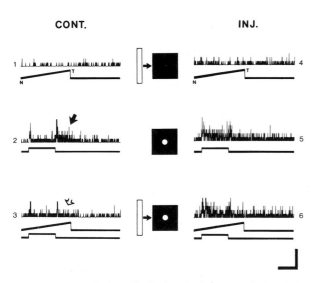

Fig. 4. Interaction between two stimuli in the visual field, processed by the superior colliculus. Traces 1 and 4: a light slit sweeping in the nasal (N) temporal (T) direction fails to modify the spontaneous activity of the geniculate neuron. The receptive field is masked by a dark board. Trace 2: an LED evokes on and off responses from the LGN cell. Note the rebound excitation at off (dark arrow). Trace 3: pairing both stimuli significantly reduces the excitation at off (arrow head). Traces under INJ: the superior colliculus has been injected with lidocaine hydrochloride. Trace 5: the on response is more tonic and no rebound excitation occurs at off. Trace 6: combining both stimuli fails to significantly modify the light response. Calibration, horizontal 300 ms, vertical 5 spikes.

belong to pulvinar receptive fields. Firstly, they are vast in area, as their elliptical circumference averaged 90.8° ± 44.2°. Secondly the majority of the LP-P units have their activity area encroaching the midline and the center of the visual field. Similar properties were described in freely behaving monkeys (Petersen et al. 1985). Thus, it seems that these peculiarities are common to LP-P cells in mammals. By comparison, LGN cells are considerably smaller (3° to 10° of arc) and their receptive fields are distributed throughout the visual field. In addition, in rabbits (Casanova 1986) and in monkeys (Petersen et al. 1985), pulvinar cells are well triggered by fairly large stationary and moving images. In general, tuning curves of the units are rather broad. These peculiarities of LP-P cells suggest that these neurons are unsuitable for discriminating small targets. Rather, LP-P cells signal to the cortex the presence of large objects which are preferably located in the visual axis: this could be the visual background. In parallel, geniculo-cortical fibers convey information about discrete objects (or contrasts) superimposed upon the background.

The superior colliculus is not only involved in visually guided behavior but many of its cells are sensitive to auditory and somesthetic stimuli. Obviously, the colliculi integrate various sensory modalities encountered in the environment. The neuronal outflow of this processing would be used simultaneously by the oculomotor network and by lemniscal neurons that receive the same incoming information.

The last figure (Fig. 5) expresses the proposed role of the tecto-thalamic paths in relation to the global frame of collicular physiology. The eye is presented with a focalized discrete image (the face) superimposed on the background. Both may be moving, or they may be stationary. Since the entire visual field is represented at both levels (i.e., the SC and the LGN), they process the same images. However, the geniculo-cortical path processes local trigger features, that is: contours, successive contrast, colors, etc. The colliculus proceeds to convert the visual map as expressed by the retinotopy of its superficial layer into an oculomotor map (Sparks and Mays 1983; Sparks and Porter 1983) in preparation for an impeding saccade.

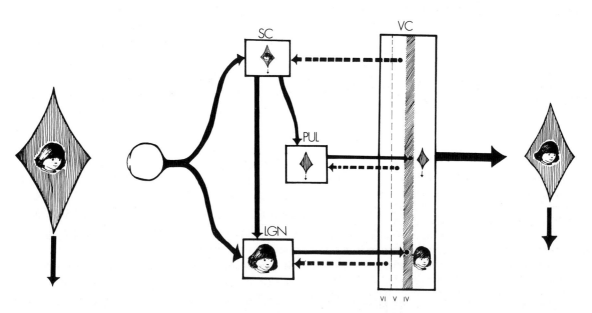

Fig. 5. Schematic diagram of the proposed role for the colliculo-thalamic pathways. The colliculo LP-P complex route deals with the background. The colliculo-geniculate route handles the focalized images. See text for further explanation.

Hence, the colliculus provides the oculomotor network with the visual map. Then, through its efferent fibers, the collicular cells operate the geniculate gate and the pulvinar excitabilities with the aim of enabling the cortex to subtract the central image from the background. For instance, it would switch off the geniculate gate to prepare the cortex for new acquisition, but it could leave the pulvinar 'switched on' in order for the cortex to evaluate the new background and to adjust the sensitivities to modified lighting conditions. It may be suggested then, that the manipulation of the thalamus by the SC allows the cortex to subtract the central image from the background. Alternatively, it could shut off all thalamic gates to prevent saccadic blur during eye displacement.

It also may be suggested that the SC establishes a hierarchy for incoming information. It has been demonstrated in monkeys (Sparks and Mays 1983; Sparks and Porter 1983) that once a movement is initiated, the program will be carried to its completion, even if during the course of the movement, the eyes are deviated. The collicular system will compensate and recalculate a new trajectory, so that in the end, the eyes fall correctly on the target. As an implicit consequence of these experiments, one may assume that once the eyes have started to acquire a new target, additional invasion of the visual field will be 'on hold' in the collicular 'memory' until the first reflex is completed.

For example, let us assume that the animal is fixating on an attractive subject, when a new disturbing stimulus invades the periphery of the visual field. This stimulus activates the collicular neurons. Depending upon its characteristics, the animal may or may not reorientate its gaze. In a sense, the colliculus acts as a multiple shutter. If the latter opens, the inflow of information would increase, such as when an animal fixates on a target while an impeding saccade will close the shutter and reduce the sensory inputs. This hypothesis is in line with the experimental observations reported on various animals. The colliculus is believed: (1) to accelerate saccades, (2) to increase their accuracies (Schiller et al. 1987), and (3) to be the site of the corollary discharge (Molotchnikoff and Lachapelle 1983). McKay (1972, 1973) has already suggested that the latter enhances as well as inhibits sensory inflow. Finally, these results may serve as a reminder that response characteristics of thalamic cells reflect as much the properties of the stimulus, as those of the cells and their neuronal environment.

Acknowledgments

This research was supported by Grants CRNSG and FCAR. We are obliged to P. Heinerman for advice on the manuscript.

References

Benevento, L. and Fallon, J.H. (1975) The ascending projections of the superior colliculus in the rhesus monkey *(Macaca mulatta). J. Comp. Neurol.,* 160: 339–362.

Casagrande, V.A., Harting, J.K., Hall, W.C., Diamond, I.T. and Martin, G.F. (1972) Superior colliculus of the tree shrew *(Tupaia glis):* evidence for a structural and functional subdivision into superficial and deep layers. *Science,* 177: 444–447.

Casanova, C. (1986) Etude des propriétés des cellules du pulvinar et de ses relations avec le collicule supérieur chez le lapin, *Ph.D. dissertation.* Depart. Biol. Sciences, Université de Montréal.

Chalupa, L.M. (1984) Visual physiology of the mammalian superior colliculus. In: Vanegas, H. (Ed.), *Comparative Neurology of the Optic Tectum,* Plenum, New York, London.

Giolli, R.A. and Pope, J.E. (1971) The anatomical organization of the visual system of the rabbit. *Doc. Ophthalmol.,* 30: 9–31.

Goodale, M.A. and Murison, R.C.C. (1975) The effects of lesions of the superior colliculus on locomotor orientation and the orienting reflex in the rat. *Brain Res.,* 88: 243–261.

Graham, J. (1977) An autoradiographic study of the efferent connections of the superior colliculus in the cat. *J. Comp. Neurol.,* 173: 629–654.

Graham, J. and Berman, N. (1981) Origins of the projections of the superior colliculus to the dorsal lateral geniculate nucleus and the pulvinar in the rabbit. *Neurosci. Lett.,* 26: 101–106.

Guitton, D., Crommelinek, T. and Roucoux, A. (1980) Stimulation of the superior colliculus in the alert cat. I. Eye movements and neck EMG activity evoked when the head is restrained. *Exp. Brain Res.,* 39: 63–73.

74

Harting, J.K., Huerta, M.F., Frankfurter, A.J., Strominger, N.L. and Royce, G.J. (1980) Ascending pathways from the monkey superior colliculus: an autoradiographic analysis. *J. Comp. Neurol.,* 192: 853 – 882.

Holstege, G. and Collewijn, H. (1982) The efferent connections of the nucleus of the optic tract and the superior colliculus in the rabbit. *J. Comp. Neurol.,* 209: 139 – 175.

Huerta, M.F. and Harting, J.K. (1983) Sublamination within the superficial gray layer of the squirrel monkey: an analysis of the tectopulvinar projection using anterograde transport methods. *Brain Res.,* 261: 119 – 126.

Huerta, M.F. and Harting, J.K. (1984) The mammalian superior colliculus: studies of its morphology and connections. In: Vanegas, H. (Ed.), *Comparative Neurology of the Optic Tectum,* Plenum Press, New York, London, pp. 687 – 773.

Jay, M.F. and Sparks, D.L. (1987) Sensorimotor integration in the primate superior colliculus. I. Motor convergence. *J. Neurophysiol.,* 57: 22 – 34.

Jeannerod, M. (1974) Les deux mécanismes de la vision. *La Recherche,* 5: 23 – 32.

Kawamura, S., Fukushima, N., Hattori, S. and Kudo, M. (1980) Laminar segregation of cells of origin of ascending projections from the superficial layers of the superior colliculus in the cat. *Brain Res.,* 184: 486 – 490.

Mackay, D.M. (1972) Voluntary eye movements as questions. In: Dichgans, J. and Bizzi, E. (Eds.), *Cerebral Control of Eye Movements and Motion Perception,* Karger, Basel, pp. 369 – 376.

Mackay, D.M. (1973) Visual stability and voluntary eye movements. In: Jung, R. (Ed.), *Handbook of Sensory Physiology, Vol. VII/3, Central Visual Information,* Springer-Verlag, Berlin, Heidelberg, New York, pp. 308 – 331.

Molotchnikoff, S. and Lachapelle, P. (1980) Evidence of collicular input to the dorsal lateral geniculate nucleus in rabbit: electrophysiology. *Exp. Brain Res.,* 40: 221 – 228.

Molotchnikoff, S. and Lachapelle, P. (1983) Local excitability in the superior colliculus influences evoked responses of lateral geniculate cells in rabbits. *Brain Res. Bull.,* 11: 533 – 545.

Molotchnikoff, S., Casanova, C., Laferriere, C. and Delaunais, D. (1983) The superior colliculus simultaneously modifies the responses of the lateral geniculate cells and of the oculomotor nuclei. *Brain Res. Bull.,* 10: 719 – 722.

Molotchnikoff, S., Delaunais, D. and Casanova, C. (1986a) Modulations of the lateral geniculate nucleus cell responses by a second discrete conditioning stimulus: implication of the superior colliculus in rabbits. *Exp. Brain Res.,* 62: 321 – 328.

Molotchnikoff, S., Delaunais, D., Casanova, C. and Lachapelle, P. (1986b) Influence of a local inactivation in the superior colliculus on lateral geniculate responses in rabbits. *Brain Res.,* 375: 66 – 72.

Petersen, S.E., Robinson, D.L. and Keys, W. (1985) Pulvinar nuclei of the behaving rhesus monkey: visual responses and their modulation. *J. Neurophysiol.,* 54: 867 – 886.

Rizzolatti, G., Camarda, R., Grupp, L.A. and Pisa, M. (1973) Inhibition of visual responses of single units in the cat superior colliculus by the introduction of a second visual stimulus. *Brain Res.,* 61: 390 – 394.

Robson, J.A. and Hall, W.L. (1976) Projections from the superior colliculus to the dorsal lateral geniculate nucleus of the grey squirrel *(Sciurus carolinensis). Brain Res.,* 113: 379 – 385.

Schiller, P.H., Sandell, J.H. and Maunsell, J.H.R. (1987) The effect of frontal eye field and superior colliculus lesions on saccadic latencies in the rhesus monkey. *J. Neurophysiol.,* 57: 1033 – 1049.

Schneider, G.E. (1969) Two visual systems. *Science,* 163: 895 – 902.

Sparks, S.L. and Mays, L.E. (1983) Spatial localisation of saccade targets. I. Compensation for stimulation-induced perturbation in eye position. *J. Neurophysiol.,* 49: 45 – 63.

Sparks, D.L. and Porter, J.D. (1983) Spatial localization of saccade targets. II. Activity of superior colliculus neurons preceding compensatory saccades. *J. Neurophysiol.,* 49: 64 – 74.

Torrealba, F., Partlow, G.D. and Guillery, R.W. (1981) Organisation of the projection from the superior colliculus to the dorsal lateral geniculate nucleus of the cat. *Neuroscience,* 6: 1341 – 1360.

Trevarthen, C.B. (1968) Two mechanisms of vision in primates. *Psychol. Forsch.,* 31: 299 – 337.

Wurtz, R.H. and Albano, J.E. (1980) Visual motor function of the primate superior colliculus. *Annu. Rev. Neurosci.,* 3:189 – 226.

T.P. Hicks and G. Benedek (Eds.)
Progress in Brain Research, Vol. 75
© 1988 Elsevier Science Publishers B.V. (Biomedical Division)

CHAPTER 7

The lateral posterior complex of the cat: studies of the functional organization

Bob Hutchins[1] and B.V. Updyke[2]

[1]*Department of Anatomy, Baylor College of Dentistry, Dallas, Texas, U.S.A., and* [2]*Department of Anatomy, Louisiana State University Medical Center, New Orleans, Louisiana, U.S.A.*

Introduction

The complex organization of the extrageniculate visual thalamus has historically resisted analysis and has inspired several sets of terminologies and divisional schemes. Rioch (1929) first proposed a thalamic organization that defined a lateral posterior, lateral intermedius, posterior, and a pulvinar nucleus in the cat and dog. Variations on Rioch's basic terminology are still used to describe the carnivore thalamus. In contemporary usage, the cat's thalamus is generally considered to have a pulvinar nucleus and a lateral posterior region which includes several lateral posterior subnuclei. The number of specific subnuclei and the terminology to be applied to these areas continue to be actively debated.

One of the major obstacles to analyzing this region has been the difficulty in identifying nuclear borders. Even with well prepared tissue that has been stained for cytoarchitectural detail, this thalamic region does not present clearly identifiable borders as compared to the dorsal lateral geniculate nucleus. Rather, much of the posterior thalamus appears as a mosaic of cellular configurations and making an analysis based purely on morphological criteria can be difficult at best. An alternative morphological approach, employing tissue stained for myelin (Fig. 1), has been used to reveal divisional boundaries for portions of the ex-

trageniculate visual thalamus (Hughes 1980; Symonds et al. 1981). Unfortunately, myelin stained sections appear to respect thalamic borders only in the very posterior regions. Investigators have also argued that topographically organized projections can be used to define functional subdivisions. When it eventually became possible to compare connectional data with Nissl stained tissue, the functionally relevant cytoarchitectural borders finally became more apparent.

It has also been felt that the functional analysis of a region must rely on a multifaceted approach, taking into account connectional, cytoarchitectural, and electrophysiological findings. In the following sections, we will offer our interpretation of these data. A discussion of the topographically organized connectional data will be presented first, followed by a description of the topographical observations as they apply to the underlying cytoarchitecture. Finally, electrophysiological data will be presented with reference to recent retinotopic mapping data and the relationship of these data to the overall functional organization of the extrageniculate visual thalamus.

Topographically organized connections of the LP complex

Initial indications that the extrageniculate visual thalamus might be topographically organized came from degeneration studies involving the visual cortex (Beresford 1961; Garey et al. 1968; Graybiel 1972; Kawamura et al. 1974). In these studies, visual cortical areas were lesioned and their fields of degeneration described, noting the topographic relationships of projections located within the lateral thalamus. However, the limitations of the technique and the lack of detailed knowledge of cortical organization made it difficult to appreciate the full significance of these findings.

Two major developments made it possible to fully exploit the connectional approach. First, electrophysiological mapping studies revealed the retinotopic organization of the lateral geniculate nucleus (Sanderson 1971), the superior colliculus (Feldon et al. 1970), and the visual cortex (Palmer et al. 1978; Tusa et al. 1978, 1979; Tusa and Palmer 1980). Second, the development and routine use of more sensitive anatomical tracers enabled investigators to design anatomical studies that could predict the general retinotopy of another area by examining connectional interrelationships. That is, it could be shown that projections from an area of known retinotopic organization preserved that retinotopic organization in their termination patterns. Using variations of this approach, studies were conducted which investigated the number of visually related structures and their retinotopic organization within the lateral posterior complex (Updyke 1977, 1981a, b; Berson

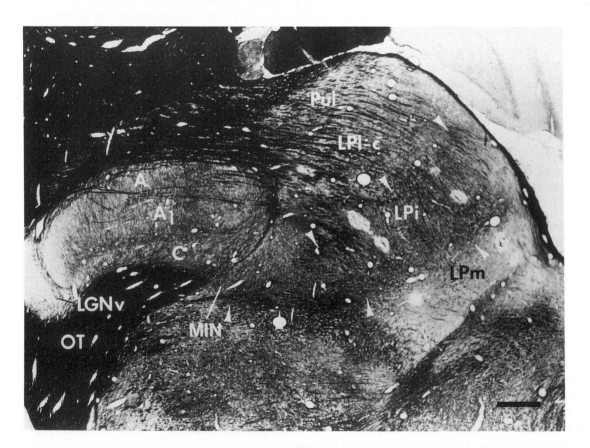

Fig. 1. A coronal section taken through the posterior region of the lateral posterior complex of the cat, stained for myelin. The borders of zone LPi are indicated by the arrows. Lesions placed during several electrode penetrations can also be seen including two lesions indicating where the representation of azimuth was determined electrophysiologically to reverse within zone LPi. Bar = 0.5 mm.

and Graybiel 1978; Hughes 1980; Symonds et al. 1981; Raczkowski and Rosenquist 1983).

The results from these studies generally agreed that there were at least three retinotopically organized areas within the LP complex (Figs. 2 and 3). Using the basic terminology adopted by Updyke (1977), the LP complex is composed of a laterally situated pulvinar (Pul) which receives a retinotopically organized projection from area 19. The lateral zone (LPl) is located adjacent and medial to pulvinar and receives retinotopically organized projections from areas 17, 18, and 19. Medial to LPl is the interjacent zone (LPi) recipient of projections from superior colliculus and bounded medially by a fourth zone, LPm. Although several investigators (Graybiel and Berson 1980; Raczkowski and Rosenquist 1983) have suggested zone LPm should not be included in the lateral posterior complex based on the absence of exclusive visual input, zone LPm has been shown to receive projections from a visually related cortical structure, the anterior ectosylvian sulcus (Mucke et al. 1982; Olson and Graybiel 1981; Updyke 1983). These cortical projections from the anterior ectosylvian sulcus have been substantiated by several additional investigators (Raczkowski and Rosenquist 1983; Roda and Reinoso-Suárez 1983; Norita et al. 1986) and it should also be noted that in one recent study (Norita et al. 1986) it was suggested the anterior ectosylvian visual cortex (AEV) projected topographically onto the medial regions of the LP complex. In these experiments, only electrophysiologically identified visual areas within the anterior ectosylvian cortex were injected with anatomical tracers, thus, the terminal topography observed was suggestive of a potential retinotopic organization within LPm.

Cytoarchitectural observations

As previously mentioned, the LP complex appears as a mosaic of subtle cytoarchitectural fields. All too often, this area has been regarded as appearing relatively featureless. Yet, when patterns of thalamic connections were compared with the cytoar-

chitecture of the lateral posterior complex (Updyke 1983), it was possible to recognize consistent cytoarchitectural boundaries (Fig. 2). In this description of the LP region, not only were the four basic subdivisions identified (i.e., Pul, LPl, LPi, and LPm), but a fifth subdivision was identified as the rostral extension of the lateral LP zone (the lateral division as originally defined by Up-

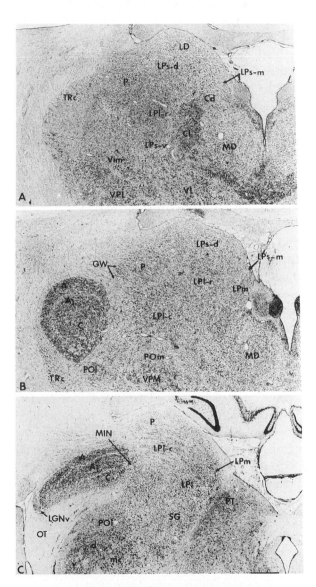

Fig. 2. Three selected coronal sections progressing from rostral (A) to caudal (C) through the lateral posterior complex. Cresyl violet. Bar = 0.5 mm.

dyke (1977) was split into a caudal zone, the LPl-c, and a rostral zone, the LPl-r) (Fig. 3). These five zones did not completely account for all of the available connectional observations, however, and Updyke (1983) further proposed the existence of a collection of cell groups which essentially surrounded the rostral one half of the complex in the form of an irregular shell (Figs. 2 and 3). These cell groups were characterized as strips or regions located peripherally to the five core zones. Of the five shell zones described, one of the more distinctive shell regions belongs to the retinorecipient area located lateral to pulvinar (GW). The dorsal shell (LPs-d) is the most extensive of the zones and is functionally defined by the projection pattern observed after injections of anterograde tracers within area 7, splenial cortex, hypothalamus, cerebellum, and area 21b (Yoshii et al. 1978; Fujii and Yoshii 1979; Itoh and Mizuno 1979; Itoh et al. 1979; Updyke 1983; Olson and Lawler 1987). The medial shell zone (LPs-m) was defined by its afferent projections from temporal, insular, and ectosylvian cortical areas (Updyke 1983). Also identified were two additional areas, the ventral (LPs-v) and rostral shell (LPs-r) zones.

All of the core zones and portions of the various shell regions were initially defined by their connectional patterns. It was only after the projection patterns were compared to the underlying cytoarchitecture that the characteristics of different LP areas were appreciated. The intention behind this attempt to reevaluate the lateral posterior cytoarchitecture was to identify the number of functional divisions. Although functional parcellation of the region by anatomical criteria has appeared to reveal the general organization of the LP complex, it was obvious that not all of the questions have been addressed. Electrophysiological mapping techniques have been successfully used to delimit visually related areas (i.e., the lateral geniculate nucleus, the superior colliculus, and the visual cortical areas) and studies using this technique within the LP region will be considered next.

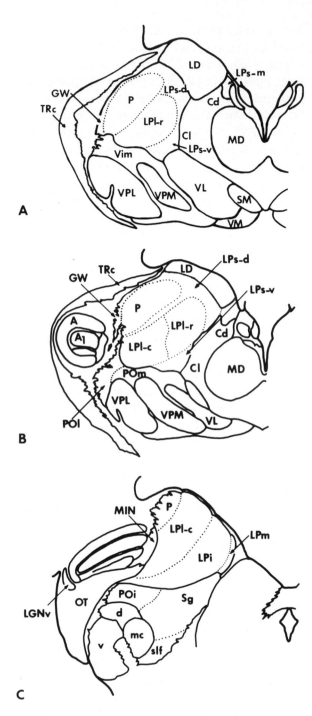

Fig. 3. Three line drawings taken from similar coronal levels as shown in Fig. 2. Note the progression of irregular shells from caudal to rostral levels.

Electrophysiological mapping in the LP complex

Initial studies employing electrophysiological techniques were concerned with investigating the response characteristics of single cells within the posterior thalamus and identifying the general location and number of cells responsive to visual stimuli (Godfraind et al. 1969, 1972; Chalupa and Fish 1978; Fish and Chalupa 1979). Although these studies were not designed to identify the overall visuotopic organization of the region, they did confirm the important role of this region in visual integration and processing. The results from two other studies (Mason 1978, 1981), however, not only related further observations concerning the response characteristics of single cells, but also supported the general retinotopic organization for pulvinar, striate-recipient, and tectorecipient subdivisions as predicted from previous anatomical studies.

The general visual topography predicted by both the anatomical and electrophysiological studies indicated a representation of the horizontal meridian running obliquely through the complex from rostrodorsal to caudoventral. The upper visual field representation was primarily located in the caudal regions and the lower visual field representation was located primarily in the rostral regions. These studies also indicated that a representation of the vertical meridian was located at the lateral edge of the pulvinar and a representation of the periphery was located between the pulvinar and the lateral division of LP. Another representation of the vertical meridian was located between the lateral division of LP and the adjacent medial zone, LPi (Updyke 1977; Mason 1978, 1981).

More recently there have been studies concerned with investigating specific subdivisions within the LP complex, the results of which are in basic agreement with earlier anatomical and electrophysiological results (Benedek et al. 1983; Chalupa et al. 1983).

Another study using multiple cell recording techniques was specifically designed to investigate the retinotopic organization of the LP complex (Raczkowski and Rosenquist 1981). Their results indicated a systematic representation of the visual field within three LP subdivisions, the pulvinar, the striate-recipient zone, and the tectorecipient zone, and effectively confirmed the general retinotopic organization for these areas. Their observations were confined to only these three areas of LP, however, and did not address questions concerning the visuotopic organization of adjacent areas.

In order to explore several additional questions, we have employed standard electrophysiological mapping techniques in paralyzed, chloralose anesthetized cats, and have examined the lateral posterior complex for visual topography. Receptive fields were sampled every 100 μm and a systematic retinotopic map was generated. Data collected thus far have reflected the basic retinotopic organization already described. That is, the pulvinar, the striate-recipient, and tecto-recipient subdivisions all respond to visual stimuli. A representation of the vertical meridian is located both on the lateral edge of the pulvinar and between striate- (LPl-c) and tecto-recipient (LPi) zones. A representation of the peripheral visual field is also found between pulvinar and striate-recipient divisions (LPl-c). However, our data revealed an unexpected finding concerning zone LPi (Hutchins and Updyke 1984). Within LPi, the representation of the azimuth was consistently found to be folded along both the dorsomedial and the ventromedial borders (Fig. 4). Thus, the representation of the vertical meridian extends for a variable distance along the LPi/LPm border and for a variable distance along the LPi/Sg border. Representations of the periphery also extend along a portion of the medial border of LPi.

Our observations indicate the existence of a visually responsive area medial to area LPi and corresponding to zone LPm. Zone LPm has a representation of the upper visual field located dorsally and posteriorly with lower visual fields appearing to be located ventrally and anteriorly.

Another very important observation has resulted from these experiments. The representation of the contralateral hemifield corresponding to zone LPm appears to be separate from the visual representation in the adjacent suprageniculate nucleus (Sg) (Hicks et al. 1984). Our observations indicate that the suprageniculate nucleus has a representation of its upper visual field anterior and medial with the representation of the lower visual field posterior and lateral. These data indicate that zone LPm contains a representation of the lower visual field which is adjacent to the representation of the upper visual field in Sg. Thus, at the LPm/Sg border there exists an abrupt discontinuity in visual representation (Fig. 4).

Additional preliminary data collected indicate separate representations of the contralateral hemifield corresponding to area LPl-r and to areas which correspond to subregions of the dorsal shell region (LPs-d) described by Updyke (1983).

These data confirm and extend previous findings concerning the functional organization of the lateral posterior complex. Despite the apparent systematic visual responsiveness of this region, there were also some additional unexpected fin-

dings. Continuity of visual representation was generally preserved across the various LP subdivisions, yet there were other areas of transition marked by major discontinuities. As mentioned above, there exists a coarse transitional area between LPm and Sg where the upper visual field in Sg is adjacent to the lower visual field of LPm. This same type of coarse transition or discontinuity was a fairly consistent feature of the border between the medial intralaminar nucleus (MIN) and zone LPl-c. Discontinuities were also observed in rostral areas between Pul and LPl-r. Our results now show these abrupt changes in representations to be a consistent finding. Moreover, this type of organization may not be so unusual when one considers that five to seven different visually organized structures are compactly arranged within the posterior thalamus. Indeed, such discontinuities between so many tightly organized areas would seem intuitively necessary.

Concluding remarks

A systematic representation of the visual world has been identified for the lateral posterior region, and this represents a further step toward understanding the integrative role of the LP complex. However, there remain many issues that have not yet been pursued. For example, studies of the connectivity of the various cortical areas in cats (Gilbert and Wiesel 1980, 1981; Montero 1981; Symonds and Rosenquist, 1984) have shown that various visual cortical areas typically project in periodic patterns to other areas in cortex and presumably correspond to a modularly based functional network. It has also been widely shown that the visual cortex and the LP complex share reciprocal projections. In fact, it has been suggested that because the LP complex shares many of the same connections as the extrastriate cortex, the LP complex may be considered an integral part of the extrastriate visual system. These observations raise several questions concerning the functional significance of corticothalamic or thalamocortical projections which do not terminate in patches, but in con-

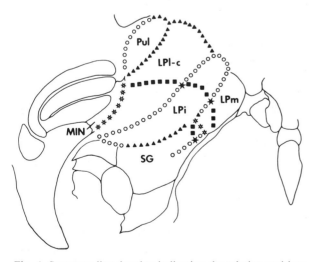

Fig. 4. Summary line drawing indicating the relative positions of the retinotopic boundaries within the lateral posterior complex at one coronal level. Note the folded representation of the vertical meridian around zone LPi and the separate retinotopic representations within SG and zone LPm. ○ = vertical meridians; ■ = horizontal meridian; ▲ = periphery; * = discontinuous visual representation; ★ = central gaze.

tinuous terminal fields (Updyke 1977, 1981a, 1983; Symonds et al. 1981; Tong et al. 1982; Raczkowski and Rosenquist 1983; Abramson and Chalupa 1985). Other considerations involve the organizational or integrational differences needed to support the coexistence of an apparent modular system with a non-modular system.

Adding to the integrative role of the LP complex is another significant and unanticipated set of projections. These thalamic connections involve a considerable portion of the LP complex and their projections to striatum (Beckstead 1984; Updyke 1986). Questions again need to be asked concerning the importance of these projections and their interaction with the visual system. Based on recent findings, it has been suggested that the LP complex may form one link in a series of pathways involving the strionigral, nigrotectal, and tectothalamic pathways (May and Hall 1986; Updyke 1986). These connections may, therefore, form the basis for a larger visuomotor control loop.

Understanding the nature of thalamic influences on these various sensory pathways, requires an interpretation of the number of functional areas in the posterior thalamus. Once the number of areas have been identified, establishing a consistent organizational format becomes important in order to facilitate the interpretation of experimental data. The correlation of several neuroscientific analyses (i.e., patterns of anatomical projections, the cytoarchitecture, and electrophysiological mapping) have collectively produced an organizational scheme that best fits the experimental observations. With the addition of a detailed retinotopic map which corresponds to these thalamic subdivisions, this work should serve as a basic framework for future studies.

Acknowledgements

The authors wish to thank Cheryl Vega and Anhmai Tran for their technical help and Wanda Jones for assisting in the typing of this manuscript. Supported by NEI grants EY05724 and EY06977.

Abbreviations

A, A$_1$	Laminae of dorsal lateral geniculate nucleus
C	Laminae of dorsal lateral geniculate nucleus
Cd	Central dorsal nucleus
Cl	Central lateral nucleus
d	Dorsal division of medial geniculate complex
Gw	Geniculate wing division of lateral posterior shell
LD	Lateral dorsal nucleus
LGNv	Ventral division of lateral geniculate complex
LPi	Interjacent zone of lateral posterior complex
LPl-c	Lateral zone of lateral posterior complex, caudal layer
LPl-r	Lateral zone of lateral posterior complex, rostral layer
LPm	Medial zone of lateral posterior complex
LPs-d	Lateral posterior shell, dorsal division
LPs-m	Lateral posterior shell, medial division
LPs-v	Lateral posterior shell, ventral division
mc	Magnocellular division of medial geniculate complex
MD	Medial dorsal nucleus
MIN	Medial interlaminar nucleus division of lateral geniculate complex
OT	Optic tract
P	Pulvinar zone of lateral posterior complex
POi	Intermediate division of posterior nuclear group
POl	Lateral division of posterior nuclear group
POm	Medial division of posterior nuclear group
PT	Pretectal complex
Sg	Suprageniculate division of posterior nuclear group

slf	Supralemniscal field division of posterior nuclear group
SM	Submedial nucleus
TRc	Thalamic reticular complex
v	Ventral lateral division of medial geniculate complex
Vim	Ventral intermediate shell
VL	Ventral lateral nucleus
VPL	Ventral posterolateral nucleus
VPM	Ventral posteriomedial nucleus

References

Abramson, B.P. and Chalupa, L.M. (1985) The laminar distribution of cortical connections with the tecto- and corticorecipient zones in the cat's lateral posterior nucleus. *Neuroscience,* 15: 81 – 95.

Beckstead, R.M. (1984) The thalamostriatal projection in the cat. *J. Comp. Neurol.,* 223: 313 – 346.

Benedek, G., Norita, M. and Creutzfeldt, O.D. (1983) Electrophysiologic and anatomic demonstration of an overlapping striate and tectal projection to the lateral posterior-pulvinar complex of the cat. *Exp. Brain Res.,* 52: 157 – 169.

Beresford, W.A. (1961) Fibre degeneration following lesions of the visual cortex of the cat. In: R. Jung and H. Kornhuber (Eds.), *Neurophysiologie und Psychophysik des visuellen Systems,* Springer-Verlag, Berlin, pp. 247 – 255.

Berson, D.M. and Graybiel, A.M. (1978) Parallel thalamic zones in the LP-pulvinar complex of the cat identified by their afferent and efferent connections. *Brain Res.,* 147: 139 – 148.

Chalupa, L.M. and Fish, S.E. (1978) Response characteristics of visual and extravisual neurons in the pulvinar and lateral posterior nuclei of the cat. *Exp. Neurol.,* 61: 96 – 120.

Chalupa, L.M., Williams, R.W. and Hughes, M.J. (1983) Visual response properties in the tectorecipient zone of the cat's lateral posterior-pulvinar complex: A comparison with the superior colliculus. *J. Neurosci.,* 3: 2587 – 2596.

Feldon, S., Felson, P. and Kruger, L. (1970) Topography of the retinal projection upon the superior colliculus of the cat. *Vision Res.,* 10: 135 – 143.

Fish, S.E. and Chalupa, M. (1979) Functional properties of pulvinar-lateral posterior neurons which receive input from the superior colliculus. *Exp. Brain Res.,* 36: 245 – 257.

Fujii, M. and Yoshii, N. (1979) Hypothalamic projections to the pulvinar-LP complex in the cat: a study by the silver impregnation method. *Neurosci. Lett.,* 12: 247 – 252.

Garey, L.J., Jones, E.G. and Powell, T.P.S. (1968) Interrelationships of striate and extrastriate cortex with the primary relay sites of the visual pathway. *J. Neurol. Neurosurg. Psychiat.,* 31: 135 – 157.

Gilbert, C.D. and Wiesel, T.N. (1980) Interleaving projection bands in cortico-cortical connections. *Soc. Neurosci. Abstr.,* 6: 315.

Gilbert, C.D. and Wiesel, T.N. (1981) Projection bands in visual cortex. *Soc. Neurosci. Abstr.,* 7: 356.

Godfraind, J.M., Meulders, M. and Veraart, C. (1969) Visual receptive fields of neurons in pulvinar, nucleus lateralis posterior and nucleus suprageniculatus thalami of the cat. *Brain Res.,* 15: 552 – 555.

Godfraind, J.M., Meulders, M. and Veraart, C. (1972) Visual properties of neurons in pulvinar, nucleus lateralis posterior and nucleus suprageniculatus thalami in the cat. I. Qualitative investigation. *Brain Res.,* 44: 503 – 526.

Graybiel, A.M. (1972) Some extrageniculate visual pathways in the cat. *Invest. Ophthamol.,* 11: 322 – 332.

Hicks, T.P., Watanabe, S., Miyake, A. and Shoumura, K. (1984) Organization and properties of visually responsive neurones in the suprageniculate nucleus of the cat. *Exp. Brain Res.,* 55: 359 – 367.

Hughes, H.C. (1980) Efferent organization of the cat pulvinar complex, with a note on bilateral claustrocortical and reticulocortical connections. *J. Comp. Neurol.,* 193: 937 – 963.

Hutchins, B. and Updyke, B.V. (1984) Retinotopic organization within the lateral posterior complex of the cat. *Soc. Neurosci. Abstr.,* 10: 727.

Itoh, K. and Mizuno, N. (1979) A cerebello-pulvinar projection in the cat as visualized by the use of anterograde transport of horseradish peroxidase. *Brain Res.,* 171: 131 – 134.

Itoh, K., Mizuno, N., Sugimoto, T., Nomura, S., Nakamura, Y. and Konishi, A. (1979) A cerebello-pulvinar-cortical and retino-pulvino-cortical pathway in the cat as revealed by the use of the anterograde and retrograde transport of horseradish peroxidase. *J. Comp. Neurol.,* 187: 349 – 358.

Kawamura, S., Sprague, J.M. and Niimi, K. (1974) Corticofugal projections from the visual cortices to the thalamus, pretectum and superior colliculus in the cat. *J. Comp. Neurol.,* 158: 339 – 362.

Mason, R. (1978) Functional organization in the cat's pulvinar complex. *Exp. Brain Res.,* 31: 51 – 66.

Mason, R. (1981) Differential responsiveness of cells in the visual zones of the cat's LP-pulvinar complex to visual stimuli. *Exp. Brain Res.,* 43: 25 – 33.

May, P.J. and Hall, W.C. (1986) The sources of the nigrotectal pathway. *Neuroscience,* 19: 159 – 180.

Montero, V.M. (1981) Topography of the cortico-cortical connections from the striate cortex in the cat. *Brain Behav. Evol.,* 18: 194 – 218.

Mucke, L., Norita, M., Benedek, G. and Creutzfeldt, O. (1982) Physiologic and anatomic investigation of a visual cortical area situated in the ventral bank of the anterior ectosylvian sulcus of the cat. *Exp. Brain Res.,* 46: 1 – 11.

Norita, M., Mucke, L., Benedek, G., Albowitz, B., Katoh, Y. and Creutzfeldt, O.D. (1986) Connections of the anterior ectosylvian visual area (AEV). *Exp. Brain Res.,* 62: 225 – 240.

Olson, C.R. and Graybiel, A.M. (1981) A visual area in the anterior ectosylvian sulcus of the cat. *Soc. Neurosci. Abstr.,* 7: 831.

Olson, C.R. and Lawler, K. (1987) Cortical and subcortical afferent connections of a posterior division of feline area 7 (area 7p). *J. Comp. Neurol.,* 259: 13 – 30.

Palmer, L.A., Rosenquist, A.C. and Tusa, R.J. (1978) The retinotopic organization of the lateral suprasylvian areas in the cat. *J. Comp. Neurol.,* 177: 237 – 256.

Raczkowski, D. and Rosenquist, A.C. (1981) Retinotopic organization in the cat lateral posterior-pulvinar complex. *Brain Res.,* 221: 185 – 191.

Raczkowski, D. and Rosenquist, A.C. (1983) Connections of the multiple visual cortical areas with the lateral posterior pulvinar complex and adjacent thalamic nuclei in the cat. *J. Neurosci.,* 3: 1912 – 1942.

Rioch, D.M. (1929) Studies on the diencephalon of Carnivora. Part I. The nuclear configuration of the thalamus, epithalamus, and hypothalamus of the dog and cat. *J. Comp. Neurol.,* 49: 1 – 119.

Roda, J.M. and Reinoso-Suárez, F. (1983) Topographical organization of the thalamic projections to the cortex of the anterior ectosylvian sulcus in the cat. *Exp. Brain Res.,* 49: 131 – 139.

Sanderson, K.J. (1971) The projection of the visual field to the lateral geniculate and medial interlaminar nuclei in the cat. *J. Comp. Neurol.,* 143: 101 – 118.

Symonds, L.L. and Rosenquist, A.C. (1984) Corticocortical connections among visual areas in the cat. *J. Comp. Neurol.,* 229: 1 – 38.

Symonds, L.L., Rosenquist, A.C., Edwards, S.B. and Palmer, L.A. (1981) Projections of the pulvinar-lateral posterior complex to visual cortical areas in the cat. *Neuroscience,* 6: 1995 – 2020.

Tong, L., Kalil, R.E. and Spear, P.D. (1982) Thalamic projections to visual areas of the middle suprasylvian sulcus in the cat. *J. Comp. Neurol.,* 212: 103 – 117.

Tusa, R.J. and Palmer, L.A. (1980) Retinotopic organization of areas 20 and 21 in the cat. *J. Comp. Neurol.,* 193: 147 – 164.

Tusa, R.J., Palmer, L.A. and Rosenquist, A.C. (1978) The retinotopic organization of area 17 (striate cortex) in the cat. *J. Comp. Neurol.,* 177: 213 – 236.

Tusa, R.J., Rosenquist, A.C. and Palmer, L.A. (1979) Retinotopic organization of areas 18 and 19 in the cat. *J. Comp. Neurol.,* 185: 657 – 678.

Updyke, B.V. (1977) Topographic organization of the projections from cortical areas 17, 18 and 19 onto the thalamus, pretectum, and superior colliculus in the cat. *J. Comp. Neurol.,* 173: 81 – 122.

Updyke, B.V. (1981a) Projections from visual areas of the middle suprasylvian sulcus onto the lateral posterior complex and adjacent thalamic nuclei in cat. *J. Comp. Neurol.,* 201: 477 – 506.

Updyke, B.V. (1981b) Multiple representations of the visual field: Corticothalamic and thalamic organization in the cat. In: C.N. Woolsey (Ed.), *Cortical Sensory Organization, Vol. 2,* Humana Press, Clifton, NJ, pp. 83 – 101.

Updyke, B.V. (1983) A re-evaluation of the functional organization and cytoarchitecture of the feline lateral posterior complex, with observations on adjoining cell groups. *J. Comp. Neurol.,* 219: 143 – 181.

Updyke, B.V. (1986) Cortical and thalamic extrastriate visual afferents to cat striatum: putative visuomotor circuits. *Soc. Neurosci. Abstr.,* 12: 1540.

Yoshii, N., Fujii, M. and Mizokami, T. (1978) Hypothalamic projections to the pulvinar-LP complex in the cat: a study by the HRP method. *Brain Res.,* 155: 343 – 346.

T.P. Hicks and G. Benedek (Eds.)
Progress in Brain Research, Vol. 75
© 1988 Elsevier Science Publishers B.V. (Biomedical Division)

CHAPTER 8

Receptive-field properties in the tecto- and striate-recipient zones of the cat's lateral posterior nucleus

Leo M. Chalupa and Bruce P. Abramson

Department of Psychology and the Physiology Graduate Group, University of California, Davis, CA 95616, U.S.A.

Introduction

The pulvinar-lateral posterior (LP) complex of the cat has been known for many years to be involved in visual function (for review, see Chalupa 1977). Almost 30 years ago it was reported that visual evoked potentials could be recorded from the cat's pulvinar-LP complex (Buser et al. 1959). Subsequently, single unit recording studies demonstrated the presence of visually responsive cells within a widespread region of the pulvinar and the LP nucleus (e.g., Godfraind et al. 1969, 1972; Veraart et al. 1972). In other neurophysiological experiments it was found that electrical stimulation of the cat's pulvinar-LP complex (Battersby and Oesterreich 1963; Chalupa et al. 1973), as well as functional blockade of this thalamic region (Chalupa et al. 1973), substantially modified visual responses in the cat's visual cortex.

With hindsight, it is now apparent that these early efforts to elucidate the functional organization of the pulvinar-LP complex were premature because they were carried out without the benefit of pertinent anatomical knowledge. The relevant anatomical information (e.g., Graybiel 1972a, b, c; Updyke 1977, 1981) delineated diverse sources of visual input to the cat's pulvinar-LP. More importantly, the results of modern tracing studies revealed that this vast region of the posterior thalamus is comprised of multiple visual areas distinguishable on the basis of their connectivity patterns.

The LP nucleus was shown initially to contain at least two visual areas: the principal tectorecipient zone in the medial LP (LPm) and a laterally adjacent striate-recipient area (LPl). In sections stained for Nissl substance it is difficult, if not impossible, to discern the boundaries of these two visual areas (see Fig. 1). In this regard, an important contribution was made by Graybiel and Berson (1980) who discovered that the tectorecipient area stained densely for acetylthiocholinesterase (ATChE), while the striate-recipient area stained poorly for this enzyme. This finding, which has been confirmed in our laboratory (Chalupa et al. 1983; Abramson and Chalupa 1985, 1988), has been used to provide a reliable and convenient means for differentiating the LPm and the LPl in conjunction with electrophysiological and anatomical studies (see Fig. 1).

In neurophysiological studies of the LP nucleus, we addressed two basic questions. First, are the visual receptive field properties of LPm cells different from those of neurons in the LPl; and second, if there are such differences, can these be related to the main sources of visual input to these two areas? In this chapter we will provide an overview of experiments that sought to answer these two questions.

Some methodological considerations

The procedures we employed to carry out extracellular recordings have been described in detail

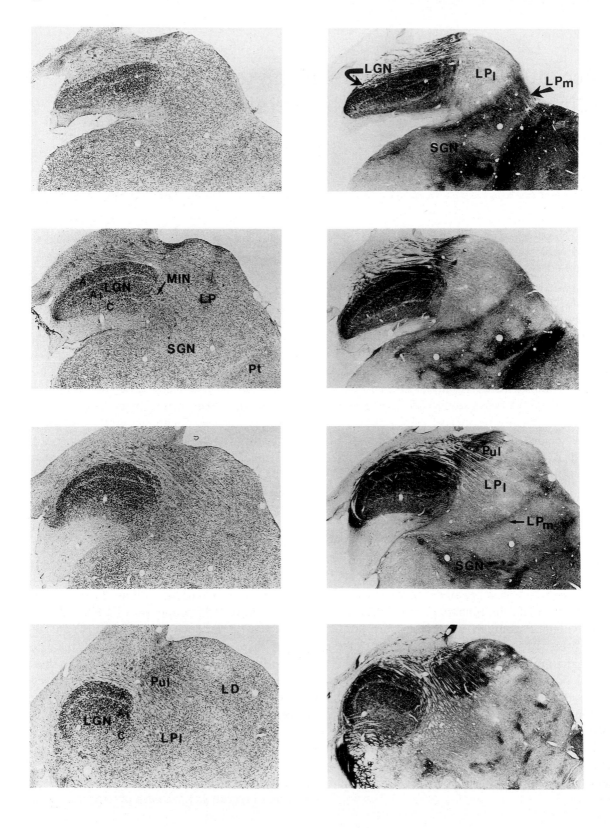

elsewhere (Chalupa et al. 1983). All recordings were from anesthetized and paralyzed animals, and both qualitative as well as quantitative procedures were used to characterize the response properties of visually responsive cells.

It should be noted that the degree to which cells in the pulvinar-LP complex respond to visual stimuli is dependent on the anesthesia used in the

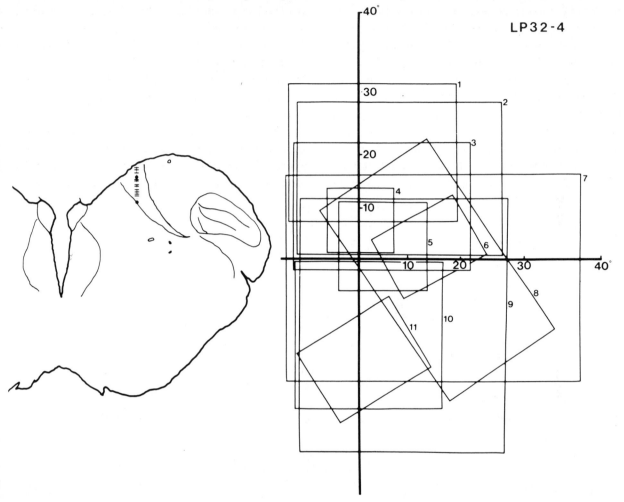

Fig. 2. The relative position of receptive fields for 11 cells recorded along a single penetration through the LPm. The receptive field labeled 1 was plotted for a cell in the most dorsal part of the track and the 11th was plotted for a neuron at the bottom of the penetration. The vertical and horizontal meridians are indicated by heavy lines. Hatch marks in the line drawing, through the LPm, denote the location of documented cells and the two solid circles along the penetration depict the marking lesions (taken from Chalupa et al. 1983).

◀ Fig. 1. Photomicrographs of coronal sections taken through the posterior thalamus. Sections at the left in each panel were stained with cresyl violet and adjacent sections at the right were stained to demonstrate acetylthiocholinesterase activity. The sections of each panel, from top to bottom, were taken at successive intervals of about 600 μm beginning at a Horsley-Clarke frontal coordinate of approx. A5.5 and continuing anteriorly. Note the clear boundaries between the major divisions of the LP nucleus distinguishable in the cholinesterase stained material. LPm, nucleus lateralis posterior, pars medialis; LPl, nucleus lateralis posterior, pars lateralis; Pul, pulvinar; LGN, lateral geniculate body; SGN, suprageniculate nucleus; LD, nucleus lateralis dorsalis; Pt, pretectal complex.

experiments. In early studies from this laboratory (Chalupa and Fish 1978; Fish and Chalupa 1979), we used a chronic preparation in which all surgical procedures were performed several days or weeks before the recording sessions. During the recordings the animals were maintained on a mixture of nitrous oxide and oxygen. In this type of preparation, most cells in the pulvinar-LP were found to respond to visual stimuli, but with few exceptions there was a great deal of response variability. To a large degree, this seemed to be due to the high and erratic pattern of spontaneous activity levels evident in many of these neurons. Particularly annoying is a 'bursty' pattern in background activity which made it very difficult to judge (without signal averaging) whether or not a given cell responded reliably. This situation seriously detracted from the enjoyment of doing such recordings. As a consequence, several years ago, we switched to an anesthetic state in which the nitrous oxide/oxygen mixture was supplemented with a low dose of chloralose (see Chalupa et al. (1983) for details). This served to effectively silence the background activity of most cells, so that the visual response patterns became readily apparent. Importantly, in several cases where recordings were made from a given cell before and after administration of chloralose, there appeared to be no appreciable change in the receptive field properties after administration of the additional anesthetic.

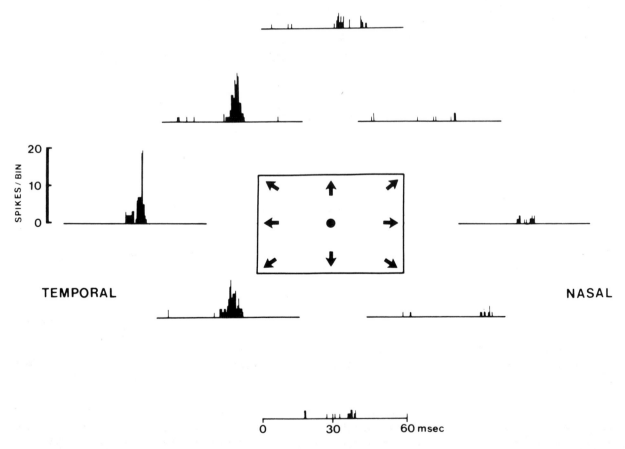

Fig. 3. Typical response of a directionally selective cell. This unit was isolated in the LPm. The different directions of stimulus movements are indicated by the arrows which point to the corresponding post stimulus time histogram (PSTH). The stimulus was a spot of light, 10° in diameter, moving at 200°/sec. The dimensions of this receptive field were 20 × 30 degrees. The PSTHs were based on 20 stimulus presentations, and the bin width was 4.8 msec (taken from Chalupa et al. 1983).

We recommend this type of preparation to colleagues who may be planning investigations of sensory properties in pulvinar-LP cells.

Visual field representations

The visual field is represented twice in the LP nucleus; once in the LPl and again in the LPm, with the vertical meridian representation corresponding to the border of these two zones (Mason 1978; Raczkowski and Rosenquist 1981; Chalupa et al. 1983; Hutchins and Updyke 1984). However, in our experience, there is generally a substantial degree of scatter in the distribution of receptive fields plotted for adjacent cells (see Fig. 2). As a consequence, in practice it is seldom possible to utilize retinal topography to pinpoint the transition from one visual area to the other in a given electrode penetration. For this reason, in all electrophysiological experiments we rely upon cholinesterase staining to localize our recordings to either the LPm or the LP1.

Similarities of response properties

Even in our first recordings it became readily apparent that most cells in the LP nucleus responded well to moving stimuli and that many of these were also directionally selective. Our criterion for directional selectivity is at least a 2 : 1 difference in the number of action potentials elicited by stimulus movement in two opposing directions. Most cells were relatively broadly tuned for the preferred direction of stimulus movement as indicated in the example provided in Fig. 3. We consider the preferred direction to be that which was in the midrange of the stimulus directions capable of activating the cell. In the principal tectorecipient zone 49% of the cells (125 of 256 tested) were found to be directionally selective. The incidence of such cells was comparable in the striate-recipient zone (130 of 221, 59%). Furthermore, as depicted in Fig. 4, the distribution of preferred directions was also similar for cells in the LPm and the LPl. In both zones, there was a preponderance

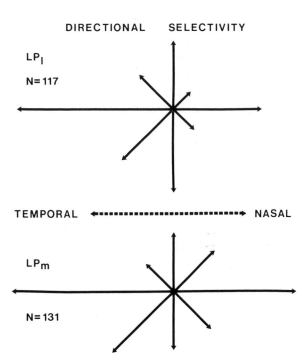

Fig. 4. The distribution of preferred directions for 131 cells in the tecto-recipient zone (LPm-lower) and 117 cells in the striate-recipient (LPl-upper) zone of the LP. Temporal is towards the periphery of the contralateral visual hemifield. The length of each arrow represents the number of cells which preferred a given direction of stimulus movement.

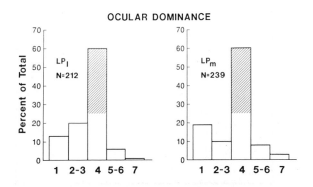

Fig. 5. The ocular dominance of cells in the LPm (n = 239) and LPl (n = 212). Cells in group 1 only responded to visual stimulation of the contralateral eye whereas those of group 7 only responded to stimulation of the ipsilateral eye. Group 4 cells responded similarly to stimulation of either eye. Cells of the BF (binocular facilitation) group responded better to binocular than monocular stimulation and are represented by the shaded portion of the graph.

of cells that preferred movement in the horizontal plane. It should also be noted that the preferred directions of these cells were not related in a clear-cut manner to the location of the receptive fields within the visual field.

The degree of binocularity exhibited by LPm neurons was also quite similar to that of LP1 cells. Figure 5 shows the ocular dominance distribution of the cells in both visual areas. An interesting binocular property exhibited by many neurons in LP is binocular facilitation. This was indicated when a given neuron responded poorly or sometimes not at all when monocular stimuli were employed, but yielded brisk responses with binocular stimulation (see Fig. 6).

Differences in response properties

While neither directional selectivity, nor the degree of binocularity differed appreciably between the populations of LPl and LPm cells, three other response properties clearly differentiated these neurons.

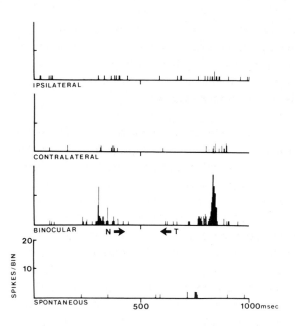

Fig. 6. An example of a cell which responded only to binocular stimulation. The stimulus was a bar of light which moved in the horizontal plane at 240°/sec. Each PSTH is based on 20 presentations and the bin width is 4 msec (taken from Chalupa et al. 1983).

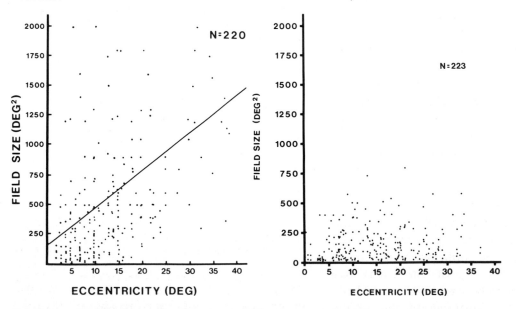

Fig. 7. Receptive field area as a function of eccentricity (distance of the receptive field center from the area centralis representation) for cells in the LPm (left graph) and LPl (right graph). For cells in the LPm there was a clear trend for the size of the receptive field to increase with eccentricity. The correlation coefficient was 0.5 which was statistically significant ($t = 8.6$, $P < 0.01$). The regression line was fit by the method of least squares. It has a slope of 32.6 and a y-intercept of 140 degrees^2. There was no correlation between receptive field size and eccentricity for cells in the LPl.

First, the size of receptive fields was significantly smaller in the striate-recipient zone than in the tectorecipient zone. This is evident from Fig. 7 which shows receptive-field size as a function of eccentricity for each population of cells. Note that for both samples of cells there is considerable variability in the dimension of receptive fields at each eccentricity. Averaged over all eccentricities the receptive field size was more than 4 times greater in LPm (645 deg^2) than in LPl (160 deg^2).

Second, the internal organization of receptive fields was also dissimilar for LP cells in the striate- and tecto-recipient zones. Many cells in both areas, even those that showed a preference for moving stimuli, responded reliably to stationary flashed spots or bars of light. In both groups of cells, virtually all of these neurons yielded phasic responses, discharging only to the onset and/or offset of the stimulus. Within the LPm, all but a few cells showed a homogenous internal organization of the receptive field. This was indicated by the observation that the response pattern (on, off, or on − off) elicited by a flashing stimulus did not change in polarity as a function of the position of the stimulus within the receptive field. In contrast, most cells in the LPl (71%, $n = 160$) showed clear changes in response polarity when the position of the stimulus was varied. The majority of such cells responded to stimulus onset and offset in the central region of their receptive field, but yielded only 'off' responses (61%) or 'on' responses (16%) at the edges. Figure 8 shows representative examples of these response patterns. In the remainder of the neurons, activation of about half of the receptive field yielded one type of response pattern, while from the other half a different pattern was elicited.

It should be noted that for most LP cells the activating region of the receptive field (i.e., that region of the visual field from which a reliable response could be obtained with a flashing or moving stimulus) was found to be flanked by a silent suppressive surround region. This was demonstrated by systematically increasing the size of the stimulus and noting the decrease in responsivity as the stimulus dimension exceeded that of the recep-

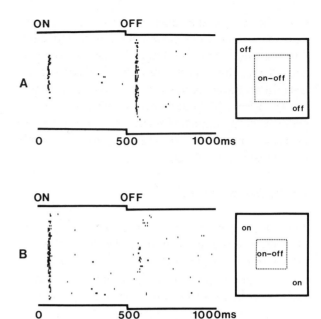

Fig. 8. Spatial-temporal maps of two cells recorded from the LPl demonstrating that response patterns varied with the locus of the stimulus within the receptive field. The stimulus was a flashing bar of light (1 × 30°) which was moved across the receptive field in 60 equally spaced steps. Time is represented on the x-axis and the normalized distance across the receptive field on the y-axis. Each dot represents a single action potential and the resolution of a raster was 4 msec. At the right, in A and B, are schematic spatial maps of the major response areas within the receptive fields taken from the data shown at the left.

tive field activating region. More than 50% of the cells in both the LPm and the LPl showed this property.

The third response characteristic that distinguished the population of LPm cells from LP1 neurons was orientation selectivity. Although oriented cells were encountered in both regions, the incidence of such neurons was substantially higher in the striate-recipient zone (46%, $n = 218$) than in the tecto-recipient region (27%, $n = 226$). Furthermore, the tuning of orientation specificities was greater in the LPl than the LPm. In the LPl, quantitative measures on 45 cells revealed that the halfwidth at half-height tuning (the angle through which the stimulus was rotated to reduce the response by half) had a mean value of 27 degrees (see Fig. 9). Similar measurements on area 17 neurons of the cat's cortex have obtained comparable values for complex cells (for reference list and further discussion, see Orban (1984) p. 153). Such quantitative assessment has not been carried out for LPm cells, but most oriented cells here respond well to bars of light that were more than 30 degrees from the preferred orientation (see Fig. 8A of Chalupa et al. 1983).

Functional implications

The foregoing observations indicate that three fundamental response properties clearly distinguish cells within two of the major visual areas of the LP nucleus. In comparison to the principal tectorecipient region, neurons in the striate-recipient zone have smaller receptive fields, an inhomogeneous rather than a homogeneous internal receptive field organization, and are more often orientation selective as well as more tightly tuned for oriented stimuli. These functional differences reflect some of the salient properties of the striate and collicular projection neurons.

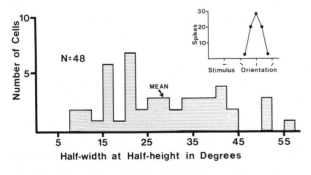

Fig. 9. The orientation selectivity for 48 cells in the striate-recipient area of the LP. An orientation-tuning curve was constructed for each cell as shown in the inset. A flashing bar of light was placed within the center of the receptive field. The number of action potentials (spikes) was counted, on-line, for 10 successive stimulus presentations at each orientation. The angle of the bar was adjusted by 15° and the procedure repeated until a response was no longer obtained. For each cell a value of half-width at half-height (the angle through which the stimulus was rotated to reduce the maximum response by half) was determined. The average value was 27°.

Superior collicular cells which project to the LPm are situated in the deep subdivision of the superficial gray layer (Abramson and Chalupa 1988). Certain receptive field properties are common to the LPm and to cells of the superficial gray (for review of collicular physiology see Chalupa (1984)). Visual cells in both structures are highly sensitive to moving stimuli, and a substantial proportion of these neurons are selective for the direction of stimulus movement. Further, virtually all neurons in the LPm as well as those in the colliculus, which can be activated by flashing stimuli, respond only in a phasic manner. The internal organization of receptive fields of these cells is homogeneous and stimuli larger than the activating region produce marked response attenuation in many LPm and collicular units.

However, not all of the response characteristics of LPm cells can be directly related to the collicular projection. One of the most obvious contrasts between LPm and superior collicular cells is their receptive field size; the average size of fields of LPm cells is at least twice that of units within the superficial strata of the superior colliculus. Further the distributions of preferred directions are also dissimilar. The vast majority of collicular cells prefer movement in the horizontal plane toward the periphery, while only a small bias for peripheral movement was found in LPm neurons (Chalupa et al. 1983). It is also the case that while 26% of the LPm cells are broadly tuned for oriented stimuli, neurons with this response property are rarely encountered in the cat's superior colliculus. Finally, cells showing binocular facilitation appear to be present in substantial number in the LPm, but not in the colliculus.

The similarities of the response properties between the superior colliculus and the LPm suggest that this tecto-thalamic pathway may be part of an ascending system concerned with localization and fixation of visual targets. On the other hand, the differences we have noted above point to a more complex role which could involve integration of visual information from tectal and extra-striate visual areas.

93

There also appear to be functional similarities between cells in the striate-recipient zone of LP and those of neurons in primary visual cortex (areas 17 and 18) that project to this region of the thalamus. It is known that these are pyramidal cells confined to layer 5 (Abramson and Chalupa 1985). While the specific receptive field properties of these cortical projection cells are yet to be determined, it is probably the case that these neurons are complex cells with response properties similar to those of corticotectal neurons that have been identified physiologically by antidromic stimulation of the colliculus (Palmer and Rosenquist 1974; Harvey 1980). In general, the response properties of LPl neurons reflect those of corticotectal cells with the notable exception that distinctive 'on−off' subregions were not seen in these cortical projection neurons, while we have observed such inhomogeneity in the receptive field organization of LPl cells. It is conceivable that such organization reflects the convergence of two or more complex cells onto a given LPl neuron. However, it is also possible that the cortical cells projecting to the LPl have different response properties than those projecting to the colliculus. This could be ascertained by determining the receptive field properties of layer 5 cells physiologically identified by antidromic stimulation of the LPl.

Studies from our laboratory, as well as those of others, indicate that the LP-pulvinar complex contains multiple visual areas. The results of the experiments we have summarized above dealt with the receptive field properties of two of the main visual zones in the LP nucleus. It would now be of interest to extend this type of analysis to the other visual regions. Recent anatomical studies from this laboratory (Abramson and Chalupa 1988) indicate that the striate-recipient zone is comprised of two visual areas. The main region, adjacent to the LPm is devoid of any collicular input, while a smaller zone bordering the pulvinar is innervated by both striate as well as tectal projections.

The results summarized above dealt only with the region of the LPl which does not receive a tectal projection, designated as the LPl-1 (Abramson 1987). Several of our electrode penetrations were in the tecto-recipient portion of the striate-recipient zone, designated the LPl-2. Here, visual receptive field properties differed markedly from those of LPl-1. Receptive fields were huge, even larger than in the LPm, and few cells were direction or orientation selective. This area appears to correspond to what Updyke (1984) has termed the 'shell' of the LP nucleus. In addition to the cortical and tectal inputs, it also receives projections from the hypothalamus as well as the cerebellum (Yoshii et al. 1978; Rodrigo-Angulo and Reinoso-Suárez 1984). The relative lack of specificity in the visual responses of these neurons suggests that this portion of the LPl may be involved in some type of visuomotor function.

The electrophysiological data we have obtained indicate that closely adjacent areas of the LP nucleus, which have been distinguished on the basis of their connectivity patterns, may subserve diverse roles in the processing of visual and visually-related information.

Acknowledgements

This work was supported by grant BNS-00807 from the National Science Foundation and grant EY-03491 from the National Eye Institute of the NIH.

References

Abramson, B.P. (1987) The functional organization of the nucleus lateralis posterior: visual response properties in the lateral zone. *Masters Thesis,* University of California, Davis.

Abramson, B.P. and Chalupa, L.M. (1985a) The laminar distribution of cortical connections with the tecto- and cortico-recipient zones in the cat's lateral posterior nucleus. *Neuroscience,* 15: 81−95.

Abramson, B.P. and Chalupa, L.M. (1985b) Two subregions within the striate-recipient area of the cat's LP complex. *Soc. Neurosci. Abstr.,* 11: 234.

Abramson, B.P. and Chalupa, L.M. (1988) Multiple pathways from the superior colliculus to the extrageniculate visual thalamus of the cat. *J. Comp. Neurol.,* in press.

Battersby, W.S. and Oesterreich, R.F. (1963) Neural limitations of visual excitability. VI. Photic enhancement following lateral thalamic stimulation. *Electroenceph. Clin. Neurophysiol.,* 15: 849 – 865.

Buser, P., Borenstein, P. and Bruner, J. (1959) Étude des systems 'associatifs' visuels et auditifs chez le chat anesthésie au chloralose. *Electroenceph. Clin. Neurophysiol.,* 11: 305 – 324.

Chalupa, L.M. (1977) A review of cat and monkey studies implicating the pulvinar in visual function. *Behav. Biol.,* 20: 149 – 167.

Chalupa, L.M. (1984) Visual physiology of the mammalian superior colliculus. In: *Comparative Neurology of the Optic Tectum,* Plenum, New York, pp. 775 – 818.

Chalupa, L.M., Battersby, W.S. and Frumkes, T.E. (1973) Some subcortical determinants of visual cortical excitability in the cat. *Intern. J. Neurosci.,* 5: 1 – 13.

Chalupa, L.M., Anchel, H. and Lindsley, D.B. (1973) Effects of cryogenic blocking of pulvinar upon visually evoked responses in the cortex of the cat. *Exp. Neurol.,* 39: 112 – 122.

Chalupa, L.M. and Fish, S.E. (1978) Response characteristics of visual and extravisual neurons in the pulvinar and lateral posterior nuclei of the cat. *Exp. Neurol.,* 36: 96 – 120.

Chalupa, L.M., Williams, R.W. and Hughes, M.J. (1983) Visual response properties in the tecto-recipient zone of the cat's lateral posterior pulvinar complex: a comparison with the superior colliculus. *J. Neurosci.,* 3: 2587 – 2596.

Fish, S.E. and Chalupa, L.M. (1979) Functional properties of pulvinar-lateral posterior neurons which receive input from the superior colliculus. *Exp. Brain Res.,* 36: 245 – 257.

Godfraind, J.M., Meulders, M. and Veraart, C. (1969) Visual receptive fields of neurons in pulvinar, nucleus lateralis posterior and nucleus suprageniculatus thalami of the cat. *Brain Res.,* 15: 552 – 555.

Godfraind, J.M., Meulders, M. and Veraart, C. (1972) Visual properties of neurons in pulvinar, nucleus lateralis posterior and nucleus suprageniculatus thalami of the cat. I. Quantitative investigation. *Brain Res.,* 44: 503 – 526.

Graybiel, A.M. (1972a) Some ascending connections of the pulvinar and nucleus lateralis posterior of the thalamus of the cat. *Brain Res.,* 44: 99 – 125.

Graybiel, A.M. (1972b) Some extrageniculate visual pathways in the cat. *Invest. Ophthalmol.,* 11: 322 – 332.

Graybiel, A.M. (1972c) Some fiber pathways related to the posterior thalamic region in the cat. *Brain Behav. Evol.,* 6: 363 – 393.

Graybiel, A.M. and Berson, D.M. (1980) Histochemical identification and afferent connections of subdivisions in the lateralis posterior-pulvinar complex and related thalamic nuclei in the cat. *Neuroscience,* 5: 1175 – 1238.

Harvey, A.R. (1980) A physiological analysis of subcortical commissural projections of areas 17 and 18 of the cat. *J. Physiol.,* 302: 507 – 534.

Hutchins, B. and Updyke, B.V. (1984) Retinotopic organization within the lateral posterior complex of the cat. *J. Neurosci. Abstr.,* 10: 727.

Mason, R. (1978) Functional organization of the cat's pulvinar complex. *Exp. Brain Res.,* 31: 51 – 66.

Orban, G.A. (1984) Neuronal operations in the visual cortex. In: V. Braitenberg, H.B. Barlow, T.H. Bullock, E. Florey, O.-J. Grusser and A. Peters (Eds.), *Studies of Brain Function,* Vol. 2, Springer-Verlag, Berlin.

Palmer L.A. and Rosenquist, A.C. (1974) Visual receptive fields of single striate cortical units projecting to the superior colliculus in the cat. *Brain Res.,* 67: 27 – 42.

Raczkowski, D. and Rosenquist, A.C. (1983) Connections of the multiple visual cortical areas with the lateral posterior-pulvinar complex in the cat. *J. Neurosci.,* 3: 1912 – 1942.

Rodrigo-Angulo, M.L. and Reinoso-Suárez, F. (1984) Cerebellar projections to the lateral posterior-pulvinar thalamic complex in the cat. *Brain Res.,* 322: 172 – 176.

Updyke, B.V. (1977) Topographic organization of the projections from cortical areas 17, 18 and 19 onto the thalamus, pretectum and the superior colliculus of the cat. *J. Comp. Neurol.,* 173: 81 – 121.

Updyke, B.V. (1981) Projections from visual areas of the middle suprasylvian sulcus onto the lateral posterior complex and adjacent thalamic nuclei in cat. *J. Comp. Neurol.,* 201: 477 – 506.

Updyke, B.V. (1983) A re-evaluation of the functional organization and cytoarchitecture of the feline lateral posterior complex, with observations of adjoining cell groups. *J. Comp. Neurol.,* 219: 143 – 181.

Veraart, C.M., Meulders, M. and Godfraind, J.M. (1972) Visual properties of neurons in pulvinar, nucleus lateralis posterior and nucleus suprageniculatus thalami in the cat. II. Quantitative investigation. *Brain Res.,* 44: 527 – 546.

Yoshii, N., Fujii, M. and Mizokami, T. (1978) Hypothalamic projections to the pulvinar-LP complex in the cat: a study by the HRP method. *Brain Res.,* 155: 343 – 346.

T.P. Hicks and G. Benedek (Eds.)
Progress in Brain Research, Vol. 75
© 1988 Elsevier Science Publishers B.V. (Biomedical Division)

CHAPTER 9

Visual function of the cat's LP/LS subsystem in global motion processing

Josef P. Rauschecker

Max-Planck-Institut für biologische Kybernetik, D-7400 Tübingen, F.R.G.

Introduction

A possible way of looking at the organization of neocortex in general and of the visual cortex in particular is to see the different areas in conjunction with their principal thalamic inputs. These inputs are bound to determine the receptive field properties of their cortical target areas to a large extent; in turn, the heavy back projections from these areas to the same thalamic nuclei suggest loops being formed that play an important role for the dynamic functioning of these systems.

In two separate but closely connected investigations we have looked at the local and global organization of receptive field properties in the cat's lateral suprasylvian cortex (PMLS and PLLS) and of its principal thalamic relay, the lateral posterior nucleus (LPl and LPm). We have found that LS and LP share a number of features in their receptive field organization. The most prominent local properties of single units in LS and in LP are their narrow directional and broad velocity tuning combined with strong binocular facilitation. Globally, direction preference (which is constant throughout the RF) is organized with a pronounced centrifugal bias, i.e., for motion away from the area centralis. Velocity preference at the same time increases with eccentricity.

These observations allow the formation of a hypothesis about the possible visual function of LS

cortex, or even better, of the LP/LS subsystem: if one looks at the total output of the system, it should be maximally activated by optic flow expanding radially from the point of fixation. Such flow fields are encountered, for example, during forward locomotion. The projection of the LS to the pontine nuclei and from there to the cerebellar vermis could form a rather direct route for visually guided movements. Alternatively, the LP/LS subsystem could be one of a whole set of subsystems involved in the perception of motion, transforming visual information from the occipital cortex to parietal areas. The two views are by no means mutually exclusive, but further testing in awake behaving animals could be useful in reaching a decision about their main emphases.

Two visual systems?

While initially most of the work in the neurobiology of vision has been devoted to the study of the geniculostriate system, *extra*geniculostriate vision has received increasing attention in recent years. One of the major outcomes of this research has been the finding of multiple representations of the retina in the cerebral cortex (see Woolsey 1981). These visual maps have their emphasis on different aspects of the visual world and seem to represent different functional specializations of visual processing (Zeki 1978). Two major branches may be discerned: one having to do with the processing of form (including color as an additional enhancing cue), the other with the processing of motion. In several species it has become possible to assign these two modes of processing to discrete anatomical structures in the cortex (Weller and Kaas 1981; Ungerleider and Mishkin 1982; Van Essen and Maunsell 1983).

This dichotomy of visual processing into 'two visual systems', as it emerges now from modern anatomy and physiology, had already been postulated 20 years ago, on the basis of behavioral experiments involving lesion studies in different species (Sprague 1966; Trevarthen 1968; Schneider 1969). In these investigations it was mainly the superior colliculus in the midbrain tectum that was

allocated to be the seat of the 'second visual system'. This was supposed to signal the 'where' in 'ambient vision', while the geniculostriate system was supposed to signal 'what', i.e., shape or form of an object, in 'focal vision'.

We now know that the superior colliculus itself, at least in higher mammals, is largely under cortical control. In turn, a number of extrastriate cortical areas receive input from the superior colliculus via the extrageniculate thalamus. Thus, we can now really suggest the existence of a 'second visual system' including structures on different brain levels, midbrain, thalamus, and cortex (Fig.1).

Thalamocortical subsystems rather than cortical maps alone determine specialized visual processing

Despite all our present enthusiasm about cortical maps it is particularly necessary, to my mind, not to underestimate the importance of thalamic nuclei for specialized visual processing. As Nissl has stated at the beginning of this century, the thalamus may be the key to understanding the cortex (Nissl 1913; see also Creutzfeldt 1983). One way of looking at the cortex and of defining a cortical area has always been to determine its main source of afferent input from the thalamus, i.e., its 'principal thalamic relay nucleus'. Von Monakow established in 1895 a scheme of thalamocortical relationships in the cat by making localized lesions in the cortex and looking at retrograde degeneration in the thalamus, a method that had been developed by von Gudden as early as 1870. Von Monakow's scheme of thalamocortical relationships is still largely valid today (see Jones 1985).

According to this view, which was advocated in recent years among others by Creutzfeldt (1983) and Jones (1985), each cortical area receives a major thalamic input from one principal relay nucleus and less important inputs from a few others. The same area of cortex sends fibers back to exactly the same thalamic nuclei it receives input from and to no others. Although the function of the corticofugal system is far from clear, this 'principle of

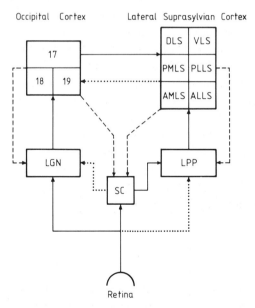

Fig. 1. Highly simplified schematic view of the 'two visual systems' in the cat. A first subsystem is formed by the geniculostriate pathway involving the occipital areas 17, 18, and 19. A second subsystem can be seen emanating from the tectofugal pathway involving the lateral posterior nuclei of thalamus (LP/pulvinar complex; LPP) and the lateral suprasylvian cortical areas (LS; for detailed nomenclature see Tusa et al. 1981). Corticofugal connections are drawn as dashed lines. Weak connections whose significance is not yet fully understood are drawn as dotted lines.

reciprocity' (Diamond et al. 1969) suggests that functional entities are formed by a cortical area *and* its thalamic relay rather than by the area of cortex alone. Some evidence for this view can be seen already from looking at primary sensory areas. New processing features are formed in the cortex by convergence and intracortical connectivity, but the similarities between cortical receptive fields and their thalamic counterparts often seem greater than their dissimilarities.

For the extrageniculate visual thalamus of the cat a clear correspondence on the basis of connec-

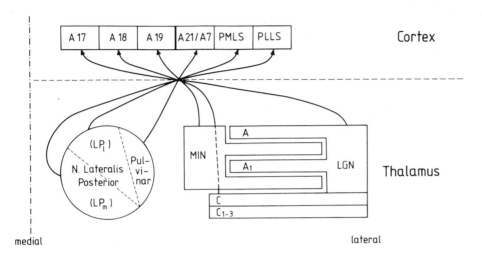

Fig. 2. Highly schematized view of some visual cortical areas and their presumed principal thalmic relays to indicate the mirror image arrangement from medial to lateral of thalamus and cortex. The scheme shown here is only a suggestion, other assignments are possible. In particular, it is not clear which cortical area should be assigned to pulvinar proper in the cat.

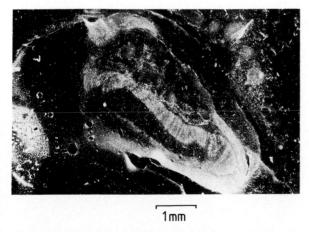

1mm

Fig. 3. Dark-field photomicrograph of a frontal section through the visual thalamus after anterograde labelling with wheat-germ agglutinin-conjugated horseradish peroxidase (WGA-HRP) injected into the contralateral eye.

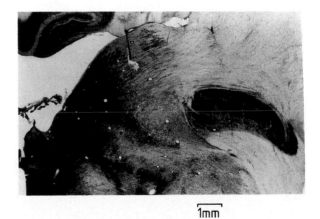

1mm

Fig. 4. Acetylcholinesterase staining of a frontal section through the visual thalamus. The lateral geniculate nucleus and the medial part of the lateral posterior nucleus (LPm) are darkly stained. LPl is only lightly stained.

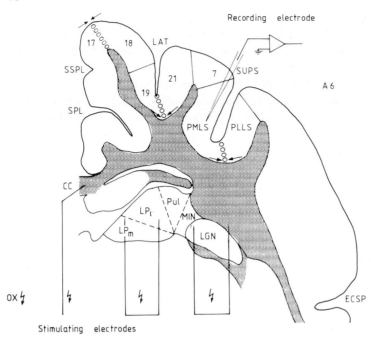

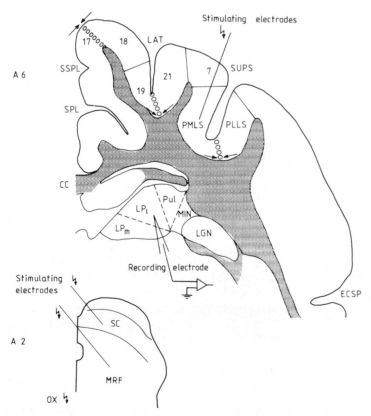

Fig. 5. Schematic view of the two experimental set-ups for recording from LP (bottom) and LS (top) including recording and electrical stimulation electrodes.

tivity has been established between the lateral and the medial subdivisions of the lateral posterior nucleus (LPl and LPm) and two areas of the lateral suprasylvian visual cortex, PMLS and PLLS (Berson and Graybiel 1978; Tong et al. 1982). This fits into the general scheme of a latero-medial succession of thalamic nuclei projecting onto a medio-lateral succession of cortical areas, and vice versa (Fig. 2). We have examined how closely the anatomical correspondence between LP and LS is matched by a physiological one in terms of receptive field organization, and whether such a correspondence would justify the view that such a thalamocortical subsystem acts as a functional entity within the visual system as a whole.

Anatomical and physiological facets of extrageni-culate visual thalamus

Different views of frontal sections through the cat's visual thalamus are shown in Figs. 3 and 4. Fig. 3 shows the results of anterograde labelling after injection of 20 μl wheat-germ agglutinin-conjugated horseradish-peroxidase (WGA-HRP; 10%) into the contralateral eye. As is well known from the use of other anterograde tracers, layers A, C and C2 of the lateral geniculate nucleus are labelled.

In Fig. 4 a section is stained for acetylcholin-esterase with the method of Graybiel and Berson (1980). The subdivisions of the LP nucleus can easily be discerned. In single unit recordings from LP (and LS) theta-glass micropipettes were used, one chamber being filled with a 5% HRP solution. Thus, electrode tracks could be reliably reconstructed and assigned to different subnuclei. In addition to the recording electrode, stimulating electrodes were implanted in several experiments to allow the electrical stimulation of various structures (Fig. 5).

Comparing the LP of the thalamus with LS cortex, two differences were most striking: (1) the generally lower proportion of units responding to visual stimuli, and (2) the higher variability of these visual responses. Two explanations for these differences can be offered, which are illustrated in Fig. 6. First, it was noted occasionally that units would respond to stimuli other than visual ones (Fig. 6B). In addition, responses seemed to be subject to the influence of arousal quite substantially, which was demonstrated by electrical stimulation of the midbrain reticular formation (MRF). An MRF stimulus given before stimulation of the optic chiasm often led to a considerable enhancement of that response (Fig. 6C).

Binocularity and directionality of cells in LP and LS

Apart from these qualitative differences, an astonishing number of similarities have been found between the lateral posterior nucleus of thalamus and the lateral suprasylvian cortex. First of all, cells in both structures were highly binocular, as can be seen from their ocular dominance distribution (Fig. 7). About 95% in LS and 90% in LP responded to stimulation of either eye. In addition, there was often remarkable binocular facilitation (Fig. 8). This even included units that would respond only when both eyes were stimulated simultaneously ('AND' units; see Rauschecker et al. 1987a).

Equally striking was the marked directionality of most cells in LP as well as in LS. About 90% of the cells in both structures showed a preference for one direction of movement of a light spot. The width of directional tuning varied greatly among cells, ranging from very narrowly tuned cells ($\pm$ 20 deg) to cells that would respond to all directions of motion.

Using antidromic stimulation, cells could be identified both in LP and in LS that were narrowly tuned for direction of motion and which projected onto LS and LP, respectively (Fig. 9). It is difficult to determine therefore, whether direction selectivity is generated first at the thalamic (or even sub-

A

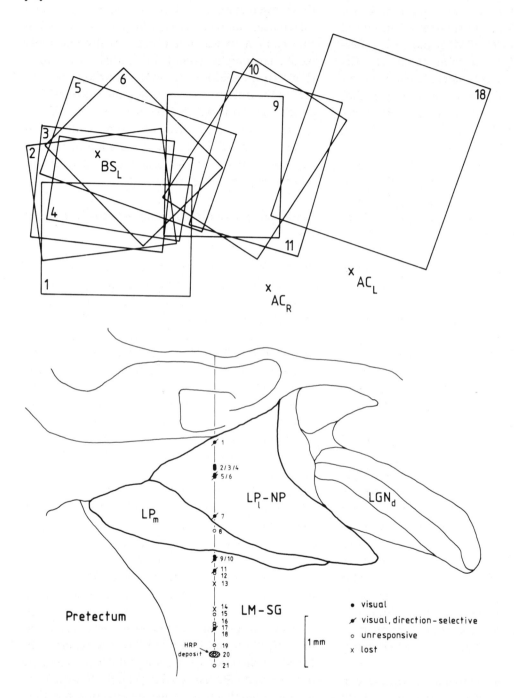

Fig. 6(A). For legend, see overleaf.

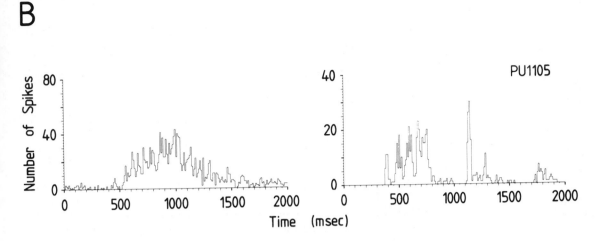

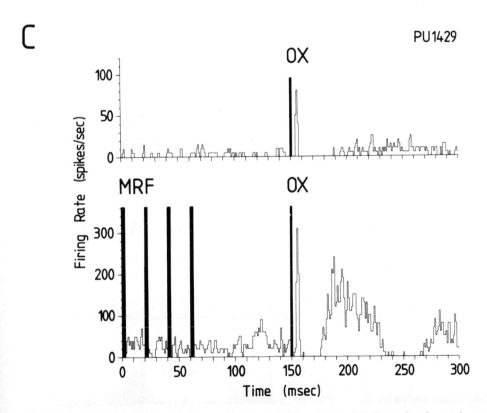

Fig. 6. Physiological recording from extrageniculate visual thalamus. (A) Example of a track reconstruction through the lateral posterior nucleus (LPl and LPm) extending deep down into the suprageniculate nucleus (LM-SG). For the following evaluation only single units recorded from LP where considered. (B) Example of a response to somatosensory stimulation of the contralateral forepaw with two different velocities recorded from the posterior part of LPm. (C) Effect of electrical stimulation of the mesencephalic reticular formation (MRF) with a pulse train beginning 150 msec before stimulation of optic chiasm (OX). The response to the OX stimulus is greatly enhanced and oscillations are evoked with a preceding MRF stimulus.

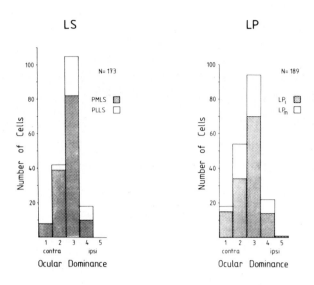

Fig. 7. Ocular dominance histograms for neurons from LP and LS. Ocular dominance classes are defined as (1)/(2) exclusively/predominantly influenced from contralateral eye, (3) equally influenced from either eye, (4)/(5) predominantly/exclusively influenced from ipsilateral eye.

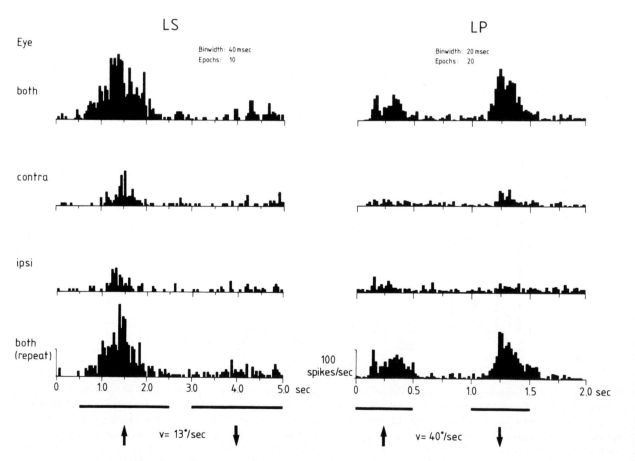

Fig. 8. Examples of binocular facilitation in LP and LS.

thalamic) level and is relayed to the cortex in an 'upstream' process, or whether it is made up cortically and imposed upon LP in 'downstream' fashion. Results from other studies (Spear and Baumann 1979; Guedes et al. 1983) conflict with each other, and so this interesting issue remains to be resolved.

Global motion processing in LP and LS

Perhaps the most intriguing similarity between LP and LS cells is their global organization of direction preferences with respect to visual field location. A large proportion of units prefer movement away from the area centralis in a fronto-parallel plane. We have previously termed this 'centrifugal' motion (Rauschecker et al. 1987a). The same tendency as is observed for cells in LS is clearly present in LP as well (Fig. 10), though not quite as pronounced. There is also a slight quantitative difference in this respect between LPl and LPm. The preponderance of cells with a 'radial' direction preference as compared to a 'circular' preference in LS is apparent in the plot of Fig. 11a.

It was stated previously that a centrifugal organization of direction preferences could be useful for the detection of expanding flow-fields of motion (Rauschecker et al. 1978a). This could be achieved by either assessing the total output of the system, or by a convergent projection of an ensemble of cells onto single units in another target area. This then could generate receptive fields displaying opponent vector organization like the ones observed in monkey parietal cortex (Motter and Mountcastle 1981; Steinmetz et al. 1987) or responding selectively to size changes and looming stimuli (Saito et al. 1986).

The mathematical analysis of velocity fields resulting from looming stimuli predicts that velocities are higher towards the periphery and are smaller around the center of fixation (their 'pole'). If one analyses the velocity preference of cells both in LP and LS, this prediction is matched exactly: velocity preference increases with eccentricity, and this is particularly clear for neurons with a preference for radial motion (Fig. 11b).

Visual function of the LP/LS subsystem

The lateral suprasylvian cortex and the lateral posterior nucleus of the thalamus both project to a number of subcortical targets, e.g., the superior colliculus and the pontine nuclei. Both these structures then give rise to a projection to the vermis of the cerebellum (Fig. 12). It was highly rewarding, therefore, to appreciate that visual cells in all of these targets of the LP/LS-system show a similar trend towards centrifugal motion preference (Vejbaesya 1967; Dreher and Hoffmann 1973; Baker et al. 1976).

Biologically, it is not surprising that a specialized system should exist for the detection of expanding velocity fields, since these occur, for example, during forward locomotion and might be used to stabilize posture during stance. It is most exciting that just these roles were assigned to the cerebellar vermis by Sprague and co-workers on the basis of brain injury and lesion studies (Chambers and Sprague 1955). The organization of the LP/LS subsystem (as part of the 'second visual system') in terms of global motion processing may thus be a good example of the way how thalamo-cortical function is organized in general: higher-order sensory processing leads to predictions about the world around us, which can then be used for the preparation of action without further delay.

Acknowledgments

The experiments described in this review were done in collaboration with A. Friederichs, M.W. von Grünau, and C. Poulin. Thanks are due to S. Hahn for preparing the figures and to M. Ghasroldashti for checking the manuscript.

A

LS

LSP109 / 3 M

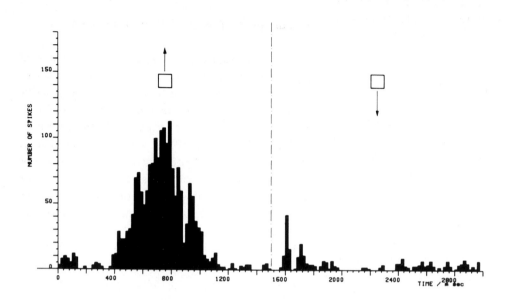

Direction Tuning

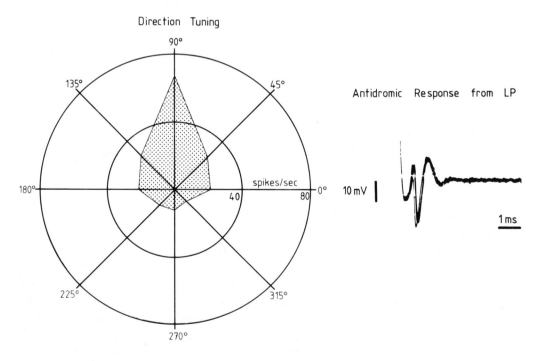

Fig. 9(A). For legend, see overleaf.

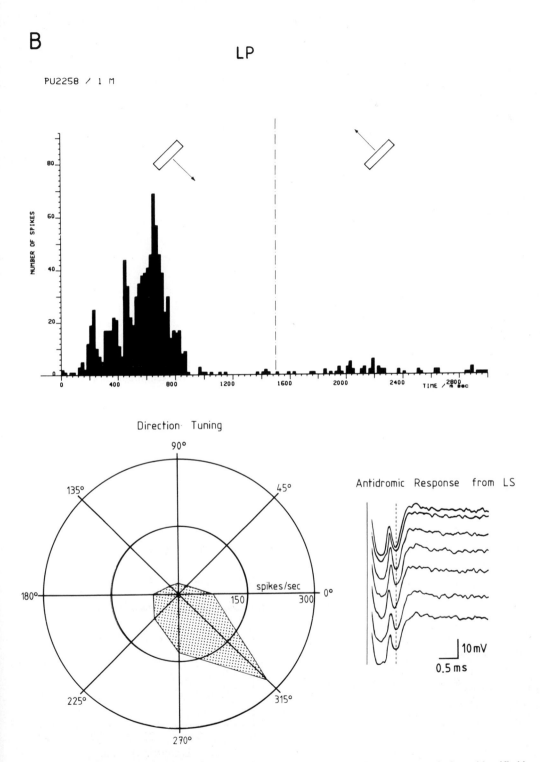

Fig. 9. Cells with narrow directional tuning projecting from LP to LS, or LS to LP, respectively, as identified by antidromic electrical stimulation (from Rauschecker et al. 1987b).

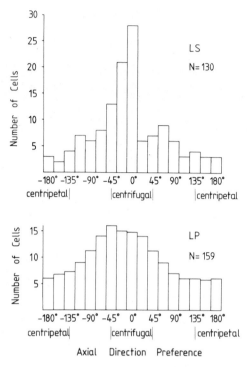

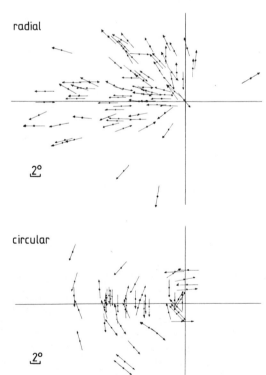

Fig. 10. Axial direction preferences in LS and LP. A clear bias for centrifugal motion can be seen in both distributions.

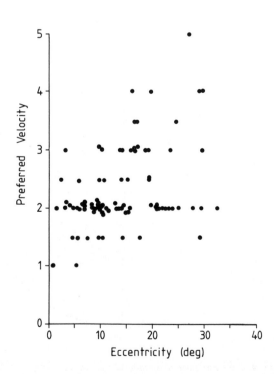

Fig. 11. (A) Plot of cells with radial and circular direction preference in LS to display their relative frequencies of occurrence in four experiments. Dots give the location of receptive field (RF) centers (or points of maximal sensitivity within the RF); arrows indicate the preferred direction of motion. (B) Velocity preference of radial cells in LS as a function of RF eccentricity (from Rauschecker et al. 1987a). A very similar relationship was found for LP.

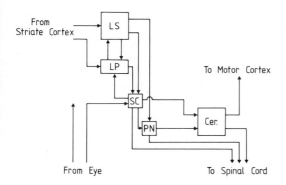

Fig. 12. Schematic wiring diagram of the LP/LS subsystem. Direct routes towards the motor output can be taken via the pontine nuclei and the cerebellar vermis. Visual cells in both these structures have been shown to possess a bias for centrifugal directions of motion.

References

Baker, J., Gibson, A., Glickstein, M. and Stein, J. (1976) Visual cells in pontine nuclei of the cat. *J. Physiol.*, 255: 415 – 433.

Berson, D.M. and Graybiel, A.M. (1978) Parallel thalamic zones in the LP-pulvinar complex of the cat identified by their afferent and efferent connections *Brain Res.*, 147: 139 – 148.

Chambers, W.W. and Sprague, J.M. (1955) Functional localization in the cerebellum. I. Organisation in longitudinal corticonuclear zones and their contribution to the control of posture, both extrapyramidal and pyramidal. *J. Comp. Neurol.*, 103: 105 – 130.

Creutzfeldt, O.D. (1983) *Cortex Cerebri*, Springer-Verlag, Berlin.

Diamond, I.T., Jones, E.G. and Powell, T.P.S. (1969) The projection of the auditory cortex upon the diencephalon and brain stem in the cat. *Brain Res.*, 15: 205 – 340.

Dreher, B. and Hoffmann, K.-P. (1973) Properties of excitatory and inhibitory regions in the receptive fields of single units in the cat's superior colliculus. *Exp. Brain Res.*, 219: 239 – 248.

Graybiel, A.M. and Berson, D.M. (1980) Histochemical identification and afferent connections of subdivisions in the LP-pulvinar complex and related nuclei in the cat. *Neuroscience*, 5: 1175 – 1238.

Guedes, R., Watanabe, S. and Creutzfeldt, O.D. (1983) Functional role of association fibres for a visual association area: the posterior suprasylvian sulcus of the cat. *Exp. Brain Res.*, 49: 13 – 27.

Jones, E.G. (1985) *The Thalamus*, Plenum Press, New York.

Motter, B.C. and Mountcastle, V.B. (1981) The functional properties of the light-sensitive neurons of the posterior parietal cortex studied in waking monkeys: foveal sparing and opponent vector organization. *J. Neurosci.*, 1: 3 – 26.

Nissl, F. (1913) Die Großhirnanteile des Kaninchens. *Arch. Psychiatr. Nervenkr.*, 52: 867 – 953.

Rauschecker, J.P., von Grünau, M.W. and Poulin, C. (1987a) Centrifugal organization of direction preferences in the cat's lateral suprasylvian visual cortex and its relation to flow field processing. *J. Neurosci.*, 7: 943 – 958.

Rauschecker, J.P., von Grünau, M.W. and Poulin, C. (1987b) Thalamocortical connections and their correlation with receptive field properties in the cat's lateral suprasylvian visual cortex. *Exp. Brain Res.*, 67: 100 – 112.

Saito, H., Yukie, M., Tanaka, K., Hikosaka, K., Fukada, Y. and Iwai, E. (1986) Integration of direction signals of image motion in the superior temporal sulcus of the macaque monkey. *J. Neurosci.*, 6: 145 – 157.

Schneider, G.E. (1969) Two visual systems: brain mechanisms for localization and discrimination are dissociated by tectal and cortical lesions. *Science*, 163: 895-902.

Spear, P.D. and Baumann, T.P. (1979) Effects of visual cortex removal on receptive field properties of neurons in lateral suprasylvian visual area of the cat. *J. Neurophysiol.*, 41: 31 – 56.

Sprague, J.M. (1966) Visual, acoustic and somesthetic deficits in the cat after cortical and midbrain lesions. In: D.P. Purpura and M.D. Yahr (Eds.), *The Thalamus*, Columbia University Press, New York, pp. 391 – 417.

Steinmetz, M.A., Motter, B.C., Duffy, C.J. and Mountcastle, V.B. (1987) Functional properties of parietal visual neurons: radial organization of directionalities within the visual field. *J. Neurosci.*, 7: 177 – 191.

Tong., L., Kalil, R.E. and Spear, P.D. (1982) Thalamic projections to visual areas of the middle suprasylvian sulcus in the cat. *J. Comp. Neurol.*, 212: 103 – 117.

Trevarthen, C.B. (1968) Two mechanisms of vision in primates. *Psychol. Forsch.*, 31: 299 – 237.

Tusa, R.J., Palmer, L.A. and Rosenquist, A.C. (1981) Multiple cortical visual areas: visual field topography in the cat. In: C.N. Woolsey (Ed.), *Cortical Sensory Organization, Vol. 2, Multiple Visual Areas*, Humana Press, Clifton, NJ, pp. 1 – 31.

Ungerleider, L.G. and Mishkin, M. (1982) Two cortical visual systems. In: Ingle, D.J., Goodale, M.A. and Mansfield, R.J.W. (Eds.), *Analysis of Visual Behaviour*, MIT Press, Cambridge. MA, pp. 549 – 586.

Van Essen, D.C. and Maunsell, H.R. (1983) Hierarchical organization and functional streams in the visual cortex. *Trends Neurosci.*, 6: 370 – 375.

Vejbaesya, C. (1967) Studies on the connections of the visual system. *Ph.D. thesis*, University of Edinburgh.

Von Gudden, B. (1870) Experimentaluntersuchungen über das

peripherische und centrale Nervensystem. *Arch. Psychiat. Nervenkr.*, 2: 693 – 723.

Von Monakow, C. (1895) Experimentelle und pathologisch-anatomische Untersuchungen über die Haubenregion, den Sehhügel und die Regio subthalamica, nebst Beiträgen zur Kenntnis früh erworbener Groß- und Kleinhirndefekte. *Arch. Psychiat. Nervenkr.*, 27: 1 – 128, 386 – 478.

Weller, R.E. and Kaas J. (1981) Cortical and subcortical con-nections of visual cortex in primates. In: C.N. Woolsey (Ed.), *Cortical Sensory Organization, Vol. 2, Multiple Visual Areas*, Humana Press, Clifton, NJ, pp. 121 – 155.

Woolsey, C.N. (1981) *Cortical Sensory Organization, Vol. 2, Multiple Visual Areas*, Humana Press, Clifton, NJ.

Zeki, S.M. (1978) Functional specialization in the visual cortex of the rhesus monkey. *Nature*, 274: 423 – 428.

PROGRESS IN BRAIN RESEARCH – VOLUME 75
VISION WITHIN EXTRAGENICULO-STRIATE SYSTEMS

edited by T.P. HICKS and G. BENEDEK

ERRATA

Chapter 10 (Norita & Katoh), pages 112 to 117:

i) Because of a printing error, part of the last sentence of the right hand column on page 112 was omitted. The sentence should read:

In the LM-Sg complex, four types of vesicle-containing profiles were observed (Fig. 5): large axon terminals containing round synaptic vesicles

ii) The right hand column on page 114 was repeated on page 117, and can therefore be deleted on page 114.

iii) **Prelims:** page v, List of Contributors:

On line 20 of that page, the correct name is:

'L.M. Chalupa'.

We apologize to the authors and to our readers for any inconvenience these errors might have caused.

The Publisher

T.P. Hicks and G. Benedek (Eds.)
Progress in Brain Research, Vol. 75
© 1988 Elsevier Science Publishers B.V. (Biomedical Division)

CHAPTER 10

Synaptic organization of the lateralis medialis-suprageniculate nuclear (LM-Sg) complex in the cat

Masao Norita and Yoshimitsu Katoh

Department of Anatomy, Fujita-Gakuen Health University, School of Medicine, Toyoake, Aichi, 470-11, Japan

Introduction

Recently, much has been learned about the 'extrageniculate' visual system. Among the thalamic nuclei, the lateralis posterior-pulvinar (LP-pulvinar) complex is known to be a principal component of the 'extrageniculate' thalamus (cf., Graybiel and Berson 1981; Updyke 1983). The most medial zone of the LP-pulvinar complex is the lateralis medialis-suprageniculate nuclear (LM-Sg) complex (Graybiel and Berson 1980). Electrophysiological studies have indicated that LM-Sg cells may have multimodal properties (Berkley 1973; Chalupa and Fish 1978), along with unimodal visually responsive properties (Suzuki and Kato 1969; Hicks et al. 1984). The aim of this article is to describe the afferent connections of the LM-Sg complex, and to point out the ultrastructural neural circuit of this complex.

Afferent connections of the LM-Sg complex

Before presenting details of the connectivity of the LM-Sg complex, we will deal briefly with the nuclear boundaries of the LP-pulvinar complex of the cat. Acetylcholinesterase (AChE)-stained sec-

Correspondence to: Masao Norita, M.D., Ph.D., Dept. of Anatomy, Fujita-Gakuen Health University, School of Medicine, Toyoake, Aichi, 470-11, Japan.

tions are very useful for determining the boundaries of the thalamic nuclei, since the cytoarchitecture of the LP-pulvinar complex is poorly differentiated in Nissl-stained sections (Fig. 1). Furthermore, as described previously by Graybiel and Berson (1981), the patterns of AChE staining in the thalamus correspond well with the input zones. Accordingly, four main subdivisions are recognized in the LP-pulvinar complex: the most lateral region, the pulvinar (Pul) is rich in AChE activity; the lateral part of the LP (LPl) including the posterior nucleus of Rioch has much weaker AChE activity; the medial part of the LP (LPm) is a zone of high AChE activity; the most medial region, the LM-Sg complex, has various-sized patches of high AChE activity. The area designated as the suprageniculate nucleus in this report may involve a considerable part of the intermediate region of the posterior thalamic nuclear group, as defined by other authors (see, e.g., Jones 1985).

The anatomical patterns of connectivity and principles of organization of the LM-Sg complex have been recently established (e.g., Berson and Graybiel 1978; Graybiel and Berson 1981; Updyke 1983). More recently, Hicks et al. (1986) demonstrated the distribution of HRP-labeled cells that send their axons to the area of the Sg containing light-sensitive cells. We also examined the afferent connections of the LM-Sg complex using the wheat germ agglutinin – horseradish peroxidase (WGA-HRP) technique (Norita et al. 1986a). Figure 2

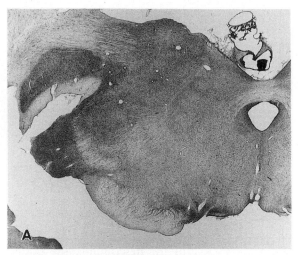

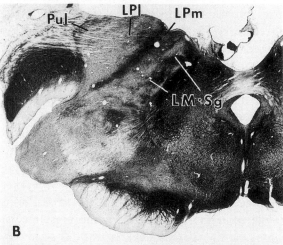

Fig. 1. Photomicrographs of representative frontal sections with the posterior thalamus that demonstrate the various subdivisions of the LP-pulvinar complex. A: a Nissl stained section. Compare with B. B: an adjacent frontal section that was stained for AChE activity. Note that the boundaries of the thalamic nuclei can be easily identified in this AChE-section. *Abbreviations:* AEs = anterior ectosylvian sulcus; AM = anterior medial nucleus; AV = anterior ventral nucleus; Cd = caudate nucleus; CL = central lateral nucleus; Cl = claustrum; CM-Pf = centromedian-parafascicular nuclear complex; LD = lateral dorsal nucleus; LGNd = dorsal nucleus of lateral geniculate body; LIc = nucleus lateralis intermedius, pars caudalis; LPl = nucleus lateralis posterior, pars lateralis; LPm = nucleus lateralis posterior, pars medialis; LS = lateral suprasylvian cortex; Ls = lateral sulcus; MD = mediodorsal nucleus; MG = medial geniculate nucleus; MSs = middle suprasylvian sulcus; Ped = cerebral peduncle; Pul = pulvinar; SC = superior colliculus; SF = suprasylvian fringe; Syls = sylvian sulcus; VA = ventral anterior nucleus; VB = ventrobasal nuclear complex; VL = ventral lateral nucleus.

shows cortical labeling following injection of WGA-HRP into the LM-Sg complex. In this case, a large number of retrogradely labeled cells were found in the granular insular cortex, with some occurring in the adjacent agranular insula. The labeled cells in the insular cortex tended to be grouped in patches. A moderate number of labeled cells were observed in the lateral suprasylvian cortex, the suprasylvian fringe and the anterior ectosylvian visual area (AEV of Mucke et al. 1982). Most labeled cells in the cortical areas were distributed in layer VI with some in layers III and V. Subcortically, a considerable number of labeled cells were detected mainly in the stratum opticum and stratum griseum intermediale of the superior colliculus (SC). Many labeled cells were seen in the thalamic reticular nucleus (TRN) in a loosely-organized topographic manner: thus, after injections into the mediodorsal or lateroventral portion of the LM-Sg complex, the labeled cells were mostly confined to the dorsal or ventral part of the TRN, respectively (Fig. 3). Fewer labeled cells were seen in the ventral thalamic nucleus, zona incerta, pretectal nuclei, substantia nigra, and periaqueductal gray.

Figure 4 shows the distribution of terminals in the LM-Sg complex labeled following an injection of tritiated amino acids into the SC, and of WGA-HRP into the AEV in the same animal. In the AEV-thalamic projections, substantial terminal labeling was found in the LM-Sg complex with some in the LPm. The AEV-LM-Sg projections seemed to terminate in a discontinuous, patchy manner. Although there were occasional matches between these patches of anterograde labeling and AChE activity, no clearly consistent relationship between them could be demonstrated. In the SC-thalamic projections, the anterograde labeling

Fig. 2. Drawings showing locations of labeled cells in the cortex ▶ ipsilateral to WGA-HRP injection in the LM-Sg complex. Each dot represents one cell. The injection site (solid black) is shown schematically on the right and above. Above: diagrammatic representation of the distribution of labeled cells in lateral view. Left and below: coronary sections showing the distribution of labeled cells in the cerebral cortex. See Fig. 1 for abbreviations.

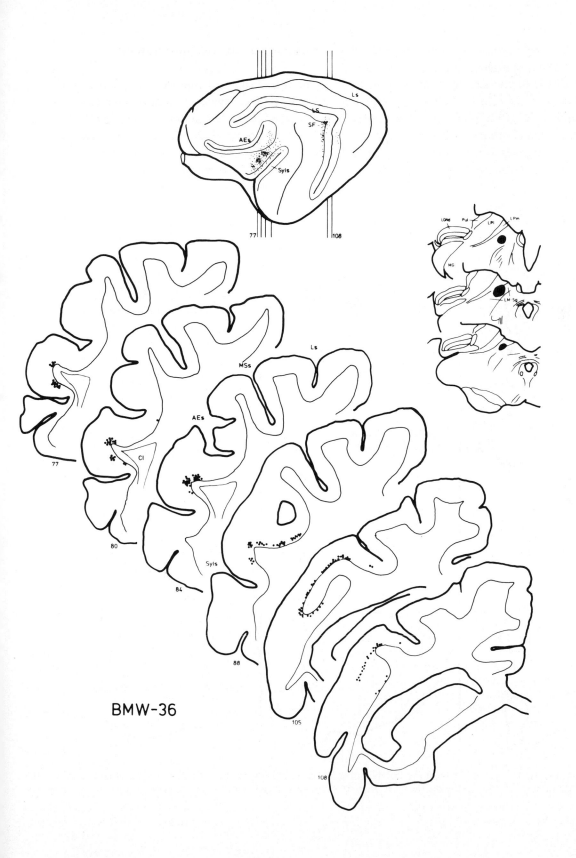

BMW-36

could be detected in three thalamic regions: the LPm, the LM-Sg complex, and the lateroventral part of the LPl. In the LM-Sg complex, the SC-thalamic labeling was also found to terminate in a patchy manner, as found in the AEV-thalamic labeling. In this combined experiment, a considerable overlap was observed between labeled AEV and SC inputs in the LM-Sg complex.

Electron microscopic observations

The ultrastructural features of synapses found in the LM-Sg complex are almost identical to those described in the LP-pulvinar complex (Hajdu et al. 1974) and other thalamic nuclei (see Madarász et al. 1981; Jones 1985, for references).

In the LM-Sg complex, four types of vesicle-

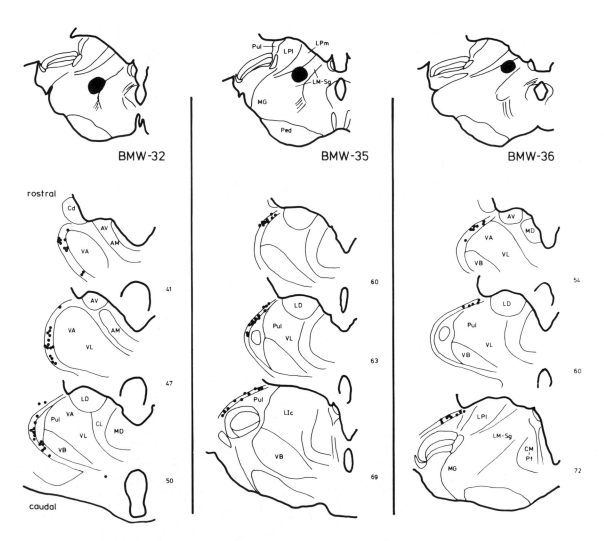

Fig. 3. Drawings of frontal sections through the thalamic reticular nucleus (TRN) to show the distributions of labeled cells in the TRN following injections of WGA-HRP into the ipsilateral LM-Sg complex. From Norita and Katoh (1987). See Fig. 1 for abbreviations.

(RL), small axon terminals filled with round synaptic vesicles (RS), axon terminals containing pleomorphic synaptic vesicles (F1), and dendritic profiles having pleomorphic synaptic vesicles (presynaptic dendrite, PSD). The PSD involves not only the dendritic trunk containing synaptic vesicles, but also dendritic appendages of the Golgi type II interneurons (F2 terminals described by Hajdu et al. (1974)).

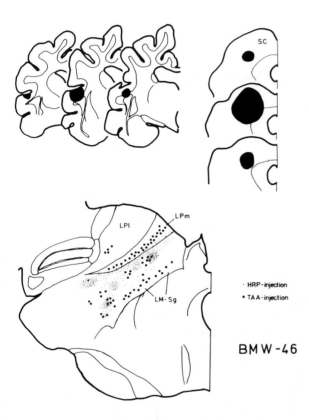

BMW-46

· HRP-injection
• TAA-injection

Fig. 4. Drawings of representative frontal sections of the cortex, the superior colliculus, and the LP-pulvinar complex, showing an injection site of WGA-HRP (2% WGA-HRP, 0.1 μl) in the AEV or a mixture of tritiated amino acids (TAA; proline and leucine 0.7 μl, 50 μCi/μl) in the SC (above), and distribution of labeled terminals in the LP-pulvinar complex (below). Small dots indicate terminals labeled by the cortical injection of WGA-HRP, large dots indicate those labeled by the tectal injection of TAA. Note a considerable overlap between labeled AEV and SC inputs in the LM-Sg complex. See Fig. 1 for abbreviations.

Groups of synapses either completely or incompletely surrounded by glial processes in a sectional plane have been found in the neuropil. This is the organization of the so-called glomerulus described in other thalamic relay nuclei (see Jones 1985, for references). In general, three different neural profiles were involved in the organization of the glomerulus: a conventional dendritic profile, the RL, and the PSD. Occasionally, F1 is found to participate in the glomerulus. The dendritic profile and the PSD are postsynaptic to the RL, and the PSD synapses upon the dendritic profile. The occurrence of the glomerulus would not seem to be distributed equally throughout the LM-Sg complex. Quantitative analysis of glomerular number in the core samples of AChE-positive patches and AChE-negative patches of the LM-Sg complex indicated that the number of glomeruli was significantly higher in the AChE-positive patches than in the AChE-negative patches (unpublished data). It is generally suggested that the presence of a glomerular arrangement may be involved in the generation of discrete responses to a stimulus as well as in the ability to perform high-fidelity synaptic activations over a wide frequency spectrum (see Steriade and Deschênes 1984, for references). Thus, it is not unreasonable to speculate that the quantitative differences in the frequencies of glomeruli found in the AChE-positive patches and in the AChE-negative patches signify that the LM-Sg complex is functionally non-homogeneous.

Sources of various types of terminals found in the LM-Sg complex have been studied using the HRP technique (Norita and Katoh 1986, 1987). Thus, after WGA-HRP injections into the AEV-insular cortex, it was possible to observe many labeled RS and a few RL mainly in the extraglomerular neuropil. Following the injection of tracer into the SC, both labeled RS and labeled RL were found (Fig. 6). The RL made multiple synaptic contacts with conventional dendrites and/or the PSD chiefly in the synaptic glomeruli. As described above, there is a considerable overlap between AEV and SC inputs in the LM-Sg complex. In

114

order to clarify whether both AEV and SC inputs terminate on the same postsynaptic profile, combined experiments, in which a lesion was produced in the AEV-insular cortex and WGA-HRP was injected into the SC, were performed (Norita and Katoh 1986). These combined studies indicated that the HRP-labeled RS and the degenerated RS were occasionally found to make synaptic contacts upon a single dendritic profile (Fig. 7), indicative of convergence of visuomotor-related signals from the AEV-insular cortex and the SC to a single LM-Sg neuron (e.g., Loe and Benevento 1969; Wurtz

and Albano 1980; Mucke et al. 1982). Following the injection of WGA-HRP into the TRN, the F1 were labeled anterogradely with the tracer. They made symmetric synaptic contacts with conventional dendrites in the extraglomerular neuropil. The TRN is known to exclusively contain inhibitory GABAergic cells (see Yen et al. 1985, for references). Thus, with regard to its visually related inputs as well as its inhibitory projections, it could be considered that the LM-Sg complex is a highly integrative structure. In order to obtain more precise information on the neural circuit of

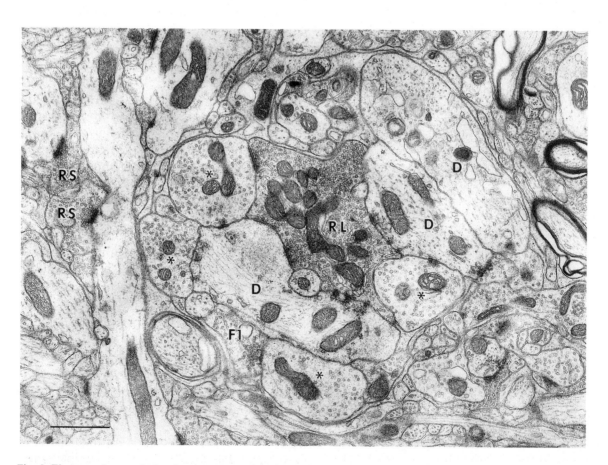

Fig. 5. Electron micrograph showing a representative synaptic glomerulus surrounded by glial processes. This glomerulus contains an RL terminal (RL), presynaptic dendrites (asterisks), a F1 terminal (F1), and conventional dendrites (D). The RL is presynaptic at multiple, moderately asymmetric contacts to the dendrites as well as a presynaptic dendrite. The presynaptic dendrites make symmetric synaptic contact with the dendrites. The F1 is presynaptic to a presynaptic dendrite with a symmetric contact. In extraglomerular neuropil, two RS are shown to make asymmetric synaptic contacts with dendrites. Bar = 1 μm.

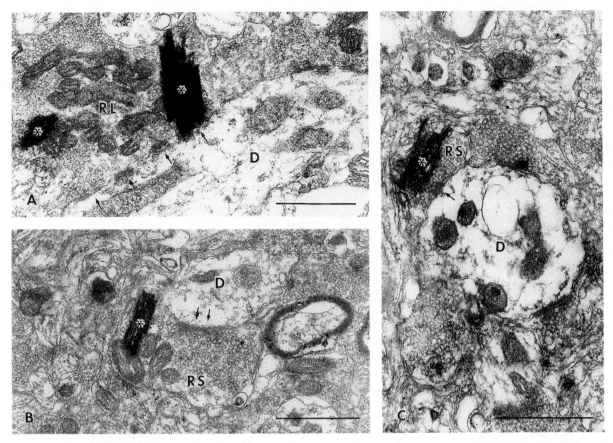

Fig. 6. Electron micrographs showing HRP-labeled axon terminals in the LM-Sg complex. TMB reaction-product crystals (asterisks) are visible. A: RL of SC derivative fiber making multiple asymmetric contacts (arrows) to a dendrite (D). B: RS of SC derivative fiber making an asymmetric contact (arrows) to a dendrite (D). C: RS of AEV derivative fiber making an asymmetric contact (arrow) to a dendrite (D). Bars = 1 μm. From Norita and Katoh (1986).

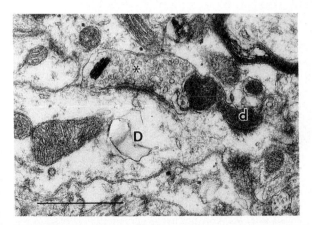

Fig. 7. Electron micrograph showing HRP-labeled terminal of SC-LM-Sg fiber (asterisk) and degenerated terminals of AEV-insular fibers (d). They form synaptic contacts upon a dendrite (D). Bar = 1 μm. From Norita and Katoh (1986).

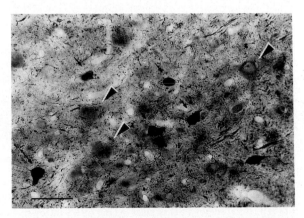

Fig. 8. Photomicrograph showing darkly stained GABA-immunoreactive cell bodies (arrows) and a high density of granular immunoreactivity in the neuropil. Note larger, nonimmunoreactive projection cells (arrowheads). Bar = 50 μm. From Norita and Katoh (1987).

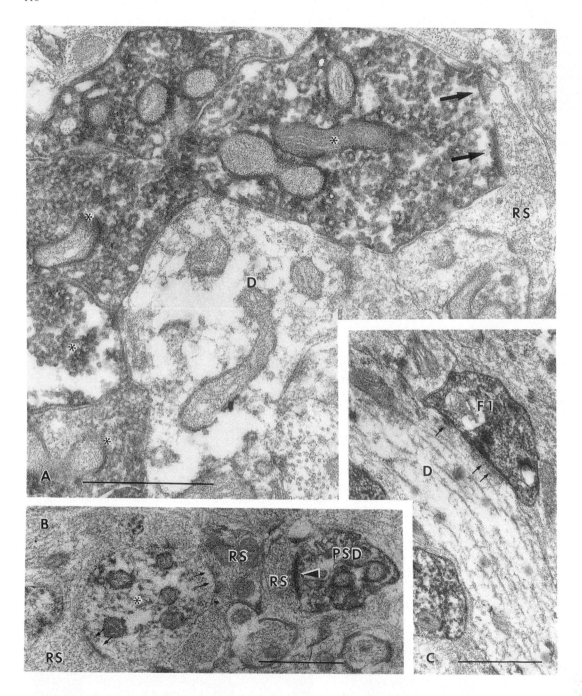

Fig. 9. Electron micrographs showing GABA-positive neural elements in a synaptic glomerulus (A) and in the extraglomerular neuropil (B, C). A: four GABA-positive presynaptic dendrites (PSD, asterisks) make symmetric contacts with a GABA-negative dendrite (D). Note one of PSD is postsynaptic to RS (arrows). B: on the left side, a GABA-positive dendrite (asterisk) receives two unlabeled RS (arrows). On the right side, RS makes an asymmetric contact (arrowhead) with GABA-positive PSD. C: GABA-positive F1 makes symmetric contacts (arrows) with GABA-negative dendrite (D). Bars = 1 μm. Modified from Norita and Katoh (1987).

and Albano 1980; Mucke et al. 1982). Following the injection of WGA-HRP into the TRN, the F1 were labeled anterogradely with the tracer. They made symmetric synaptic contacts with conventional dendrites in the extraglomerular neuropil. The TRN is known to exclusively contain inhibitory GABAergic cells (see Yen et al. 1985, for references). Thus, with regard to its visually related inputs as well as its inhibitory projections, it could be considered that the LM-Sg complex is a highly integrative structure. In order to obtain more precise information on the neural circuit of the LM-Sg complex, we (Norita and Katoh 1987) used a GABA-immunocytochemical method (Montero and Zempel 1985). Small immunoreactive cells, identified as Golgi type II interneurons, were found throughout the LM-Sg complex (Fig. 8). The PSD and the F1 were identified as the immunoreactive neural profiles. The GABAergic PSD were involved mostly in synaptic glomeruli, while GABAergic F1 formed symmetric axodendritic synaptic contacts mainly in the extraglomerular neuropil (Fig. 9). The F1 appeared to correspond to either axon terminals from the TRN or the axon terminals of interneurons (cf., Hajdu et al. 1974).

Conclusions

There are certain differences in connective pattern between the LM-Sg complex and other subdivisions of the LP-pulvinar complex. Thus, the visually related cortices, the suprasylvian fringe and the AEV-insular cortex (Mucke et al. 1982; Olson and Graybiel 1983; Hicks et al. 1986; Norita et al. 1986b) that project to the LM-Sg complex are known to be non-retinotopically ordered areas (e.g., Minciacchi et al. 1987). The deeper collicular layers sending axons to the LM-Sg complex contain neurons that respond to visual, somatic and auditory, and/or multimodal stimuli (Meredith and Stein 1986), while other subdivisions (Pul,

LPl, LPm) connect with the retinotopically ordered cortical areas (e.g., areas 17, 18, 19, the Clare-Bishop area, and/or area 20). Furthermore, the LPm receives inputs from the superficial tectal layers responsive only to visual stimuli. Thus, according to the visual processing, the LM-Sg complex might be a unique structure within the LP-pulvinar complex.

From the results of these ultrastructural findings, we concluded that (1) small GABA-immunoreactive neurons in the LM-Sg complex, together

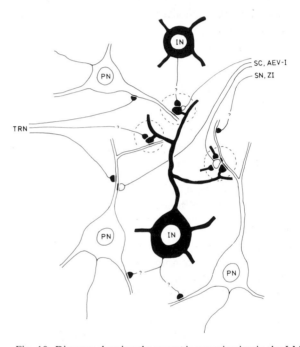

Fig. 10. Diagram showing the synaptic organization in the LM-Sg complex. GABA-positive neural elements are blackened. Synaptic glomeruli are indicated by dotted circles. The TRN afferent fibers form synaptic contacts mainly with the dendrites of the projection neurons (PN) in the extraglomerular neuropil. Afferent fibers from the AEV-insular cortex (AEV-I) make synaptic contacts with the projection cell dendrites. Some of the deep collicular afferents (SC) participate in the synaptic glomerulus. The presynaptic dendrites from GABA-positive interneurons participate in the synaptic glomerulus. Axons of the GABA-positive interneurons (IN) might make contact with the dendrites of the projection neurons. Fibers from the substantia nigra (SN) and zona incerta (ZI) may be possible candidates for GABAergic afferents. From Norita and Katoh (1987). See Fig. 1 for abbreviations.

with GABAergic fiber projections from the TRN, are the two main inhibitory sources influencing the LM-Sg projection neurons; (2) GABAergic interneurons receive the deep collicular afferents, which in turn may inhibit the neural activity of the LM-Sg projection neurons through the dendrodendritic synapses in the synaptic glomeruli; (3) GABAergic TRN axons also inhibit the LM-Sg projection neurons mainly in the extraglomerular neuropil. Furthermore, (4) the GABAergic LM-Sg interneurons and other extrinsic GABAergic neurons such as those in the substantia nigra (Di Chiara et al. 1979), might inhibit the LM-Sg projection neurons exclusively in the extraglomerular neuropil (Fig. 10).

References

Berkley, K.J. (1973) Response properties of cells in ventrobasal and posterior group nuclei of the cat. *J. Neurophysiol.*, 36: 940–952.

Berson, D.M. and Graybiel, A.M. (1978) Parallel thalamic zones in the LP-pulvinar complex of the cat identified by their afferent and efferent connections. *Brain Res.*, 147: 139–148.

Chalupa, L.M. and Fish, S.E. (1978) Response characteristics of visual and extravisual neurons in the pulvinar and lateral posterior nuclei of the cat. *Exp. Neurol.*, 61: 96–120.

Di Chiara, G., Porceddu, M.L., Morelli, M., Mulas, M.L. and Gessa, G.L. (1979) Evidence for a GABAergic projection from the substantia nigra to the ventromedial thalamus and to the superior colliculus of the rat. *Brain Res.*, 176: 273–284.

Graybiel, A.M. and Berson, D.M. (1980) Histochemical identification and afferent connections of subdivisions in the lateralis posterior-pulvinar complex and related thalamic nuclei in the cat. *Neuroscience*, 5: 1175–1238.

Graybiel, A.M. and Berson, D.M. (1981) Families of related cortical areas in the extrastriate visual system: summary of an hypothesis. In: C.N. Woolsey (Ed.), *Multiple Cortical Sensory Areas: Somatic, Visual and Auditory*, The Humana Press, Clifton, NJ.

Hajdu, F., Somogyi, Gy. and Tömböl, T. (1974) Neuronal and synaptic arrangement in the lateralis posterior-pulvinar complex of the thalamus in the cat. *Brain Res.*, 73: 89–104.

Hicks, T.P., Stark, C.A. and Fletcher, W.A. (1986) Origins of afferents to visual suprageniculate nucleus of the cat. *J.*

Comp. Neurol., 246: 544–554.

Hicks, T.P., Watanabe, S., Miyake, A. and Shoumura, K. (1984) Organization and properties of visually responsive neurones in the suprageniculate nucleus of the cat. *Exp. Brain Res.*, 55: 359–367.

Jones, E.G. (1985) *The Thalamus*, Plenum Press, New York.

Loe, P.R. and Benevento, L.A. (1969) Auditory-visual interaction in single units in the orbito-insular cortex of the cat. *Electroenceph. Clin. Neurophysiol.*, 26: 395–398.

Madarász, M., Tömböl, T., Hajdu, F. and Somogyi, Gy (1981) Some comparative quantitative data on the different (relay and associative) thalamic nuclei in the cat. A quantitative EM study. *Anat. Embryol.*, 162: 363–378.

Meredith, M.A. and Stein, B.E. (1986) Visual, auditory, and somatosensory convergence on cells in superior colliculus results in multisensory integration. *J. Neurophysiol.,* 56: 640–662.

Minciacchi, D., Tassinari, G. and Antonini, A. (1987) Visual and somatosensory integration in the anterior ectosylvian cortex of the cat. *Brain Res.*, 410: 21–31.

Montero, V.M. and Zempel, J. (1985) Evidence for two types of GABA-containing interneurons in the A-laminae of the cat lateral geniculate nucleus: a double-label HRP and GABA-immunocytochemical study. *Exp. Brain Res.*, 60: 603–609.

Mucke, L., Norita, M., Benedek, G. and Creutzfeldt, O. (1982) Physiologic and anatomic investigation of a visual cortical area situated in the ventral bank of the anterioir ectosylvian sulcus of the cat. *Exp. Brain Res.*, 46: 1–11.

Norita, M. and Katoh, Y. (1986) Cortical and tectal afferent terminals in the suprageniculate nucleus of the cat. *Neurosci. Lett.*, 65: 104–108.

Norita, M. and Katoh, Y. (1987) The GABAergic neurons and axon terminals in the lateralis medialis-suprageniculate nuclear complex of the cat: GABA-immunocytochemical and WGA-HRP studies by light and electron microscopy. *J. Comp. Neurol.*, 263: 54–67.

Norita, M., Katoh, Y. and Hida, T. (1986a) Afferent connections of the suprageniculate nucleus of the cat: WGA-HRP study. *Neurosci. Lett.*, Suppl., 3: S184.

Norita, M., Mucke, L., Benedek, G., Albowitz, B., Katoh, Y. and Creutzfeldt, O.D. (1986b) Connections of the anterior ectosylvian visual area (AEV). *Exp. Brain Res.*, 62: 225–240.

Olson, C.R. and Graybiel, A.M. (1983) An outlying visual area in the cerebral cortex of the cat. In: J.-P. Changeux et al. (Eds.), *Molecular and Cellular Interactions Underlying Higher Brain Functions, Progress in Brain Research, vol. 58*, Elsevier, Amsterdam, pp. 239–245.

Steriade, M. and Deschênes, M. (1984) The thalamus as a neuronal oscillator. *Brain Res. Rev.*, 8: 1–63.

Suzuki, H. and Kato, H. (1969) Neurons with visual properties in the posterior group of the thalamic nuclei. *Exp. Neurol.*, 23: 353–365.

Updyke, B.V. (1983) A reevaluation of the functional organization and cytoarchitecture of the feline lateral posterior complex, with observations on adjoining cell groups. *J. Comp. Neurol.*, 219: 143 – 181.

Wurtz, R.H. and Albano, J.E. (1980) Visual-motor function of the primate superior colliculus. *Annu. Rev. Neurosci.*, 3: 189 – 226.

Yen, C.T., Conley, M., Hendry, S.H.C. and Jones, E.G. (1985) The morphology of physiologically identified GABAergic neurons in the somatic sensory part of the thalamic reticular nucleus in the cat. *J. Neurosci.*, 5: 2254 – 2268.

T.P. Hicks and G. Benedek (Eds.)
Progress in Brain Research, Vol. 75
© 1988 Elsevier Science Publishers B.V. (Biomedical Division)

CHAPTER 11

The role of the primate lateral terminal nucleus in visuomotor behavior

Michael J. Mustari[1], Albert F. Fuchs[1], Thomas P. Langer[1], Chris Kaneko[1] and Josh Wallman[2]

[1]*Regional Primate Research Center, University of Washington, Seattle, WA 98195, and* [2]*Department of Biology, CUNY, New York, NY 10031, U.S.A.*

Introduction

When the head moves the vestibulo-ocular reflex (VOR) generates an oppositely directed eye movement whose gain (eye velocity divided by head velocity) in the dark is typically less than one. In the light, therefore, this mismatch between the eye velocity generated by the VOR and head velocity creates a slip of the image of the entire visual world across the retina. Such full field visual motion is the adequate stimulus for the optokinetic system which drives the eyes in the direction of visual motion with a gain near one for velocities up to 90 deg/sec in humans (Cohen et al. 1977). Therefore, the optokinetic system contributes substantially to visual image stabilization during lower velocity or constant velocity head movements where the VOR is inadequate (Simpson 1984).

The neural pathways subserving the optokinetic reflex and its interaction with the VOR are not fully understood, but they are thought to involve the accessory optic system (AOS). In the cat and rabbit, the AOS consists of three terminal nuclei (lateral, medial and dorsal; LTN, MTN, DTN) distributed along the mesencephalic brainstem (Hayhow 1966) and the nucleus of the optic tract (NOT) located in the pretectum (Collewijn 1975). AOS nuclei all receive direct retinal inputs from the contralateral eye as well as projections from

the ipsilateral visual cortex (Berson and Graybiel 1980; Marcotte and Updyke 1982). Each AOS nucleus contains neurons that encode a particular direction of visual movement. In the cat (Hoffmann 1981; Grasse and Cynader 1982, 1984), the preferred directions appear to be predominantly horizontal (DTN and NOT) or vertical (LTN and MTN). In the rabbit (Collewijn 1975; Simpson et al. 1979), the preferred directions appear to be aligned with the planes of the semicircular canals, presumably to facilitate visuo-vestibular interactions. This interaction could be subserved by AOS connections with the dorsal cap of the inferior olive, which sends visual climbing fiber activity to the cerebellar flocculus (Maekawa and Simpson 1973). The flocculus in turn projects to the vestibular nuclei.

A similar circuitry seems to exist in the monkey. Although there is some debate as to the existence of the MTN, both the LTN and DTN do exist and, along with the NOT, receive direct retinal input (Itaya and van Hoesen 1983; Weber 1985; Weber and Giolli 1986). Also, our preliminary data (see below) indicate that the LTN and NOT project to the dorsal cap. As in the cat and rabbit, the dorsal cap projects to the flocculus (Langer et al. 1985) which in turn projects to the vestibular nucleus (Brodal 1978; Langer et al. 1985). That the monkey flocculus is necessary for a normal VOR and optokinetic response has been shown by lesion studies (Zee et al. 1981).

Although the anatomical organization of the monkey AOS has received some attention, relatively little is known about the signals it carries. Recently, it has been shown that single NOT units (Hoffmann 1985; Mustari et al. 1985) encode the direction of visual movement and that electrical stimulation of the primate NOT elicits a horizontal optokinetic nystagmus (OKN) with most of the classic features present in visually induced OKN (Schiff and Cohen, 1986). Nothing, however, is known about the behavior of the various terminal nuclei. To rectify this situation, we recorded the activity of single LTN units in the alert primate. A preliminary report of these data has been presented (Mustari et al. 1985).

Methods

Single unit activity was recorded from the LTN of four juvenile rhesus monkeys *(Macaca mulatta)* trained to make eye movements in a variety of visual environments. The aseptic surgical procedures, performed under deep anesthesia, have been described in detail elsewhere (Fuchs and Luschei 1970). Briefly, a scleral search coil for measuring eye movements was placed under the insertions of the four rectus muscles (Fuchs and Robinson 1966). A stainless steel recording chamber was stereotaxically implanted on the skull and three dental acrylic lugs were attached to the skull to hold the head. During behavioral training and subsequent single unit recording sessions, the monkeys sat facing a tangent screen with their heads stabilized. Each monkey was trained to fixate a stationary target spot and to track a jumping or smoothly moving target spot over a patterned background or in the dark. The targets moved in various directions and velocities (0 – 60 degrees/sec) with either sinusoidal or ramp trajectories.

Visual receptive fields were plotted while the monkey fixated a small (0.25 deg) stationary target spot. Two separate x/y mirror galvanometer systems (General Scanning) allowed independent control of the target spot and visual test stimuli by either a waveform generator (Wavetech) or a computer (PDP 11-73). The visual test stimuli were either a textured full field (70 × 50 deg) or small spot (1 – 5 degree diameter). Both galvanometer systems were equipped with electronic shutters.

Single units were recorded extracellularly with tungsten microelectrodes using conventional methods (Fuchs and Luschei 1970). Target and eye position signals, unit discharge and other relevant signals were saved on analog tape (Honeywell 5600) for subsequent computer (PDP 11-73) digitization and quantitative data analysis.

Electrolytic lesions were placed on electrode tracks where responsive units were encountered. At the conclusion of the experimental series, each animal was given a lethal dose of barbiturate and perfused with saline followed by 10% formalin. Frozen sections were cut every 40 μm, mounted on microscope slides, and stained for histological reconstruction of electrode tracks and cell locations.

Results

All of the units ($n = 67$) described in this study were confirmed histologically to be located in the LTN. Figure 1 shows a photomicrograph of a histological section containing marking lesions. Two lesions were placed on one track (solid arrows) above (1 and 2 mm) the location where units that discharged with background movement were encountered. One lesion (open arrow) was placed on another track at the exact depth of responding units.

Unit classification

Units were classified according to their response during visual stimulation, saccades and smooth pursuit of a small target spot against a patterned background or in the dark (hereafter called smooth pursuit in the dark). Almost 70% of the units responded during smooth pursuit in the dark and during background movement while the monkey fixated a stationary spot; such units were preliminarily classified as tracking and visual. To determine whether their response during smooth pursuit might reflect a visual response due to imperfect tracking, the spot was extinguished for a brief time during which the monkey was able to continue his smooth movement. For 15 tracking and visual units so tested, 11 continued their enhanced discharge during the blank and therefore had a sensitivity to eye movement per se; therefore, they were classified as eye movement and visual units. For the remaining four, the unit discharge fell to its resting rate during the target blank, indicating that the enhanced discharge had a visual

origin; therefore, they were classified as visual tracking units. Of the remaining 30% of the units, 12% discharged during smooth pursuit but had no evidence of visual sensitivity and were classified as eye movement, whereas 19% did not discharge during smooth pursuit but did have visual sensitivity and were classified as visual.

The response of a typical tracking and visual unit during three test conditions is shown in Fig. 2. With the animal fixating a stationary target spot (Fig. 2A, V_E) full field visual background movement (V_B) produced a brisk increase in unit firing rate for upward movement. During smooth pursuit in the dark, the same unit showed a weak and

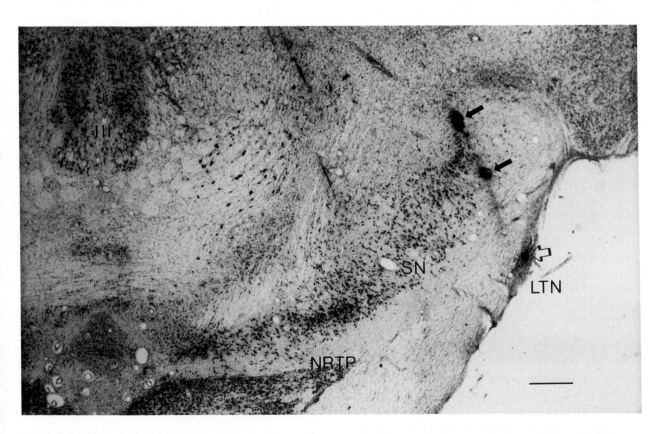

Fig. 1. Photomicrograph of a Nissl-stained section, cut in the stereotaxic plane. Two electrode tracks are shown with marking lesions placed either above (solid arrows) or at the location (i.e., in the LTN, open arrow) of units that responded to vertical background movement. Abbreviations: LTN, lateral terminal nucleus; SN, substantia nigra; NRTP, nucleus reticularis tegmenti pontis; III, oculomotor nucleus. Stereotaxic level is equivalent to A6 of the *Stereotaxic Atlas of the Monkey Brain* by Snider and Lee (1961). Scale bar = 1 mm.

124

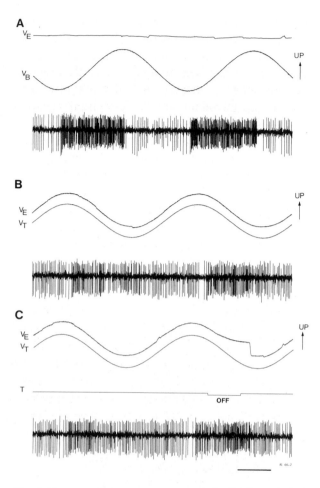

Fig. 2. Response of an eye movement and visual unit to vertical background movement (A), during smooth pursuit in the dark (B) and during smooth pursuit with the target spot turned off briefly (C). Vertical eye, target and background (V_E, V_T and V_B, respectively). Target spot (T) is turned off during smooth pursuit in (C) for 500 msec. Sinusoidal movement is ± 10 degrees for all conditions; scale bar = 500 msec.

variable response during downward smooth pursuit (Fig. 2B). The weak downward smooth pursuit response persisted during the target blank (Fig. 2C, OFF) placing this unit in the eye movement and visual category.

The visual receptive field of this unit was mapped with a small (1 deg diameter) test spot and found to be 10×10 degrees and centered on the fovea. Visual receptive fields were plotted with a one to five degree spot for 12 additional units and found

to range in size from 5×5 to 70×50 degrees (i.e., the entire tangent screen). Of the 5 units tested, all were binocular.

LTN units are often dominated by their visual inputs. Figure 3 illustrates this domination by plotting the sensitivity of units to visual background movement against their sensitivity during smooth pursuit in the dark. The sensitivity (spikes/sec in the preferred direction minus spikes/sec in the non-preferred direction) of each unit was calculated from firing rates averaged from at least 10 cycles in each condition. The majority of units lie above the line of equal sensitivity and therefore are visually dominated.

The response characteristics of a visual unit are shown in Fig. 4. Like the unit in Fig. 2, this unit also exhibits a robust response to upward background movement (Fig. 4A) but unlike the unit in Fig. 2, it exhibits no change in firing during smooth pursuit in the dark (Fig. 4B). About half of the units had no modulation during smooth pursuit in the dark. However, all visual units were modulated during smooth pursuit over a textured visual background.

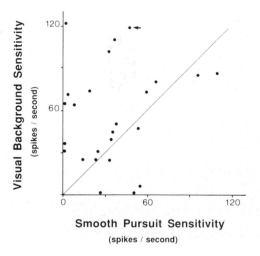

Fig. 3. Relative sensitivity of tracking and visual units during background movement and during smooth pursuit in the dark. Sensitivity was defined as firing rate in the preferred minus firing rate in the non-preferred direction. Arrow, data point from the unit illustrated in Fig. 2.

Like the unit in Fig. 2, the response for this unit during background movement is characterized by a rapid rise to peak firing rate as the visual background (V_B) changes direction. This abrupt change of unit firing at the change in stimulus direction was typical for all units and can be seen very clearly in the instantaneous firing rate histogram (FR) of Fig. 4. The firing rate for this and other units typically stays constant or actually decreases as the background goes from 0 through

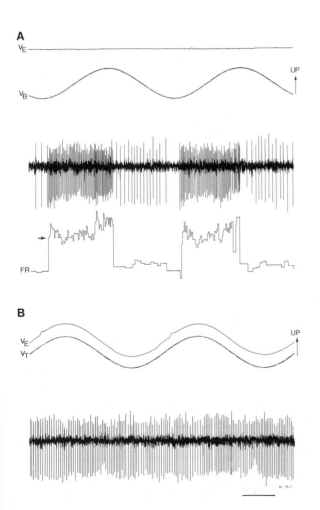

Fig. 4. Response of a visual unit during vertical background movement (A) and smooth pursuit in the dark (B). Note that the unit is not modulated during smooth pursuit in the dark. The arrow on the instantaneous firing rate (FR) trace corresponds to 50 spikes/sec. Other conventions are as in Fig. 2.

30 deg/sec and back to 0, suggesting that they are most sensitive to the direction and not the velocity of background movement.

Direction selectivity

The majority (98%) of LTN units that responded to movement of the full field visual stimulus preferred movement with a vertical component. The preferred direction of units was determined by moving the background horizontally, vertically and obliquely (± 45 degrees from horizontal) while the monkey fixated a stationary target spot. The best direction was determined aurally for 32 (Fig. 5C, open arrows) of 37 units. As can be seen in Fig. 5C the majority of these units preferred vertical background movement. In 5 units, complete tuning curves were obtained by recording activity during all 8 directions of movement and fitting curves (e.g. Fig. 5A,B) to averaged firing rates using a FFT algorithm (Wallman and Valez 1985). This procedure calculates a preferred direction which was often one not actually tested (Fig. 5A and B, solid arrows). Nevertheless, for these units, the preferred direction determined by ear was very close to that determined quantitatively. LTN units typically had rather broad directional tuning curves (e.g. Fig. 5A,B).

Visual velocity sensitivity

The lack of velocity sensitivity in LTN units is documented in Fig. 6, where peak firing rate is plotted against the peak stimulus velocity ($3-60$ deg/sec) of a sinusoidally moving background. The velocity data for the unit illustrated in Fig. 4 are indicated by an asterisk. Most units show no relation between firing rate and visual background velocity.

Anatomical connections of the LTN

To place the LTN within the circuitry believed to be involved in eye movement control, we have begun studies of its afferent and efferent connec-

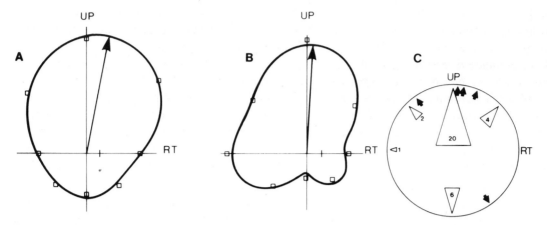

Fig. 5. Directional tuning curves for full field background movement during fixation for two different units (A and B) and directional preferences for all tested units as described in the text (C). The solid arrows are the computed preferred direction of each unit. The number inside each arrow (C) represents different individual units with approximately the same direction preference (see text). Direction of background movement is indicated (Up and Right, RT). Tic mark = 10 spikes/sec.

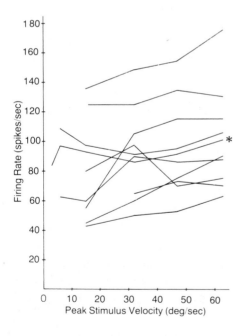

Fig. 6. The firing rate of units with visual sensitivity is plotted against the peak stimulus velocity. Animals fixated a stationary target spot while the full field background was moved sinusoidally (±10 deg) at frequencies ranging from 0.1 to 1.0 Hz. The asterisk marks the velocity sensitivity data for the unit illustrated in Fig. 4.

tions. The pattern of retinal termination in the LTN was determined by monocular intraocular injection of tritiated amino acids in two animals. One animal had a 1-day and the other a 5-day post-injection survival time. In both animals the autoradiographic label was confined to the LTN contralateral to the injected eye. Label was not above background in the LTN ipsilateral to the injected eye or in the neuropil surrounding either LTN. Autoradiographic label was also found over the pretectum bilaterally.

In two additional animals we placed medullary brainstem horseradish peroxidase (HRP) injections which included the dorsal cap of the inferior olive. In both cases, cells in the LTN ipsilateral to the HRP injection were retrogradely labelled (TMB-reacted). Even though one of these injections appeared to be rather large, not all of the neurons in the LTN were labelled, suggesting that the primate LTN projects to regions other than the dorsal cap.

Discussion

The direction selectivity of monkey LTN units is their most conspicuous property. LTN units start to discharge immediately after stimulus turn-around (Figs. 2A, 4A) and continue discharging as long as the visual background moves in the preferred direction. Like that of lower mammals, the primate LTN encodes the vertical direction of full-field background motion. A majority (78%) of our LTN units preferred upward visual motion. A similar directional bias was found neither in the cat, where units preferring up or down movement were equally represented (Grasse and Cynader 1984) nor in rabbit, where units with down and posterior preferences predominated (Simpson et al. 1979).

Primate LTN units do not signal the velocity of the visual background. The firing rate envelope during sinusoidal background movement in the preferred direction tends to be flat-topped (Fig. 4A), even when the peak velocity of the sinusoidal movement was only 3 deg/sec. Therefore, monkey LTN units signal primarily the direction of visual motion and not its velocity. Consistent with this conclusion is the lack of a monotonic change in peak firing rate with peak eye velocity for most LTN units (Fig. 3). In contrast, both rabbit (Simpson et al. 1979) and cat (Grasse and Cynader 1984) LTN units do show a monotonic relationship between firing rate and background velocity over part of their velocity range.

The typical primate LTN unit responds to all velocities in the range tested (0 – 60 deg/sec) with no decrement at higher stimulus velocities. This lack of high velocity cut-off is like that obtained in the monkey NOT (Mustari et al. 1985; Hoffmann and Distler 1986), cat NOT (Hoffmann and Schoppmann 1981) and in the cat terminal nuclei (Grasse and Cynader 1982, 1984) where some units were tuned to 100 deg/sec. In contrast, rabbit MTN units cease to respond to velocities greater than 6 deg/sec (Simpson et al. 1979).

In addition to responding to full-field visual motion, many of our LTN units discharged to movement of a small (0.25 – 1 deg diameter) spot. This ability to respond to small visual stimuli has also been reported in the primate NOT (Mustari et al. 1985; Hoffmann and Distler 1986). In contrast,

LTN units in the rabbit (Collewijn 1975; Simpson et al. 1979) and cat (Hoffmann and Schoppmann 1981; Grasse and Cynader 1984) require large field stimuli.

Twelve percent of the units in the LTN responded during smooth pursuit in the dark but evinced no visual sensitivity. This is the first demonstration of AOS units with activity related specifically to voluntary eye movements. Eleven of 15 tracking and visual units also continued their increased discharge when the target spot was turned off during smooth pursuit in the dark, suggesting that they too had an eye movement sensitivity. Such eye movement modulation presumably reflects the existence of non-retinal afferents to the LTN and suggests that the LTN is more than a simple visual nucleus.

Acknowledgements

This study was supported by grants EY0075, EY0609, and RR00166.

References

Berson, D.M. and Graybiel, A.M. (1980) Some cortical and subcortical fiber projections to the accessory optic nuclei in the cat. *Neuroscience*, 5: 2203 – 2217.

Cohen, B., Matsuo, V. and Raphan, T. (1977) Quantitative analysis of the velocity characteristics of optokinetic nystagmus and optokinetic after-nystagmus. *J. Physiol.*, 270: 321 – 344.

Collewijn, H. (1975) Direction-selective units in the rabbit's nucleus of the optic tract. *Brain Res.*, 100: 489 – 508.

Fuchs, A.F. and Luschei, E.S. (1970) Firing patterns of abducens neurons of alert monkeys in relationship to horizontal eye movement. *J. Neurophysiol.*, 33: 382 – 392.

Fuchs, A.F. and Robinson, D.A. (1966) A method for measuring horizontal and vertical eye movement chronically in the monkey. *J. Appl. Physiol.*, 21: 1068 – 1070.

Giolli, R.A., Blanks, R.H.I. and Torigoe, Y. (1984) Pretectal and brain stem projections of the medial terminal nucleus of the accessory optic system of the rabbit and rat as studied by anterograde and retrograde neuronal tracing methods. *J. Comp. Neurol.*, 227: 228 – 251.

Grasse, K.L. and Cynader, M.S. (1982) Electrophysiology of the medial terminal nucleus of the accessory optic system in the cat. *J. Neurophysiol.*, 48: 490 – 504.

Grasse, K.L. and Cynader, M.S. (1984) Electrophysiology of

128

the lateral and dorsal terminal nuclei of the cat accessory optic system *J. Neurophysiol.*, 51: 276 – 293.

Hoffmann, K.P. and Distler, C. (1986) The role of direction
selective cells in the nucleus of the optic tract of cat and
monkey during optokinetic nystagmus. In: Keller and Zee
(Eds.), *Adaptive Processes in Visual and Oculomotor
Systems, Advances in Bioscience*, Vol. 57 p. 261 – 266,
Pergamon Press, Oxford.

Hoffmann, K.P. and Schoppmann, A. (1981) A quantitative
analysis of the direction-specific response of neurons in the
cat's nucleus of the optic tract. *Exp. Brain Res.*, 51:
236 – 246.

Itaya, S.K. and van Hoesen, G.W. (1983) Retinal axons to the
medial terminal nucleus of the accessory optic system in Old
World monkeys. *Brain Res.*, 331: 150 – 154.

Langer, T.P., Fuchs, A.F., Scudder, C. and Chubb, M.C.
(1985) Efferents to the flocculus of the cerebellum in the
Rhesus Macaque as revealed by retrograde transport of
horseradish peroxidase. *J. Comp. Neurol.*, 235: 1 – 25.

Maekawa, K. and Simpson, J.I. (1973) Climbing fiber responses evoked in the vestibulo-cerebellum of the rabbit
from the visual system. *J. Neurophysiol.*, 36: 649 – 666.

Maekawa, K. and Takeda, T. (1979) Origin of descending afferents to the rostral part of the dorsal cap of inferior olive
which transfers contralateral optic activities to the flocculus:
a horseradish peroxidase study. *Brain Res.*, 77: 385 – 395.

Marcotte, R.R. and Updyke, B.V. (1982) Cortical visual areas

of the cat project differentially onto the nuclei of the accessory optic system. *Brain Res.*, 242: 205 – 217.

Mustari, M.J., Fuchs, A.F. and Wallman, J. (1985) Visual and
oculomotor response properties of single units in the pretectum of the behaving rhesus monkey. *Soc. Neurosci. Abstr.*,
11: 78.

Schiff, D., Cohen, B. and Raphan T. (1986) Stimulation of the
nucleus of the optic tract (NOT) induces nystagmus in the
monkey. *Developments in Oculomotor Research*, IUPS
XXX International Congress.

Simpson, J.I. (1984) The accessory optic system. *Annu. Rev.
Neurosci.*, 7: 13 – 41.

Simpson, J.I., Soodak, R.E. and Hess, R. (1979) The accessory
optic system and its relationship to the vestibulo-cerebellum.
In: R. Granit and O, Pompeiano (Eds.), *Reflex Control of
Posture and Movement, Progress in Brain Research, vol. 50*,
Elsevier, Amsterdam, pp. 715 – 724.

Snider and Lee (1961) *Stereotaxic Atlas of the Monkey Brain*,
University of Chicago Press, Chicago, IL.

Weber, J.T. (1985) Pretectal complex and accessory optic
system of primates. *Brain Behav. Evol.*, 26: 117 – 140.

Weber, J.T. and Giolli, R.A. (1986) The medial terminal
nucleus of the monkey: evidence for a complete accessory optic system. *Brain Res.*, 365: 164 – 168.

Zee, D.S., Yamazaki, A., Butler, P.H. and Gücer, G. (1981)
Effects of ablation of flocculus and paraflocculus on eye
movements in primate. *J. Neurophysiol.*, 46: 878 – 899.

T.P. Hicks and G. Benedek (Eds.)
Progress in Brain Research, Vol. 75
© 1988 Elsevier Science Publishers B.V. (Biomedical Division)

CHAPTER 12

Visual projections induced into auditory thalamus and cortex: implications for thalamic and cortical information processing

Mriganka Sur

Department of Brain and Cognitive Sciences, Massachusetts Institute of Technology, Cambridge, Massachusetts, U.S.A.

The issue

A central question in visual development and processing is: what is intrinsically 'visual' about visual thalamus and cortex? Does visual function derive from specific inputs (and outputs), or from intrinsic organization and specific microcircuitry in central visual structures independent of input and output? In other words, what makes visual thalamus or cortex 'visual?'

To answer these questions, we have followed up, in ferrets, observations made earlier in hamsters by Schneider (1973) and Frost (1981, 1986). When we ablate central retinal targets in newborn animals and create alternative terminal space for retinofugal fibers by deafferenting the auditory thalamus, the retina develops projections to the auditory thalamus (Sur and Garraghty 1986; Sur et al. 1988). The auditory thalamus retains its projections to auditory cortex. We can now ask how similar to normal visual thalamus (and cortex) is the auditory thalamus (and cortex) with visual inputs. Major differences in the structural organization of visual projections and functional properties of visual cells would argue that intrinsic properties

of central visual structures are crucial to determining their function. But essential similarities between visual and nonvisual thalamus (and cortex) would argue that a key property determining visual function is the appropriate input at least early in development.

There are many examples of redirecting connections in the mammalian brain following early or late surgical manipulations (Jacobson 1978; Lund 1978), but nearly all examples of a major rearrangement are in rodents. These include rerouting of retinal axons that normally terminate in the thalamus or midbrain to adjacent or contralateral and homotopic visual loci (Cunningham 1976; Lund and Lund 1976; Finlay et al. 1979; Thompson 1979). Importantly for our purpose, when normal axon targets in the visual or olfactory system are ablated in rodents, and alternative terminal space made available in other structures by partial deafferentation, ingrowing axons establish connections in these new structures (Schneider 1973; Devor 1975; Graziadei et al. 1979; Frost 1981). Ablation of a principal site of termination of retinal axons, the superior colliculus, in neonatal hamsters, combined with sectioning of the major input to either the medial geniculate nucleus, the principal auditory thalamic nucleus, or the ventrobasal nucleus, the principal somatosensory thalamic nucleus, leads to aberrant, ectopic,

Correspondence to: Mriganka Sur, Ph.D., Department of Brain and Cognitive Sciences, M.I.T., E25-618, Cambridge, MA 02139, U.S.A.

retinal projections to the medial geniculate or the ventrobasal nucleus respectively (Schneider 1973; Kalil and Schneider 1975; Frost 1981, 1986). The ectopic projections to the ventrobasal nucleus in hamsters can show some retinotopic order (Frost 1981), exhibit synaptic organization characteristic of somatosensory inputs to the ventrobasal nucleus (Campbell and Frost 1985), and lead to visual responses from neurons that project to somatosensory cortex (Frost and Metin 1985).

Our interest is specifically in the functional consequences of visual projections to nonvisual structures, and their implications for normal and abnormal development. For the studies described here, we chose for a variety of reasons to use ferrets, which are carnivores with well developed visual pathways much like those of cats (Law and Stryker 1985; Zahs and Stryker 1985). Ferrets are born very early in development (after 41 days of gestation, compared to 63 days for cats). At birth, the ferret retina has invaded the thalamus but retinogeniculate fibers have not segregated into laminae (Linden et al. 1981; cf. Shatz 1983; Cucchiaro and Guillery 1984), and we reasoned that it would be relatively easy to promote plasticity in the retinothalamic projection by surgery at birth rather than complicated prenatal surgery. Finally, the stimulus features and response properties of cells in visual thalamus (Stryker and Zahs 1983) and visual cortex (Law and Stryker 1985) of ferrets are well developed and are very similar to those in cats, which have been studied extensively (Sherman and Spear 1982).

Experimental procedure and results

The experimental design to induce visual projections to the auditory system in ferrets is illustrated in Fig. 1. Retinal targets are reduced in newborn ferrets by ablating the superior colliculus and visual cortical areas 17 and 18 of one hemiphere; ablating visual cortex causes the lateral geniculate nucleus (LGN) in the ipsilateral hemisphere to atrophy severely by retrograde degeneration. Concurrently, alternative target space for ingrowing

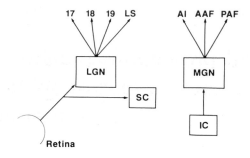

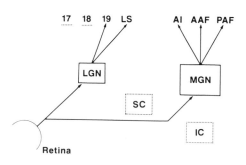

Fig. 1. The experimental design to induce visual projections to the auditory system in ferrets. Top: projections in normal animals. The retina projects to the lateral geniculate nucleus (LGN) and superior colliculus (SC). The LGN projects to cortical areas 17 (primary visual cortex) and 18 as well as to other extrastriate areas including area 19 and the lateral suprasylvian (LS) cortex. In the auditory system, the inferior colliculus (IC) projects to the medial geniculate nucleus (MGN). The ventral division and the deep dorsal division of the MGN project heavily to primary auditory cortex (AI), as well as to other cortical areas including the anterior auditory field (AAF) and the posterior auditory field (PAF) in cortex. Bottom: if cortical areas 17 and 18 are ablated in neonatal ferrets, the LGN atrophies severely by retrograde degeneration. Ablating the superior colliculus as well, and creating alternative terminal space in the medial geniculate nucleus by ablating the inferior colliculus or sectioning fibers ascending from it, causes the retina to project to the MGN and hence to auditory cortex. We have not been able to induce retinal projections into somatosensory thalamic nuclei in ferrets, as is possible in hamsters (Frost 1981). We have also been unable to induce retinal projections into either the auditory or somatosensory thalamus in cats by neonatal surgery, perhaps because by birth, in cats, retinal axons have already grown into their target visual structures. If temporal factors play a role in the retinofugal plasticity we describe, W cells, born last in the retina (Walsh et al. 1983), would be the most likely to innervate novel targets in ferrets. Reprinted from Sur et al. (1988).

retinal afferents is created in the medial geniculate nucleus (MGN) by ablating either the inferior colliculus or sectioning fibers ascending to the MGN in the brachium of the inferior colliculus (Schneider 1973). Operated animals are reared to adulthood for further anatomical and physiological experiments.

In these animals, the retina projects to normal thalamic targets, including the surviving, shrunken LGN, as well as aberrantly to the lateral posterior nucleus (LP) and to auditory thalamic nuclei (Fig. 2). The new retinal projections to the auditory thalamus include patches of label in the dorsal, medial and ventral divisions of the MGN along

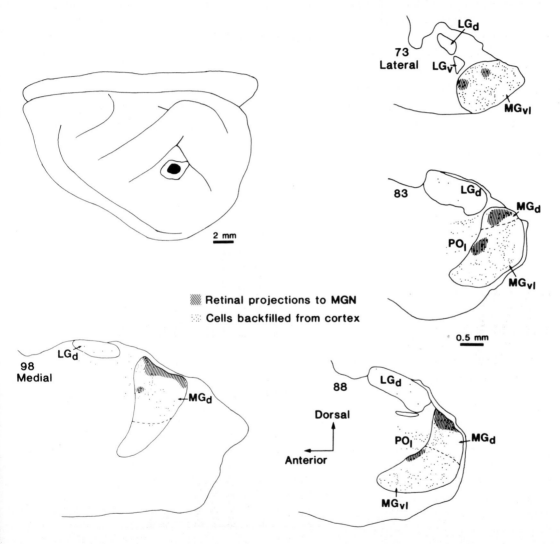

Fig. 2. Anatomy of retinal projections induced into the auditory system. Results from an experiment demonstrating experimentally induced retinal projections to the auditory thalamus, and the connections of auditory thalamus with auditory cortex. The eye contralateral to the experimentally altered hemisphere is seen here as projecting to patches or lamellae in the dorsal and ventral divisions of the MGN (MGd and MGvl, respectively). The figure shows numbered parasagittal sections of the thalamus. The retinal projections to the surviving dorsal LGN (LGd) and ventral LGN (LGv) are not shown. In the same animal, cells projecting from the thalamus to primary auditory cortex (shown at top left) lie in auditory thalamic nuclei MGvl, MGd, and the lateral division of the posterior complex (POl). Many cells in MGd and MGvl overlie the retinal projection zone. Reprinted from Sur et al. (1988).

132

sions of the MGN along with the lateral part of the posterior nuclear complex adjacent to the MGN, a region closely associated with the MGN in auditory inputs and cortical projections (Merzenich and Kaas 1980; Aitkin et al. 1984). The retinal projections to the MGN complex are sparse to moderate in intensity and the projections from one eye cover up to a third of the area of the MGN. We have confirmed that the MGN in operated animals projects normally to auditory cortex (Fig. 1), both by the (rather weak) transneuronal label in auditory cortex following intraocular injections of wheat germ agglutinin – horseradish peroxidase (WGA-HRP) or [^{35}S]methionine and by extensive retrograde labeling of cells in the MGN following

restricted injections of HRP into primary auditory cortex (Fig. 2).

In electrophysiological recordings from the auditory thalamus in operated animals, we have compared visual responses in the MGN with responses from the surviving LGN in the same animals as well as from the LGN in normal animals. We classify cells as receiving retinal W, X or Y cell input based on a battery of tests, including receptive field size, latency to optic chiasm stimulation and linearity of spatial summation (Enroth-Cugell and Robson 1966; Hochstein and Shapley 1976). In auditory thalamus or cortex, we first test cells for electrical activation through the stimulating electrodes placed at the optic chiasm,

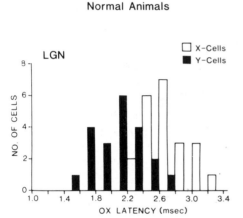

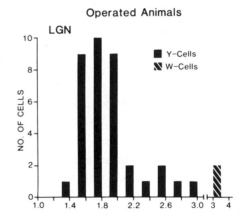

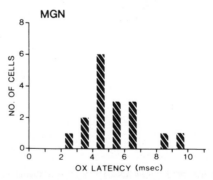

Fig. 3. Electrophysiological results from the thalamus of operated animals, and comparison with normal animals. In the LGN of normal animals, X and Y cells (and W cells) can be readily identified (top, left). In operated animals, the atrophied LGN contains only Y cells and W cells (top, right), while visual input to the MGN appears to arise from retinal W cells (bottom, right; note that the scale on the abscissa is compressed here). Visual cells in the MGN, like W cells in the normal or surviving LGN, respond rather poorly to visual stimulation, and have large receptive fields that are on-, off-, or on/off center and circular. Adapted from Sur et al. (1988).

then their visual responsiveness. We also test the auditory responses of cells in the auditory thalamus or cortex with click or tone stimuli delivered through earphones.

In the LGN of normal animals, we record briskly driven X and Y cells in the A laminae (Fig. 3) as well as Y and W cells in the C laminae (Esguerra et al. 1986). In the LGN of operated animals, we record almost exclusively Y cells in the A laminae and Y and W cells in the C laminae. We ascribe the loss of X cells in the A laminae of operated animals to the retrograde degeneration of geniculate X cells following ablation of visual cortex, in particular area 17 (Humphrey et al. 1985). A similar result has been shown in cats after neonatal ablation of visual cortex (McCall et al. 1986); in cats, this also leads to transneuronal retrograde loss of X cells in the retina (Tong et al. 1982), and we have confirmed a reduction in medium sized retinal ganglion cells in ferrets with neonatal ablation of visual cortex (Sur et al. 1988).

In the MGN of operated animals, we record only cells with long latencies to optic chiasm stimulation (mean latency, 5.5 msec; Fig. 3). The visual responses of these cells are weak and 'sluggish' (Sur and Sherman 1982). Cells respond best to large, flashing or moving spots of light, with responses that are often quite variable from trial to trial. Receptive fields, for cells for which fields can be ascertained, are large, with diameters 4–5 times the diameters of X and Y cell receptive fields at similar eccentricities. Receptive fields are on-, off-, or on/off-center and concentric. Visually driven cells are not obviously orientation or direction selective.

In primary auditory cortex of operated animals, visual cells again have long latencies to optic chiasm stimulation, with a mean latency of 9.5 msec. The separation of latencies between cells in primary auditory cortex and the MGN (Fig. 3) is consistent with the notion that most of the cortical cells receive visual input through the ipsilateral MGN. Latencies to optic chiasm stimulation in area 17 of normal animals, which is dominated by the X and Y pathways through the LGN, are much shorter (mean latency 4.2 msec). Visual cells in auditory cortex have large receptive fields, and prefer slowly flashing or moving large spots or bars (Table 1). Receptive fields, when they can be ascertained, are in the contralateral hemifield, indicating that the cortical visual responses arise from input through the ipsilateral, operated hemisphere and not through the intact hemisphere via the corpus callosum. Of our sample so far, about 25% of the cells that we could drive visually (10 of 38) have been direction selective. About 20% of cells have shown evidence of orientation selectivity (Table 1); we qualitatively judge the orientation tuning of these cells to be broader than that of oriented cells in normal area 17. All the oriented cells responded to light onset and offset, or to moving light and dark bars, and we have classified them as complex (Hubel and Wiesel 1962).

We have not been able to reliably drive neurons either in the MGN or in primary auditory cortex of the operated hemisphere with acoustic stimuli. This is consistent with the fact that we deafferentated the auditory thalamus in the operated hemisphere. As a control for our results on visual responses from auditory structures in operated animals, we have not been able to elicit responses from cells in the MGN or primary auditory cortex in normal animals to either electrical stimulation of the optic tract or visual field stimulation.

W cell input to auditory thalamus and cortex

These results demonstrate that, as in hamsters, retinal projections can be induced into nonvisual

TABLE 1

Visual cells in auditory cortex

Driven electrically from optic chiasm	57
Driven visually	38
Oriented receptive fields	6
Non-oriented receptive fields	23
Full field flashes	9

134

thalamus in ferrets, and these projections can impart visual function (viz. visual driving and discernible receptive field properties) to cells in nonvisual thalamus and cortex. How comparable to 'normal' are the visual responses in the auditory pathway? Many of the response features of cells in the MGN are similar to those of cells in the C-laminae of the LGN (Sur and Sherman 1982) or in the superficial layers of the superior colliculus (Hoffman 1973; Sherk 1979) that receive input from retinal W cells (Stanford 1987). While we cannot rule out input from other cell classes in abnormal synaptic configurations (Campbell and Frost 1985), the electrophysiological results suggest that retinal W cells provide the sole or major input to the MGN in operated animals. Experiments involving retrograde labeling of retinal ganglion cells following HRP injections in the thalamus (Roe et al. 1987) support this suggestion: while retinal input to the thalamus in normal animals arises from small ($<$ 200 μm^2) medium (200 – 350 μm^2) and large ($>$ 350 μm^2) retinal ganglion cells, the aberrant projection to the MGN arises only from the small ganglion cells.

It is more difficult to compare the visual responses from auditory cortex, since a pure W cell thalamocortical pathway is difficult to demonstrate in normal animals (Sherman and Spear 1982). Still, it is clear that many visual cells in auditory cortex do show integrative properties characteristic of cells in visual cortex (Hubel and Wiesel 1962; Sherman and Spear 1982).

Implications for the organization of sensory thalamus and cortex

Our results, while still mostly qualitative, suggest a transformation of visual response properties in the auditory pathway of operated ferrets that is similar to the transformation that occurs along the visual pathway of normal ferrets and cats. That is, the thalamus appears to relay receptive field properties that are generated in the retina, and new properties are generated in at least some cells in the cortex.

How does the auditory cortex carry out this transformation? One possibility is that visual inputs direct the development of intrinsic connectivity in auditory cortex, which then comes to resemble that in visual cortex. A second possibility, not entirely separable from the first, is that the intrinsic connectivity of auditory cortex is similar in certain, perhaps essential, aspects to that in visual cortex. Intracortical information flow paths in primary visual cortex (Gilbert and Wiesel 1979; Ferster and Lindstrom 1983) and primary auditory cortex (Mitani et al. 1985) deduced from intracellular physiology and anatomy do indeed share remarkable similarities. On this view, one function of sensory cortex would be to perform stereotypical transformations of input akin to the 'direction', 'orientation' or 'complex' transformations done by visual cortex. (See, for example, Whitfield and Evans (1965) for 'directionality' in auditory cortical units in frequency space, and Hyvärinen and Poranen (1978) for direction and orientation selective units in somatosensory cortex.)

Finally, our experiments implicate possible similarities in axon guidance cues across thalamic nuclei, but raise new questions about how target recognition occurs during normal retinothalamic development (that is, why do retinal W axons not normally innervate the MGN?). Perhaps the earliest retinofugal fibers, the X axons (Walsh et al. 1983), recognize specific cues in the LGN (Sur et al. 1987) and later axons, particularly the W axons which are among the last to grow out of the retina (Walsh et al. 1983), follow the earlier fibers. If retinal X axons are removed early enough in development, as with a neonatal ablation of visual cortex in ferrets, the late developing W fibers can seek out 'new' targets.

Acknowledgements

I thank Preston Garraghty and Anna Roe for their contributions to this study, and Martha MacAvoy and Theresa Sullivan for excellent technical assistance. Supported by NIH grant EY 07023,

BRSG RR07047, March of Dimes grant 1-1083 and the Whitaker Fund.

References

Aitkin, L.M., Irvine, D.R.F. and Webster, W.R. (1984) Central neural mechanisms of hearing. In: *Handbook of Physiology: The Nervous System III*, Amer. Physiol. Soc. Bethesda, MD, pp. 675 – 737.

Campbell, G. and Frost, D.O. (1985) Synaptic organization of anomalous retinal terminations within somatosensory thalamus after neonatal brain lesions in hamsters. *Soc. Neurosci. Abstr.*, 11: 977.

Cucchiaro, J. and Guillery, R.W. (1984) The development of the retinogeniculate pathways in normal and albino ferrets. *Proc. R. Soc. Lond. B*, 223: 141 – 164.

Cunningham, T.J. (1976) Early eye removal produces extensive bilateral branching in the rat. *Science*, 194: 857 – 859.

Devor, M. (1975) Neuroplasticity in the sparing or deterioration of function after early olfactory tract lesions. *Science*, 190: 998 – 1000.

Enroth-Cugell, C. and Robson, J.G. (1966) The contrast sensitivity of retinal ganglion cells of the cat. *J. Physiol. (Lond.)*, 187: 516 – 552.

Esguerra, M., Garraghty, P.E., Russo, G.S. and Sur, M. (1986) Lateral geniculate nucleus in normal and monocularly sutured ferrets: X- and Y-cells and cell body size. *Soc. Neurosci. Abstr.*, 12: 10.

Ferster, D. and Lindstrom, S. (1983) An intracellular analysis of geniculocortical connectivity in area 17 of the cat. *J. Physiol. (Lond.)*, 342: 181 – 215.

Finlay, B.L., Wilson, K.G. and Schneider, G.E. (1979) Anomalous ipsilateral retinotectal projections in Syrian hamsters with early lesions: topography and functional capacity. *J. Comp. Neurol.*, 183: 721 – 740.

Frost, D.O. (1981) Ordered anomalous retinal projections to the medial geniculate, ventrobasal and lateral posterior nuclei. *J. Comp. Neurol.*, 203: 227 – 256.

Frost, D.O. (1986) Development of anomalous retinal projections to nonvisual thalamic nuclei in Syrian hamsters: a quantitative study. *J. Comp. Neurol.*, 252: 95 – 105.

Frost, D.O. and Metin, C. (1985) Induction of functional retinal projections to the somatosensory system. *Nature*, 317: 162 – 164.

Gilbert, C.D. and Wiesel, T.N. (1979) Morphology and intracortical projections of functionally characterized neurones in cat visual cortex. *Nature*, 3: 120 – 125.

Graziadei, P.P.C., Levine, R.R. and Monti-Graziadei, G.A. (1979) Plasticity of connections of the olfactory sensory neuron: regeneration into the forebrain following bulbectomy in the neonatal mouse. *Neuroscience*, 4: 713 – 727.

Hochstein, S. and Shapley, R. (1976) Quantitative analysis of retinal ganglion cell classifications. *J. Physiol. (Lond.)*, 262: 237 – 264.

Hoffmann, K.P. (1973) Conduction velocity in pathways from retina to superior colliculus in the cat: a correlation with receptive field properties. *J. Neurophysiol.*, 36: 409 – 424.

Humphrey, A.L., Sur, M., Uhlrich, D.J. and Sherman, S.M. (1985) Projection patterns of individual X- and Y-cell axons from the lateral geniculate nucleus to cortical area 17 in the cat. *J. Comp. Neurol.*, 233: 159 – 189.

Hubel, D.H. and Wiesel, T.N. (1962) Receptive fields, binocular interaction and functional architecture in the cat's visual cortex. *J. Physiol. (Lond.)*, 160: 106 – 154.

Hyvärinen, J. and Poranen, A. (1978) Movement-sensitive and direction and orientation-sensitive receptive fields in the hand area of the postcentral gyrus in monkeys. *J. Physiol. (Lond.)*, 283: 523 – 537.

Jacobson, M. (1978) *Developmental Neurobiology*, 2nd edn., Plenum, New York.

Kalil, R.E. and Schneider, G.E. (1975) Abnormal synaptic connections of the optic tract in the thalamus after midbrain lesions in newborn hamsters. *Brain Res.*, 100: 690 – 698.

Law, M.I. and Stryker, M.P. (1985) The projection of the visual world onto area 17 of the ferret. *Invest. Ophthalmol. Vis. Sci.*, Suppl., 24: 227.

Linden, D.C., Guillery, R.W. and Cucchiaro, J. (1981) The dorsal lateral geniculate nucleus of the normal ferret and its postnatal development. *J. Comp. Neurol.*, 203: 189 – 211.

Lund, R.D. (1978) *Development and Plasticity of the Brain*, Oxford University Press, New York.

Lund, R.D. and Lund, J.S. (1976) Plasticity in the developing visual system: the effects of retinal lesions made in young rats. *J. Comp. Neurol.*, 169: 133 – 154.

McCall, M.A., Tumosa, N., Guido, W. and Spear, P.D. (1986) Responses of residual neurons in the lateral geniculate nucleus after long-term visual cortex damage in kittens and adult cats. *Soc. Neurosci. Abstr.*, 12: 591.

Merzenich, M.M. and Kaas, J.H. (1980) Principles of organization of sensory-perceptual systems in mammals. *Prog. Psychobiol. Physiol. Psychol.*, 9: 1 – 42.

Mitani, A., Shimokouchi, M., Itoh, K., Nomura, S., Kudo, M. and Mizuno, N. (1985) Morphology and laminar organization of electrophysiologically identified neurons in the primary auditory cortex in the cat. *J. Comp. Neurol.*, 235: 430 – 447.

Roe, A.W., Garraghty, P.E. and Sur, M. (1987) Retinotectal W cell plasticity: experimentally induced retinal projections to auditory thalamus in ferrets. *Soc. Neurosci. Abstr.*, 13: 1023.

Schneider, G.E. (1973) Early lesions of the superior colliculus: factors affecting the formation of abnormal retinal projections. *Brain Behav. Evól.*, 8: 73 – 109.

Shatz, C.J. (1983) The prenatal development of the cat's retinogeniculate pathway. *J. Neurosci.*, 3: 482 – 499.

Sherk, H. (1979) A comparison of visual-response properties in cat's parabigeminal nucleus and superior colliculus. *J. Neurophysiol.*, 42: 1640 – 1655.

Sherman, S.M. and Spear, P.D. (1982) Organization of visual pathways in normal and visually deprived cats. *Physiol. Rev.*, 62: 738 – 855.

Stanford, L.R. (1987) W-cells in the cat retina: correlated morphological and physiological evidence for two distinct classes. *J. Neurophysiol.*, 57: 218 – 244.

Stryker, M.P. and Zahs, K.R. (1983) ON and OFF sublaminae in the lateral geniculate nucleus of the ferret. *J. Neurosci.*, 3: 1943 – 1951.

Sur, M. and Garraghty, P.E. (1986) Experimentally induced visual responses from auditory thalamus and cortex. *Soc. Neurosci. Abstr.*, 12: 592.

Sur, M., Garraghty, P.E. and Roe, A.W. (1988) Experimentally induced visual projections into auditory thalamus and cortex, submitted for publication.

Sur, M., Roe, A.W. and Garraghty, P.E. (1987) Evidence for early specificity of the retinogeniculate X cell pathway. *Soc.*

Neurosci. Abstr., 13: in press.

Sur, M. and Sherman, S.M. (1982) Linear and nonlinear W cells in C-laminae of the cat's lateral geniculate nucleus. *J. Neurophysiol.*, 47: 869 – 884.

Thompson, I.D. (1979) Changes in the uncrossed retinotectal projection after removal of the other eye at birth. *Nature*, 279: 63 – 66.

Tong, L., Spear, P.D., Kalil, R.E. and Callahan, E.C. (1982) Loss of retinal X-cells in cats with neonatal or adult visual cortex damage. *Science*, 217: 72 – 75.

Walsh, C., Polley, E.H., Hickey, T.L. and Guillery, R.G. (1983) Generation of cat retinal ganglion cells in relation to central pathways. *Nature*, 302: 611 – 614.

Whitfield, I.C. and Evans, E.F. (1965) Responses of auditory cortical neurons to stimuli of changing frequency. *J. Neurophysiol.*, 28: 655 – 672.

Zahs, K.R. and Stryker, M.P. (1985) The projection of the visual field onto the lateral geniculate nucleus of the ferret. *J. Comp. Neurol.*, 241: 189 – 211.

T.P. Hicks and G. Benedek (Eds.)
Progress in Brain Research, Vol. 75
© 1988 Elsevier Science Publishers B.V. (Biomedical Division)

CHAPTER 13

Influence of moving textured backgrounds on responses of cat area 18 cells to moving bars

G.A. Orban, B. Gulyás and W. Spileers

Laboratory for Neuro- and Psychophysiology, Faculty of Medicine, University of Leuven, Herestraat, B-3000 Leuven, Belgium

Introduction

Most neurophysiological studies on mechanisms involved in motion analysis have used a single stimulus such as a moving bar, grating or random dot pattern. The visual world in which humans, monkeys, and cats live is far more complex than these simple stimuli. If the visual system of these species is designed to analyse the complex environment in which they live, it is likely that earlier studies missed much of the processing capacities of the visual system. In order to fill this void we have embarked upon a systematic study of responses of early visual processing levels in cat and monkey brains to complex moving stimuli. The first series of these studies looked at the modulation of responses to a moving bar by a moving textured background. Such a background motion strongly influenced area 17 and geniculate cells in the cat (Gulyás et al. 1987a; Orban et al. 1987a). The response of both geniculate and striate neurons was strongly suppressed by motion of the textured background (Gulyás et al. 1987a). In addition, the direction selectivity of striate neurons was strongly modulated by background motion giving rise to six different relative direction selectivity types. All geniculate cells were non-direction selective and remained so in all conditions, independently of background motion (Orban et al. 1987a, b). Extension of these studies to V1 and V2 of the monkey revealed that the suppressive influence of the

background motion was much weaker in the monkey than in the cat. While the direction selectivity of only one quarter of the cells was modulated in V1, about one half was modulated in V2 of the monkey (Gulyás et al. 1987b; Orban et al. 1987b).

In the present report we extend the study to area 18 of the cat. Area 18 of the cat is considered to be a second primary area (Tretter et al. 1975; Orban 1984), and has been implicated in the analysis of moving objects (Orban et al. 1981a, b). Comparison of the interactions in areas 17 and 18 should reveal further differences between these areas and could therefore further test the hypothesis that area 17 is involved in the analysis of stationary objects and area 18 in the analysis of moving objects (Orban et al. 1981a, b).

Preliminary testing

The methods used for this study are exactly the same as those used by Gulyás et al. (1987a) and Orban et al. (1987a). Cats were anaesthetized (70%/30% N_2O/O_2, and Nembutal 1 mg/kg/h) and paralyzed (Flaxedil and (+)-tubocurarine). Visual cortical cells were recorded with glass-coated tungsten electrodes. Only cells positively identified in histological sections as belonging to area 18 are included in this report. All cells had receptive fields within 10° from the fixation point. After the initial handplotting to localise the receptive field in both eyes and to determine the optimal length and orientation of the moving bar, cortical cells were tested with a light and dark bar velocity multihistogram (contrast: log $\Delta I/I = -0.09$, background illumination: 4.9 cd/m², speeds ranging from 0.5 to 512 deg/sec). This test provides quantitative information of RF structure, direction selectivity and velocity characteristics. This test was used to select the optimal speed and optimal contrast polarity. The results of this test confirmed our previous observations (Orban et al. 1981a, b) that area 18 contains more cells responsive to fast

speeds, more velocity tuned cells and more direction selective cells than area 17.

The second test performed on the cortical cells was a bar-contrast multihistogram, using the optimal speed and contrast polarity. The background was a stationary white noise pattern, kindly provided by P. Hammond. The noise pattern had pixels of 0.04° in size, a black-to-white ratio of 1, and the contrast within the pattern was 0.82. Two-dimensional Fourier analysis showed that its power distribution was flat with equal energy at all orien-

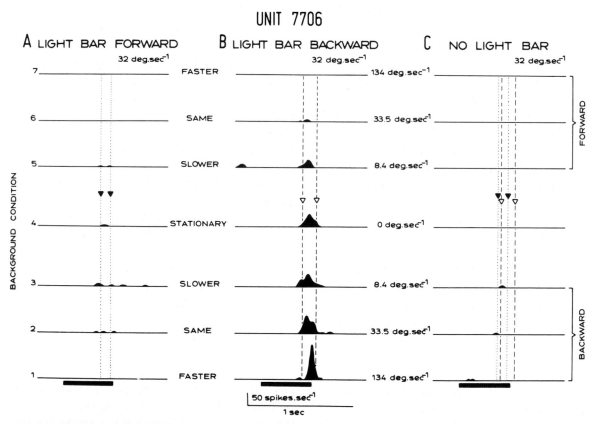

Fig. 1. Peristimulus time histograms (PSTHs) representing the average response ($n = 21$) of cell 7706 to the light bar moving forward over the background (A), to the light bar moving backward over the background (B), and to the background moving on its own (C). This velocity broad band A cell was recorded in layer 2–3 and had a RF at 5.7° from the fixation point. Each row of the PSTHs correponds to a background condition indicated by a number between 1 and 7. Conditions 1–3 correspond to background motions in the backward direction, condition 4 corresponds to a stationary background, and conditions 5–7 to the background moving forwards. In the conditions 2 and 6, the background moves at the same speed as the bar (33 deg/sec); in conditions 3 and 5 it moves slower than the bar (8.5 deg/sec); and in conditions 1 and 7 it moves faster than the bar (134 deg/sec). The solid and open arrows indicate the limits between which the response to the forward and backward motions of the bar are calculated. In order to obtain the net responses to the bar, in, for instance, condition A3, the average firing rate between the solid arrows in C3 is subtracted from the average firing rate between the same arrows in A3. The horizontal bars below the PSTHs indicate the movement period.

tations for spatial frequencies up to 2 cycles/degree. The contrast multihistogram was used to select for further testing the contrast that produced 50% of the maximum response.

The bar-background interaction multihistogram

The modulatory influence of the moving textured background on the bar response was tested in the bar-background interaction multihistogram. This multihistogram comprised 3 × 7 conditions which were presented in interleaved and random order. The bar either moved in one direction (forward), in the opposite direction (backward), or was absent (Fig. 1). The background was stationary, moved forward or backward. The background moved forward or backward at the same speed as the bar, 4 times slower or 4 times faster. For the cell in Fig. 1, the bar speed was 32 deg/sec, and the background speeds were 8.4 deg/sec, 33.5 deg/sec and 134 deg/sec, respectively. The conditions of these multihistograms were analyzed in blocks of seven conditions corresponding to a single direction of motion of the bar. The PSTH corresponding to the zero background speed, in which the bar moved on its own over the stationary background, served as reference for a block. The response to the moving bar was localized by a peak-detecting algorithm providing the limits of the response at 10% level of the maximum in the peak. These limits were then used to evaluate the response, in terms of average firing rate, for the 7 background conditions of the block corresponding to a single bar direction. Since the bar and the background moved together in the interaction series and we were interested only in the changes in the responses to the bar induced by the background motion, we had to subtract the responses to the moving background from the responses to the combined stimulation. Therefore we measured in the PSTH corresponding to the background moving on its own at the same speed and in the same direction as in the combined stimulation, the average firing rate between the same limits as used in the PSTH corresponding to

the combined stimulation, and subtracted this firing rate from the average firing rate measured in the PSTH corresponding to the combined stimulation. The net average firing rate obtained in this way represents the response to the bar provided that for the combined stimulation the responses to the bar and the background add linearly. Given the relative low contrast of both patterns this is a reasonable assumption, as was proven by the fact that the interactions were found to be similar whether or not the noise moving on its own elicited a response. The subtraction to obtain the net average firing rate removed the contribution of the spontaneous activity and therefore the significance level simply equals $2\sqrt{2}$ times the standard deviation of the spontaneous average firing rate evaluated from the different 250 msec epochs preceding the motion in the different stimulus conditions.

In order to evaluate the significance of the changes induced by the background motion, the six conditions in which the background moved in addition to the bar, were compared with the seventh condition (the reference condition) in which the background was stationary. Therefore a run-by-run analysis was performed to measure, per stimulus presentation of a given condition, the net number of spikes (the number for the combined stimulation minus the number for the noise alone) occurring between the limits of the response to the bar determined in the average histogram for that condition. The distribution of these numbers of spikes in the 6 conditions in which the background moved were then compared with the distribution of the number of spikes obtained in the reference condition in which the background was stationary. The comparison was done with a nonparametric Mann-Witney U test and the significance level was set at 5% (two-tailed).

The cell shown in Fig. 1 was a direction selective, velocity broad band, A cell (wide RF width, non-overlapping ON-OFF subregions), recorded in the superficial layers (2–3) of area 18. It clearly preferred the backward motion of the bar, and kept this preference when the background moved backward. Forward motion of the background, especially at 33 and 134 deg/sec, strongly suppressed the response to the preferred direction of the bar. This is a clear example in which the direction selectivity depended upon the background condition. The cell is direction selective only for a stationary background and for in-phase motion of the background. This relative direction selectivity was observed in none of the 118 area 17 cells tested and is exactly opposite to what we called conditional direction selectivity in our previous publication (Orban et al. 1987a). Therefore we now introduce the terms anti-phase and in-phase conditional direction selectivity, and the cell of Fig. 1 is a typical case of in-phase conditional direction selectivity.

The average interaction profiles: a measure of suppression

In order to represent the modification of the bar response by the background motion, the response to the bar in net average firing rate was plotted as a function of the background conditions for each direction of bar motion. This plot represents an interaction profile of a single cell for a given direction of motion. If the MDI* of the cell was larger than 33, the interaction profile of the preferred direction was considered representative of the cell; otherwise the mean of the profiles in both directions was taken as representative.

In order to represent the interaction in a group of neurons, an average interaction profile was constructed in the following way. The representative interaction profile of each cell was normalized with respect to the reference condition (zero background motion) and the median, and the first and third quartiles of these normalized profiles were calculated. Figure 2 compares the average interac-

tion profiles for areas 17 and 18. Since our area 18 sample only included cells with RFs within 10° of the area centralis, the area 17 sample was limited to the same range of eccentricities. In both areas, responses were suppressed by background motion, especially when the background moved at the same speed as, or faster than, the bar. In both areas the suppression was somewhat stronger when the background moved in-phase than when it moved anti-phase with the bar. However, in neither area was this tendency significant. Average interaction profiles of 2 groups of neurons were compared by testing for each background condition (except the reference condition) the difference between the distributions of normalized responses in both neuronal samples with a nonparametric Mann-Whitney U test. Comparison of the average profiles of areas 17 and 18 revealed no significant difference. Hence area 18 cell responses are equally strongly suppressed as those of area 17 cells. This

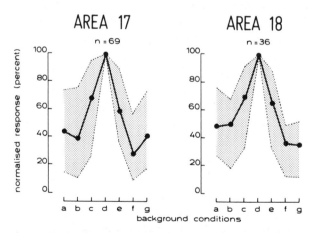

Fig. 2. Average interaction profiles of area 17 cells (left) and area 18 cells (right). The solid lines represent the medians, the dashed lines the quartiles. The background conditions are expressed in relative terms. In conditions a – c the background moves in anti-phase with the bar, in condition d the background is stationary; in conditions e – g the background moves in-phase with the bar. In conditions b and f background moves at the same speed as the bar, in conditions c and e it moves four times slower than the bar, and in conditions a and g the background's speed is four times faster than that of the bar. The numbers indicate the sample sizes.

---

* MDI is defined as the weighted average of the DIs obtained at different speeds where DI is $(1 - RNP/RP) \times 100$, with RP the response in the preferred direction and RNP the response in the nonpreferred direction.

is in keeping with our previous findings (Gulyás et al. 1987a) that the suppression is a very general phenomenon at the cortical level and probably reflects the suppression already present at the LGN level.

Relative direction selectivity types

In area 17 we described 6 relative direction selectivity types. Four types were direction selective when the background was stationary: absolutely, conditionally direction selective, differencing and limited direction selective cells. Two types were not direction selective when the background was stationary: anti-phase direction selective and relative non-direction-selective cells. No anti-phase direction selective cell was observed until now in area 18, and only a few area 18 cells were relative non-direction-selective (3/36), or differencing direction selective (1/36). Figure 3 shows typical examples of

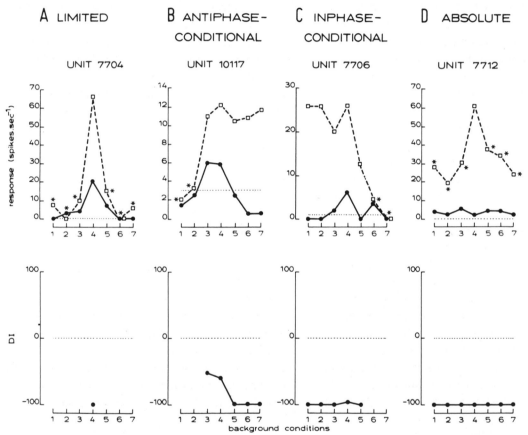

Fig. 3. Examples of limited direction selectivity (A), anti-phase conditional direction selectivity (B), in-phase conditional direction selectivity (C), and absolute direction selectivity (D). The net responses to the bar moving in the preferred direction (dashed lines) and in the non-preferred direction (solid lines) are plotted as a function of background conditions in the upper row; the corresponding direction indices are plotted as a function of background conditions in the lower row. In this figure, just as in Fig. 1, the background conditions are expressed in absolute terms. The asterisks in the upper row indicate the conditions for which responses to the preferred direction are significantly different from the control response (condition 4). The horizontal dashed lines indicate the significance levels. In the lower row, direction indices were calculated only when at least one of the responses exceeded 25% of the control response in condition 4. Unit 7704 was a velocity tuned S cell (narrow RF with non-overlapping ON and OFF subregions), recorded in layers 2 – 3, with an RF at 3.9° for the fixation point. Unit 10117 was a velocity tuned HS cell (endstopped, narrow RF with non-overlapping ON and OFF subregions), recorded in layers 2 – 3, with a RF at 3.4° from the fixation point. Unit 7706 is the same cell as in Fig. 1. Unit 7712 was a velocity tuned A cell (wide RF with non-overlapping ON and OFF subregions) recorded in layer 6, with a RF at 5.6° from the fixation point.

the 4 main relative direction selectivity types observed in the present area 18 sample. The anti-phase conditionally direction selective cells correspond to the conditionally direction selective cells reported in our previous study of area 17. The cell of Fig. 1 was an in-phase conditionally selective cell. Table 1 compares the proportion of the different types in area 17 and 18. The main differences between the 2 areas are a higher proportion of absolutely direction selective cells, and a lower proportion of relative non-direction-selective cells in area 18 compared to area 17. Furthermore the area 18 sample includes in-phase conditionally direction selective cells and no anti-phase direction selective cells, while the reverse is true for the area 17 sample.

Relative direction selectivity and disparity

In the conclusion of our area 17 studies (Orban et al. 1987a) we argued that some of the relative direction selectivity types could subserve functions other than the measurement of object motion. Anti-phase, conditionally, and differencing direction selective cells could segregate the visual scene by measuring differences in direction or speed of motion while limited direction selective cells could extract depth from motion. In-phase conditionally direction selective cells cannot subserve motion segregation, since they respond with maximal optimalization when both patterns move in the same direction and at the same speed. On the other hand, they form a pair with the anti-phase conditionally direction selective cells, and by the same

reasoning as was used to suggest that limited direction selective cells could signal positions of the noise pattern around the fixation plane, one could suggest that conditionally direction selective cells signal that the noise pattern is located in front (in-phase conditional cells) or behind (anti-phase conditional cells) the fixation plane. The conditionally direction selective cells would then be the analogues of near and far cells (Poggio and Fisher 1978) for motion parallax signals, just as limited direction selective cells are the analogues of tuned excitatory cells. The observation that in-phase conditionally direction selective cells occur only in area 18 would then fit with the finding that far and near cells are more abundant in area 18 than in area 17 (Ferster 1981; Spileers, Orban, Gulyás and Bishop, unpublished). In order to further test these conjectures, we assessed in the same cells the interactions between moving bar and background, and binocular disparity tuning. If our hypothesis was correct, one would expect a correlation between relative direction selectivity types and stereotypes. Ideally, one would expect to find neurons which belong to analogous types in the two domains (stereo and motion parallax) and which indicate the same position in depth by the two mechanisms.

Position disparity response curves were generated by keeping the movement trajectory in the dominant eye fixed, and shifting the movement trajectory in the non-dominant eye. Monocular control conditions were randomly interleaved with the binocular conditions in the multihistograms.

For 23 of the 36 cells in area 18, both types of

TABLE 1

Proportion (%) of relative direction selectivity types

	Absolute	Anti-phase	Conditional phase	Conditional in-phase	Differencing	Limited	Non-direction selective	Unclassified	Total
Area 18 (n = 36)	36	0	14	14	3	25	8	0	100
Area 17 (n = 69)	13	6	20	0	0	26	29	6	100

TABLE 2

Correlation between disparity types and relative direction selectivity types

Disparity	Relative direction selectivity				
	Unmodulated	Limited	Conditioned	Differencing	Total
Unmodulated	3	2	1	0	6
Tuned excitatory	4	2	0	0	6
Broad inhibition	0	0	2	1	3
Near-far	4	0	4	0	8
Total	11	4	7	1	23

multihistograms were collected. The disparity response curves could be classified into 6 classes: cells without disparity tuning (unmodulated), tuned excitatory and tuned inhibitory, far and near cells, and cells with a broad inhibition in the position disparity domain. The latter are selective for direction in depth (Cynander and Regan 1978; Orban et al. 1986). Table 2 shows the correlation between disparity types and relative direction selectivity types. Absolutely direction selective cells and relative non-direction selective cells have been put into one category labelled as 'unmodulated' and both conditionally direction selective cells have also been put into a single category. Very significantly, tuned excitatory cells were either unmodulated by the background, or limited direction selective, and the near and far cells were either unmodulated by the background motion, or conditionally direction selective. This suggests that some area 18 cells carry not only stereo signals or only motion parallax signals but that a number of area 18 cells receive analogous signals from stereo and motion parallax. Given the methodological difficulties involved in estimating the absolute disparity in paralyzed animals, it is difficult to show that cells which are both tuned excitatory and limited direction selective, carry signals about the same position in depth for both domains (stereo and motion parallax). However, for far and near cells it is possible in paralyzed animals to decide whether they signal that objects are in front or behind the fixation plane. In fact, for all 4 cells which were far or near for stereo and conditionally direction selective, there was an agreement between the position in depth indicated by the stereo and the motion parallax. One of these cells is

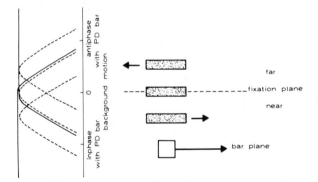

Fig. 4. Coding of position in depth of the background with respect to the fixation plane and the bar. Limited direction selectivity cells signal that the background is near the fixation plane (those tuned to slow in-phase signal that is just in front of the fixation plane; those tuned to zero background motion, on the fixation plane; those tuned to slow anti-phase, just behind the fixation plane). In a previous study (Orban et al. 1987a) we showed that only a small patch of the noise is required to observe the limited direction selectivity. Anti-phase conditionally direction selective cells signal that the background is behind the fixation plane (far). In-phase conditionally direction selectivity cells signal that the background is in front of the fixation plane (near). Hence the limited, anti-phase conditionally and in-phase conditionally direction selective cells are the analogues in the motion parallax domain of the tuned excitatory, far and near cells, respectively, in the stereo (position disparity) domain.

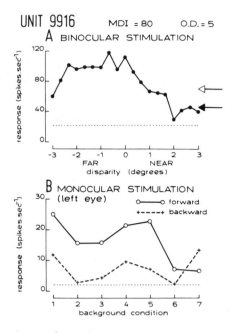

UNIT 9916   MDI = 80   O.D. = 5

Fig. 5. An area 18 cell signalling 'far' both by stereo and motion parallax. A: Disparity response curve for the preferred direction of motion (forward). The arrow indicates the monocular response levels (open arrow, left eye; solid arrow, right eye). The dashed line indicates the significance level. B: The net responses to movement of the bar in forward and backward directions plotted as a function of background conditions. Same conventions as in Fig. 3. Unit 9916 was a velocity tuned HA cell (endstopped, wide RF with non-overlapping ON and OFF subregions) recorded in layers 2 – 3 with a RF at 4.7° from the fixation point. The MDI of the cell was 80 and the cell belonged to ocular dominance class 5.

shown in Fig. 5. This cell was a direction selective binocular cell, recorded in layers 2 – 3. The cell responded optimally for negative disparities (far) and the response dropped steadily between zero and +2 degrees disparity (Fig. 5A). At this disparity the response was close to the significance level and the response remained low between 2 and 3 degrees disparity. This cell was classified as a far cell, although the response dropped only gradually around zero disparity. When tested in the bar-background interaction test (Fig. 5B), the cell was anti-phase conditionally direction selective, although the response for the slow in-phase motion of the background (compared to the preferred direction of the bar) was as strong as the response

for antiphase motion between bar and background. This cell thus signalled 'far' including in fact on, and just in front of, the fixation plane) by both the stereo and the motion parallax cues.

Summary and conclusion

1) These experiments confirm that a moving textured background exerts a powerful influence on responses of cortical cells to a moving bar. Responses of area 18 cells to moving bars are suppressed by the background motion at the same speed as, or faster than, the bar's, just as those of area 17 and geniculate cells. The direction selectivity of over half of the area 18 cells is modulated by background motion, and this proportion is similar to that in area 17.

2) These experiments suggest that areas 17 and 18 have the machinery not only to analyse object motion (absolutely direction selective cells), but to segregate scenes by motion (anti-phase, anti-phase conditionally and differencing direction selective cells), and to extract depth from motion (limited, in-phase and anti-phase conditionally direction selective cells).

3) These experiments confirm and extend our previous observations on the specialization of areas 17 and 18. Area 17 could participate in the analysis of stationary objects (relative non-direction-selective cells), and in motion segregation (anti-phase, anti-phase conditionally and differencing direction selective cells), and in the signalling of depth near the fixation plane (limited direction selective cells). Area 18 could participate in the analysis of object motion (absolutely direction selective cells) and in the extraction of depth from motion (conditionally and limited direction selective cells).

4) Finally, our experiments suggest that signals of different type (stereo and motion) can converge onto the same visual cortical cells. Hence, some cortical cells, even at the primary level, can represent relatively high level visual information. Furthermore, it suggests that the processing of visual information at the cortical level may not solely be

divergent (Zeki 1978). A possible solution to the discrepancy between the perceptual unity of objects and the likelihood that the different aspects of these objects are processed in different cortical areas would be that the convergence of the different types of visual information is distributed amongst different pools of cells each exhibiting a limited convergence.

Acknowledgements

The technical help of G. Vanparrijs, P. Kayenbergh and G. Meulemans as well as the computerized typing of Y. Celis is kindly acknowledged. The authors are indebted to P.O. Bishop for his help in developing the computerized disparity testing, and to H. Maes for help with the software controlling the equipment. This study was supported by a grant from the Ministry of Science Policy (GOA 84/88).

References

Cynader, M. and Regan, D. (1978) Neurones in the cat parastriate cortex sensitive to the direction of motion in three-dimensional space. *J. Neurophysiol.*, 274: 549 – 569.

Ferster, D. (1981) A comparison of binocular depth mechanisms in areas 17 and 18 of the cat visual cortex. *J. Physiol.*, 311: 623 – 655.

Gulyás, B., Orban, G.A., Duysens, J. and Maes, H. (1987a) The suppressive influence of moving textured backgrounds on responses of cat striate neurons to moving bars. *J. Neurophysiol.*, 57: 1767 – 1792.

Gulyás, B., Orban, G.A. and Spileers, W. (1987b) A moving noise background modulates the responses of striate neurones to moving bars in the cat but not in the monkey. *J. Physiol.*, 390: 28.

Orban, G.A., Kennedy, H. and Maes, H. (1981a) Response to movement of neurons in areas 17 and 18 of the cat: velocity sensitivity. *J. Neurophysiol.*, 45: 1043 – 1057.

Orban, G.A., Kennedy, H. and Maes, H. (1981b) Response to movement of neurons in areas 17 and 18 of the cat: direction selectivity. *J. Neurophysiol.*, 45: 1059 – 1073.

Orban, G.A. (1984) *Neuronal Operations in the Visual Cortex,* Springer, Berlin, 367 pp.

Orban, G.A., Spileers, W., Gulyás, B. and Bishop, P.O. (1986) Motion in depth selectivity of cortical cells revisited. *Soc. Neurosci. Abstr.,* 12: 584.

Orban, G.A., Gulyás, B. and Vogels, R. (1987a) Influence of a moving textured background on direction selectivity of cat striate neurons. *J. Neurophysiol.*, 57: 1792 – 1812.

Orban, G.A., Gulyás, B. and Spileers, W. (1987b) A moving noise background modulates responses to moving bars of monkey V2 cells but not of monkey V1 cells. *Suppl. Invest. Ophthalmol. Vis. Sci.,* 28: 197.

Poggio, G.F. and Fischer, B. (1977) Binocular interaction and depth sensitivity in striate and prestriate cortex of behaving rhesus monkey. *J. Neurophysiol.*, 40: 1392 – 1405.

Tretter, F., Cynader, M. and Singer, W. (1975) A comparative analysis of cat striate and parastriate cortex. *Brain Res.,* 85: 180 – 181.

Zeki, S. (1978) Functional specialization in the visual cortex of the rhesus monkey. *Nature,* 274: 423 – 428.

T.P. Hicks and G. Benedek (Eds.)
Progress in Brain Research, Vol. 75
© 1988 Elsevier Science Publishers B.V. (Biomedical Division)

CHAPTER 14

The patchy intrinsic projections of visual cortex

Simon LeVay

Robert Bosch Vision Research Center, Salk Institute for Biological Studies, P.O. Box 85800, San Diego, California 92138,
U.S.A.

Introduction

In 1982 Rockland and Lund noticed a curious pattern of labeling that was produced by injections of horseradish peroxidase (HRP) into the primary visual cortex of the tree shrew. Spreading for 2 – 3 mm from the injection sites were patches of peroxidase labeling, spaced at intervals of about 0.5 mm, and separated by regions of unlabeled or lightly labeled tissue. The patches consisted of neuronal cell bodies, presumably labeled by retrograde axonal transport, and axon terminals, presumably labeled by anterograde transport. Since this initial description comparable findings have been reported for a variety of visual areas in several species. The purpose of this review is to summarize what is known about these patchy local projections and to discuss their functional significance.

Where have patches been seen?

By making extracellular injections of tracers such as HRP, peroxidase-conjugated wheat-germ agglutinin (WGA-HRP), [3H]proline or fluorescent beads, investigators have demonstrated intrinsic patchy projections in area 17 of the tree shrew (Rockland and Lund 1982; Rockland et al. 1982; Sesma et al. 1984), ferret (Rockland 1985a), cat (Luhmann et al. 1986), and the macaque and squirrel monkey (Rockland and Lund 1983; Livingstone and Hubel 1984a). They have been seen in area 18 of cats (Matsubara et al. 1985, 1987; Price 1986;

LeVay 1988) and macaque and squirrel monkeys (Rockland and Lund 1983; Livingstone and Hubel 1984a; Rockland 1985b), area MT of macaque monkeys (Maunsell and van Essen 1983), and the Clare-Bishop area of cats (LeVay, unpublished observations). In fact, there are no convincing examples of areas lacking these intrinsic projection systems.

Shape and layout of the patches

According to most descriptions the patches have a columnar organization – they extend vertically from the pial surface to the white matter. Often, however, certain layers (especially layers 2 and 3) are more heavily labeled than others. Sometimes the patchiness is more evident in some layers than others: in area 17 of the tree shrew, for example, very sharply-defined patches in layers 2 and 3A overlie a much more continuous distribution of label in layer 3C (Rockland et al. 1982). Values for the widths of individual patches range from about 250 to 500 μm, and are not obviously correlated with the size of the injection sites. The gaps between the patches are comparable in width to the patches themselves, so that the overall periodicity is in the range of 0.5 – 1.0 mm.

The shape of the patches as seen in surface view has generally been described as round or irregular. In area 17 of the tree shrew (Rockland et al. 1982) and the ferret (Rockland 1985a), however, they take the form of bands, with some indication of beading along the bands. The bands are oriented orthogonal to the 17 – 18 border. In areas 17 and 18 of primates relatively large tracer injections give rise to labeling which, especially in the immediate neighborhood of the injection site, has the form of a lattice enclosing 'holes' of unlabeled tissue (Rockland and Lund 1983; Rockland 1985b). Smaller injections in the same areas give rise to patches of label within an unlabeled matrix (Livingstone and Hubel 1984b).

How far do the patches extend?

In most descriptions, the patches closest to the injection site are the most heavily labeled, and they become progressively fainter with increasing distance. Thus the absolute tangential spread of the patches can be hard to determine, and may be influenced by the sensitivity of the methods as much as by the actual limits of the projection. Nevertheless figures of 1 – 4 mm (as measured from the center of the injection site) are common.

It is striking that the extent of the patches is no greater in area 17 of the macaque monkey than it is in that of the tree shrew (2 – 3 mm in both cases: Rockland and Lund 1982, 1983), in spite of the large difference in the size of this area in the two species. This observation suggests that the extent of the patchy projections is scaled to the cellular or columnar dimensions of the cortex – dimensions that vary only modestly from species to species – rather than to the size of the cortical area or the magnification of the retinal image on it. As far as one can tell from the published reports, the extent of the patches is also more or less invariant with retinotopic location, again suggesting a scaling to the dimensions of the cortical processing machinery, not to visual field dimensions.

It is nevertheless important to consider what the extent of the patchy projections means in terms of receptive-field dimensions. The question here is whether the projections can be interpreted as interconnecting cells with overlapping receptive fields, or whether they interconnect the representations of entirely separate regions of visual space. Because of the size of individual receptive fields, and the scatter in the receptive field positions of neighboring cells, the representation of a single point in the visual field is spread over a cortical distance of 2 – 3 mm, according to measurements by Hubel and Wiesel (1974) in monkey area 17. This distance is invariant with retinotopic location. The similarity of this figure to that given for the spread of the patches in the same species (Rockland and Lund 1983) is striking. When one considers that Hubel and Wiesel used the conservative 'minimum response' method to plot receptive field size, and that the estimate of the spread of patches may be over-generous, given that transport could have been from the edges rather than the centers of the injection sites, it seems safe to conclude that, in monkey area 17, the patchy projections interconnect regions containing cells with overlapping receptive fields. One might, in fact, suggest that the total area containing labeled patches corresponds to the total cortical mapping of the aggregate receptive fields of a column of cells at the injection site (what one might term a 'column image' by analogy with the 'point image' and 'receptive field image' of McIlwain (1976). Of course, the patchy projections may themselves contribute to the size of the column image.

Nelson and Frost (1985) have addressed the same question for cat striate cortex by comparing three pieces of data: estimates of cortical magnification factor derived from the mapping studies of Tusa et al. (1978), measurements of receptive-field dimensions from their own experiments and from studies of Kato et al. (1978) and Orban et al. (1979), and an estimate of 6 mm for the length of the intrinsic axon collaterals of cortical neurons, derived from the intracellular HRP-filling studies of Gilbert and Wiesel (1979). They concluded that some cell types (end-stopped cells in particular) were likely to receive inputs, via the tangential axons, from cortical regions representing visual space outside of their excitatory receptive fields. There are several reasons for doubting this conclusion, however. It takes no account of scatter in receptive-field position, or of the possibility that the longest axons may synapse specifically on those cell types with the largest fields. Also, the figure of 6 mm seems to be excessive; although Gilbert and Wiesel (1979) described the axon of one cell (their Fig. 4) as extending 6 – 8 mm from the cell body, direct measurements from that figure gives a value of 3.1 mm. (Foreshortening may account for part of the discrepancy, but there also seems to be a confusion between the total (bidirectional) spread of the arbor and its maximum extent in one direction from the cell body.) This was a cell whose axon ramified in layer 6, where cells have very long receptive fields (Gilbert 1977). A more typical value for the maximum reach of an axon from its parent cell body (in cat striate cortex) seems to be 1.5 – 2.0 mm (Gilbert and Wiesel 1979, 1983), a value comparable to the extent of labeling seen with extracellular HRP injections (Luhmann et al. 1986). If this figure is used in Nelson and Frost's (1985) calculation, the tangential projections remain within the column image in the cat just as they appear to do in the monkey.

Evidence bearing on the same question has been obtained with quite different methods by Ts'o et al. (1986a). These authors used cross-correlation analysis to study connections between pairs of neurons situated at various horizontal distances from each other in area 17 of the cat. They observed positive correlations between pairs of cells that were separated by 2 – 3 mm and that had non-overlapping receptive fields. They concluded that the long intrinsic projections of area 17 serve to provide cortical neurons with information from regions of visual space outside of their 'classical' receptive fields. The conclusion is weakened, however, by the fact that most if not all of the long-range effects seen by Ts'o et al. were suggestive of common activation of the 2 neurons by a third (unrecorded) cell, rather than monosynaptic connections between them. This third cell (which need not even have been in area 17) might well have had a large receptive field centered between the two recorded cells, and partially overlapping both of them.

For most of the species and areas where patchy projections have been described, insufficient infor-

mation is available to decide whether they extend beyond the 'column image'. Even if they do so, however, it should still be borne in mind that the labeling is always most intense in the immediate vicinity of the injection site. It is therefore reasonable to think that the bulk, at least, of the patchy projections mediate interactions between cells with overlapping receptive fields. If one defines a receptive field in more generous fashion than by the 'minimum response' method (by estimating receptive-field width on the basis of a length summation test, for example), this conclusion becomes even more assured.

'Fixed' or 'sliding' patches?

In their studies of patchy projections in area 17 of the tree shrew Rockland et al. (1982) interpreted the observed labeling pattern to mean that there were fixed, stripe-like zones of cortex that were interconnected over considerable tangential distances, while between them lay another set of stripe-like zones which either had much shorter tangential connections or else lacked them entirely. Their reason for reaching this conclusion was that the injection sites were much larger than the individual patches; if there was an underlying continuum of tangential projections, any detailed patchiness should have been smeared out.

A quite different interpretation of the same findings was offered by Mitchison and Crick (1982). They suggested that the intrinsic tangential connections of cortical neurons do indeed form a continuum. The patchiness seen after HRP injections arises, according to their hypothesis, from the following connectivity rule: a given cortical cell connects only to other cells of the same or similar orientation preference, and only along an axis in visual space that is functionally significant for that cell (for example, along the axis defined by the cell's orientation preference). Their computer simulation showed that, given a stripe-like layout of orientation columns, such as is thought to exist in the tree-shrew's striate cortex (Humphrey and Norton 1980; Humphrey et al. 1980), and an orderly, undistorted representation of the visual field (Kaas et al. 1972), this connectivity rule will lead to stripe-like labeling after local injections of HRP, even when the effective injection site occupies an entire hypercolumn. (Whether it will lead to patchy projections of sufficiently widespread distribution when the injection site occupies several hypercolumns, was not investigated.) The stripes will follow a direction on the cortical surface that is similar though not identical to that of the orientation stripes. This was, roughly, the direction of the HRP stripes actually observed by Rockland et al. (1982).

Whether the patchy projections are in fact related to the orientation system, and if so in what particular manner, will be discussed in more detail below. The important point for the moment is that Mitchison and Crick's model involves 'sliding' patches: the intrinsic connections as a whole completely and uniformly fill the tangential extent of area 17, and presumably of any other area where they occur.

One approach to deciding between fixed and sliding patches has been to make two or more injections at nearby locations. Thus Rockland (1985b) made pairs of injections of HRP, spaced 1.5 – 2.5 mm apart, in area 18 of squirrel monkeys. She reported that in the zone between the two sites the lattice-like patterns 'superimposed without losing periodicity' – a finding taken to support the idea of fixed patches. It should be noted, however, that Mitchison and Crick's 'sliding' model also predicts superimposition of the label in some regions, especially on the direct line between the two injection sites. Also, since the same tracer was used for both injections, it was difficult to draw firm conclusions about how closely the two patterns superimposed.

Matsubara et al. (1987) have performed similar experiments in area 18 of the cat, but using two different tracers (HRP and concanavalin A) for the two injections. They also mapped the distribution of preferred orientations in the region of the injections. In one case there was partial interdigitation of the two sets of patches, a finding that the authors interpreted to mean that the patchy projections do 'slide' and form, in toto, a continuous system. In two other cases there was considerable overlap between the two sets of patches. According to Matsubara et al., the variable determining the degree of overlap was the relationship between the preferred orientations represented at the two injection sites: when they were the same, the patches overlapped, and when they differed, the patches interdigitated. The relationship between the patches and the orientation system is considered further below. As to the issue of fixed versus sliding patches, Matsubara et al.'s experiments certainly indicate that the patches slide; whether they do so enough to form a completely continuous, uniform projection system, however, is left unclear.

Punctate injections are by their nature unsuitable for testing the continuity or otherwise of a projection system. Another difficulty has been the lack of fixed landmarks in the tissue that might permit correlations between the results of separate experiments. This second difficulty has been overcome, in the case of monkey striate cortex, by the discovery of the system of patches that stain densely with cytochrome oxidase (CO) histochemistry (Humphrey and Hendrickson 1980; Horton and Hubel 1981; Horton 1984). These patches, drolly named 'blobs' by Livingstone and Hubel (1984a), are spaced about 350 μm apart and line up with the ocular dominance stripes. In the supragranular layers, where the blobs are most prominent, they are also physiologically distinct: there is a high proportion of non-oriented, color-coded cells within them as compared with the inter-blob regions, which are rich in orientation-selective neurons (Livingstone and Hubel 1984a).

Both Rockland and Lund (1983) and Livingstone and Hubel (1984a,b) have attempted to correlate the layout of the projection patches with the blobs, with somewhat different results. Rockland and Lund found no consistent relationship between the two sets of patches, although near the injection site, where the HRP-labeling formed a lattice enclosing unlabeled 'holes', the blobs tended to lie in the walls of the lattice rather than in the holes. In their first report Livingstone and Hubel (1984b) described the HRP patches furthest from the injection sites as lying exclusively in register with the blobs. In their second study (Livingstone and Hubel 1984a) they described the results of making very small iontophoretic deposits of HRP (comparable in size to a single blob). In cases where the injection sites were within blobs, the transported label was also found within blobs, while injections of regions between blobs led to patchy labeling that also fell between blobs. They concluded that the patchy intrinsic projections of monkey striate cortex are likely to be, in toto, a continuous system, but that this system contains at least two independent sets of connections, one joining blobs with each other, and the other interconnecting the non-blob regions.

In this second study there was no obvious difference in the extent of the patchy connections of blob and non-blob regions, in contrast to the earlier study which indicated longer connections for the blobs. It seems most likely that the conclusion of the earlier study was correct, and that the very small injections used in the second study simply did not reveal the far patches in the cases of blob-centered injections.

There may be further subtleties to the blob/patch relationship. Although Livingstone and Hubel (1984b) reported that *all* the blobs surrounding a (blob-centered) injection site were labeled, this is not very evident in their figures; some blobs lying well within the zone of patchy labeling seem to be unlabeled. This question deserves further study, particularly since blobs can differ from each other in ocularity (Hendrickson et al. 1981; Horton and Hubel 1981) and possibly also in the color properties of the cells they contain (Ts'o et al. 1986b). Also, since the non-blob injections gave rise to labeling of patches, rather than to a lattice with holes, the question of continuity within this subsystem of projections remains open. One obvious possibility is that the patchy projections of the non-blob regions are equivalent to the entire patchy projections seen in species, such as the cat, that lack blobs. Thus a plausible (but as yet unproven) organizing principle for monkey striate cortex is that it contains two independent sets of 'sliding' patches, laid out within the fixed confines of the blob and non-blob tissue.

In monkeys, area 18 (or V2) also has fixed landmarks revealed by cytochrome oxidase (CO) histochemistry. These take the form of CO-dense stripes separated by light 'interstripes'. The dense stripes can further be subdivided into 'thin' and 'thick' stripes, which alternate with each other (Horton and Hubel 1981; Humphrey and Hendrickson 1983; Tootell et al. 1983; Horton 1984; Wong-Riley and Carroll 1984). The three types of stripe (thin, thick and interstripe) differ from each other in their connections (Curcio and Harting 1978; Livingstone and Hubel 1982; Livingstone and Hubel 1984a; DeYoe and van Essen 1985; Shipp and Zeki 1985) as well as in the response properties of the neurons within them (DeYoe and van Essen 1985; Hubel and Livingstone 1985, 1987; Shipp and Zeki 1985). Rockland (1985b) reported that the intrinsic patchy labeling produced by HRP injections into monkey area 18 had no consistent relationship with the CO stripes in the same tissue. Livingstone and Hubel (1984a), whose injections were smaller, reported that the patchy projections did align with the CO stripes: if the injection was in a dense stripe the patches were also in dense stripes, and if the injection was in an interstripe the patches were also in interstripes. Curiously, the patchy projections appeared to ignore the differences between the two types of dense stripe. At any event, there seem to be two interdigitating sets of fixed connections in monkey area 18, as in area 17. Whether each set itself contains 'sliding' elements remains to be explored.

To summarize this complex issue, it seems likely that much more of the cortex participates in the intrinsic tangential projection system than just those patches that are labeled by a single injection. To decide whether the projection system is completely uniform and continuous, however, would require the application of new methods, such as the development of antibodies specific for this set of axons. Examination of the relationship between the patchy inter-areal projections and the intrinsic projections (see below) may also throw light on the issue.

The cells of origin of the patchy projections

Do all kinds of cortical neurons participate in the patchy projections, or only certain types? The most global distinction one can make among cortical neurons is between those possessing spine-laden dendrites and those whose dendrites have few or no spines (Lund 1973). Spiny neurons include pyramidal cells, spiny stellate cells, and intermediate forms. All the axons leaving a given cortical area, whether destined for other cortical areas, for the opposite hemisphere, or for subcortical targets, are thought to arise from these cells (for cat area 17, for example, see Gilbert and Kelly 1975; Shatz 1977; Albus and Meyer 1981; Cohen et al. 1981; LeVay and Sherk 1981, 1983; Katz et al. 1984), although not all spiny neurons have axons that leave the area (Lund 1973; Gilbert and Wiesel 1983). Spiny neurons also provide the major interlaminar connections (Gilbert and Wiesel 1979). Spine-free cells include a multitude of subtypes defined on the basis of dendritic or axonal morphology: spine-free stellate cell, bipolar cell, granule cell, chandelier cell, basket cell, and so on (for cat area 17, see O'Leary 1941; Peters and Regidor 1981; Meyer 1983). It has long been suspected that spiny and spine-free neurons are respectively excitatory and inhibitory in function. The most persuasive evidence for this correlation is that most, if not all spine-free cells can be labeled with antibodies to GABA, the major cortical inhibitory transmitter, or to glutamic acid decarboxylase, the enzyme responsible for synthesis of GABA from glutamate (Ribak 1978; Freund et al. 1983; Somogyi et al. 1983a; Somogyi and Hodgson 1985), while spiny neurons are not labeled with these markers. It would not be surprising, however, if there eventually turned out to be some exceptions to this generalization.

Several lines of evidence point to spiny neurons as being the cells of origin of the patchy intrinsic projections. First, several investigators have mentioned that many of the retrogradely labeled cells in the patches have pyramidal-shaped cell bodies (e.g., Rockland and Lund 1982). Second, the pattern of synaptic inputs onto these retrogradely labeled cell bodies, as seen in EM sections, is characteristic of spiny neurons, at least in the case of cat area 18 (LeVay 1988). Third, experiments combining retrograde transport of fluorescent beads with GABA immunocytochemistry indicate that the cells do not contain this transmitter (LeVay 1987).

The same conclusion has been drawn from examination of the axonal arborizations of individual cortical neurons stained by intracellular injection of HRP (Gilbert and Wiesel 1979, 1983, 1985; Martin and Whitteridge 1984). Some pyramidal and spiny stellate cells have axon collaterals that run tangentially for distances comparable with the extent of the patchy projections. The terminal branches of these collaterals that carry the synaptic boutons, are often aggregated into clusters with a periodicity comparable to that of the patches. The numbers of boutons in each cluster is very small – a tiny fraction of the numbers of boutons in a patch labeled by HRP transport. Thus the clusters belonging to many neurons would have to lie in register to produce the 'macroscopic' patches.

Generally speaking, the axonal arborizations of the spine-free neurons are much more limited in their tangential spread. Many, indeed, have axonal arbors whose dimensions are similar to those of the cells' dendritic trees. The one cell which might make a claim to involvement in the patchy projections is the basket cell (Marin-Padilla 1969), whose axonal arbor, in cat area 17, can spread 1.5 mm from the cell body, and whose axon terminals show some clustering (Martin 1984). This cell is unlikely to make a significant contribution to the patchy projections, however, because it is thought to be a GABAergic neuron (Freund et al. 1983), and because the types of synaptic connections formed by its axon (Somogyi et al. 1983b) are different from those formed by labeled axons in the patches (see below). Most probably, the tangential collaterals of basket cells and other spine-free cells contribute only to the 'halo' of label seen around an HRP injection site, not to the remote patches.

Synaptic connections

Just as cortical neurons can be divided into two broad morphological classes, so can cortical synapses (Gray 1959; Colonnier 1968). The type 1 or 'asymmetrical' synapses are characterized by pronounced cytoplasmic dense material associated with the postsynaptic membrane, while the type 2 or 'symmetric' synapses have only slight postsynaptic densities. The synaptic vesicles at the type 2 synapses are also somewhat smaller than at type 1 synapses, and with some fixation conditions take on a flattened or pleomorphic shape. The axons of spiny neurons form type 1 synapses, while those of spine-free neurons form type 2 synapses (LeVay 1973; Somogyi 1977; Peters and Fairen 1978; McGuire et al. 1984, 1985; Saint-Marie and Peters 1985; Gabbott et al. 1987). Only one exception to this rule has been reported, a subtype of spine-free bipolar cells in the rat's visual cortex that apparently forms type 1 synapses (Peters and Kimerer 1981). Axon terminals that form type 1 synapses are not immunoreactive with antisera to GAD or GABA while type 2 synapses do react with these antibodies (Ribak 1978; Freund et al. 1983; Lavie and Hendrickson 1986). This and other less direct lines of evidence suggest that type 1 synapses are excitatory and type 2 synapses inhibitory.

In an EM study of patchy intrinsic projections of cat area 18 (LeVay 1988) it was found that nearly all (at least 96%) of the labeled axon terminals in the patches formed type 1 synapses. This finding supports the conclusion that the cells giving rise to the patchy projections are spiny neurons. The synapses were formed predominantly (86%) onto dendritic spines, with most of the remainder being made onto dendritic shafts. These numbers are similar to those reported for synapses formed by the intrinsic axon collaterals of individual, HRP-filled pyramidal cells (McGuire et al. 1985; Gabbott et al. 1987). They indicate that the patchy projections not only arise from, but also predominantly synapse on, neurons with spiny dendrites. Thus the synaptic arrangements favor the interpretation that a major function of the patchy projections is to mediate mutual excitation between groups of pyramidal or spiny stellate neurons.

The patches and ocular dominance columns

The intrinsic patches are quite similar in appearance to the patches produced, in the visual cortex of several species, by transneuronal transport of tracers injected into one eye (cat, Shatz et al. 1977; mink, McConnell and LeVay 1986; galago, Hubel et al. 1975; spider monkey, Florence and Casagrande 1978; macaque monkey, Wiesel et al. 1974; chimpanzee, Tigges and Tigges 1979). This transneuronal labeling pattern corresponds to the physiologically-defined ocular dominance columns, as has been demonstrated by combined autoradiographic/recording experiments in macaque monkey (LeVay et al. 1980) and cat (Shatz and Stryker 1978). The question therefore arises whether there is any systematic relationship between the two systems of patches.

Clearly there is none in the tree shrew, because this species lacks ocular dominance columns (Casagrande and Harting 1975). Squirrel monkeys also lack ocular dominance columns, or at least they cannot be demonstrated by transneuronal autoradiography (Hubel et al. 1975), yet they have intrinsic patches. There are also prestriate cortical areas in the macaque monkey, such as area MT, that lack ocular dominance columns but have intrinsic patchy projections (Rockland and Pandya 1979; Maunsell and van Essen 1983). In area 17 of the macaque monkey, however, the relationship of the intrinsic patchy projections to the cytochrome oxidase blobs implies that the periodicity of the patchy projections is exactly matched to that of the ocular dominance columns. As mentioned earlier, it is unclear whether all nearby blobs are interconnected, or only some of them. If the latter, the projections might serve to interconnect cell groups of the same ocularity, or of opposite ocularity.

In area 17 of the cat the results of the cross-correlation study by Ts'o et al. (1986a) suggest that the long-distance tangential connections are preferentially between cells of the same ocularity. In cat area 18 Matsubara et al. (1987) looked at the same question by comparing the distribution of the intrinsic patches with the functional architecture of the same piece of tissue as mapped in multiple electrode penetrations. They found no systematic relationship between the ocular dominance of neurons at the injection site and of those in the labeled patches. Obviously, more data are needed to resolve this question.

The patches and orientation columns

This is the issue which has engendered the most interest and controversy within the entire topic of intrinsic projections. Various investigators have offered evidence that these projections interconnect cells of like orientation, cells of unlike orientation, oriented cells as opposed to unoriented cells, and unoriented cells as opposed to oriented cells. There is even the view that they have nothing to do with orientation.

In their study of the tree shrew's striate cortex Rockland and Lund (1982) noted the similarity of the intrinsic patches (which are band-like in this species) to the band-like pattern of 2-[^{14}C]deoxyglucose (2DG) labeling that is produced by exposing the animal to stripes of a single orientation (Humphrey et al. 1980). They speculated that the intrinsic projections and the regions of 2DG labeling occupied the same fixed, stripe-like zones, and that these zones represented the entire set of orientation-selective neurons; between them would be zones of cells with entirely different properties. They did not, however, perform double-label experiments to test this idea. Mitchison and Crick (1982), as described earlier, suggested that the patchy projections interconnected columns of like orientation (but only in certain specific directions). This hypothesis gained support from Ts'o et al.'s

(1986) cross-correlation study in cat area 17. They observed correlated firing between widely-spaced pairs of neurons when the two members of the pair shared a common orientation preference, but not otherwise (see also Michalski et al. 1983).

Matsubara et al.'s (1985, 1987) findings in cat area 18 were quite the reverse: they reported that the patchy projections were between cell groups whose preferred orientations were different, and on average orthogonal. They suggested that the function of the patchy projections was to mediate cross-orientation inhibition, a type of inhibition that has been thought, on various lines of evidence, to be responsible for sharpening or even generating the orientation selectivity of cortical neurons (e.g., Sillito 1979; Sillito et al. 1980). This hypothesis seems improbable, however. The orientation selectivity of cells in cat area 18 is affected little, if at all, by iontophoresis of the GABA antagonist n-methylbicuculline (Vidyasagar and Heide 1986). There is also morphological and immunocytochemical evidence, discussed above, that the patchy projections in cat area 18 are excitatory in function. Even disynaptic inhibition seems not to be a major function of the patchy projections, given that the great majority of the synapses appear to be made onto pyramidal or spiny stellate neurons. The notion of cross-orientation inhibition appears itself to be in trouble, given the finding that EPSPs and IPSPs recorded in cortical neurons are both well-tuned to the cell's preferred orientation (Ferster 1986, 1987).

It seems unlikely that the patchy projections would follow opposite rules of connectivity in areas 17 and 18, connecting like orientation columns in area 17 and unlike columns in area 18. Therefore, while one can think of possible functions for excitatory connections between cells of opposite orientation preference (Maffei and Fiorentini, 1976), it seems more plausible that the differences between the two sets of findings are due to methodological factors. Either the cross-correlation technique yields incomplete information about the pattern of connectivity, or (perhaps more likely) the difficulties inherent in matching electrode tracks to patterns of peroxidase labeling has caused problems in inferring the orientations represented in the labeled patches.

In monkey area 17 the finding that the longest patchy projections are made between blobs (see above) suggests a preferential involvement with the non-oriented, color-coded system. The shorter patchy projections of the non-blob tissue may still harbor an orientation-specific projection system within it, however.

Directional preference

In some cortical areas there is a columnar organization for the preferred direction of movement. In areas where cells are orientation-selective, such as cat area 18, directionality columns, if they exist at all, are simply subsets of the orientation columns (Payne et al. 1980; Swindale et al. 1987), but in other areas, such as the lateral suprasylvian areas in the cat and area MT in monkeys, directionality has a columnar organization in its own right (Hubel and Wiesel 1969; Zeki 1974; Spear and Baumann 1975). There is one report, for cat area 18, that a cell's directional selectivity is reduced or abolished by inactivation of a region of cortex near the recorded cell − specifically, the region representing visual space in the cell's preferred direction of motion (Eysel and Wörgötter 1986). This finding was interpreted to mean that, as a stimulus moves across the animal's field of view, a wave of inhibition moves in a corresponding direction across the cortical surface, and blocks the responses of cells whose null directions correspond to that direction of movement. Such a mechanism would undoubtedly require patchy tangential connections. However, a problem with this model is the evidence mentioned above favoring an excitatory role for the patchy projections. Perhaps the proposed mechanism operates over a relatively short range, corresponding to the axonal arborizations of the basket cells. This would be consistent with the observation that directional selectivity is present even for movements that are small with

respect to the dimensions of the cell's receptive field (Goodwin et al. 1975).

Non-classical receptive fields

Some cortical cells can be influenced from regions of the visual field well beyond their 'classical' receptive fields (e.g., Nelson and Frost 1978, 1985; Zeki 1980; Allman et al. 1985; Tanaka et al. 1986). This influence is seen as a modulation of the cell's responses to stimulation within its classical field. Often, these non-classical effects are complementary to the classical responses (opposite in directionality, for example). Cells in extrastriate cortical areas seem to display these effects more commonly than those in area 17.

One phenomenon of this type of particular interest in the context of patchy projections is a facilitatory (or disinhibitory) effect observed in some cells in cat area 17 by Nelson and Frost (1985). This facilitation was elicited by stimulation of zones beyond the ends of the receptive field (along the cell's orientation axis), and was tuned to the cell's preferred orientation. Nelson and Frost suggested that the facilitation was mediated by patchy projections that were selective for orientation and for visual field direction in the manner proposed by Mitchison and Crick (1982; see above). This interpretation seems very plausible. It is not completely clear, however, that the effect described by Nelson and Frost was a distinct 'non-classical' response, rather than simply reflecting the tail-end of the cell's length-summation curve.

It is worth pointing out that there are other pathways, besides the tangential intrinsic projections, that may be capable of mediating the non-classical effects. Feedback connections from higher areas may well play a role. Another candidate is the cortico-claustral loop; cells in the visual claustrum are orientation-selective and exhibit summation up to stimulus lengths of 40 degrees or more (LeVay and Sherk 1981). They project retinotopically to most visual cortical areas including area 17 (LeVay and Sherk 1981). Thus they may well contribute to wide-field orientation-dependent effects of the type described by Nelson and Frost (1978, 1985).

Patchy extrinsic projections

Many of the projections linking one visual area with another are also patchy (e.g., Gilbert and Kelly 1975; Rockland and Pandya 1979; Montero 1981; Tigges et al. 1981; Bullier et al. 1984; Livingstone and Hubel 1984a; Symonds and Rosenquist 1984; McConnell and LeVay 1986; Sherk 1986; Van Essen et al. 1986). It would seem plausible that the intrinsic and extrinsic projections are patchy for the same reason, and that the two sets of patches are spatially related (coinciding or interdigitating with each other, for example).

The one clear example in this respect is the projection from area 17 to area 18 in the monkey. The evidence that the intrinsic projections within these two areas respect the landmarks provided by cytochrome oxidase histochemistry (blobs in 17, stripes in 18) has been described above. The projections between the two areas respect the same landmarks: the blobs in 17 project to the thin CO-dense stripes in 18, and the non-blob regions project to the interstripes (Livingstone and Hubel 1984a).

The situation in the cat may be analogous. There is evidence (Gilbert and Wiesel 1987) from combined transport-2DG experiments that the patchiness of the projection from area 17 to area 18 is due to its orientation-specificity (columns of like orientation in the two areas being interconnected). This principle is the same as that thought to govern the intrinsic patchy projections of area 17 (Ts'o et al. 1986a). Hence cells in interconnected patches in area 17 appear to project to the same set of patches in area 18.

One should caution, however, that patchy extrinsic projections may not always form continuous systems when viewed as a whole. The projections from area 18 to areas MT and V4 in the monkey each arise from discrete, fixed sets of patches (DeYoe and van Essen 1985; Shipp and Zeki 1985). There may well be examples of similar noncontinuous projection systems in the cat, but,

hindered by the lack of intrinsic landmarks comparable to the cytochrome oxidase patches, efforts to verify or disprove their existence have yielded inconclusive or contradictory results (Gilbert and Wiesel 1981; Bullier et al. 1984; Sherk 1986). Until this issue has been resolved, the relationship between the intrinsic and extrinsic patchy projections must remain uncertain.

General considerations

As noted by Barlow (1981), the striking character of cortical connectivity is not its exuberance but its poverty: the chances of any randomly-selected pair of cells being directly connected is almost negligible, and those that are connected generally lie very close to each other. Hence it is likely that the minimization of the number and length of connections is an important principle of cortical design. Do the patchy intrinsic projections follow or flout this principle?

Seen in isolation, they evidently flout it, since they connect non-adjacent regions of cortex. Presumably, though, they represent part of a total design which does approach minimal connectivity. Take, for example, the blob and non-blob systems in monkey area 17. These appear to represent parallel channels in which information relevant to the perception of contour and color are independently processed (Livingstone and Hubel 1984a). If these channels were embodied in separate areas (say areas 17 and 18), rather than parcellating both of these areas between them, the intrinsic projections of each area could be shorter and non-patchy. The fact that this solution is not adopted suggests that the two channels are not independent; rather, that they are interconnected or share common inputs or outputs. These interchannel connections would be greatly extended by placing the channels in separate areas, to a degree (one guesses) that would match or outweigh the savings in *intra*-channel connections. (The two channels very likely do share a common input from the nonoriented cells of layer 4C-beta (Hubel and Wiesel 1968; Lund 1973; Michael 1986), even though the blobs have their own private thalamic inputs as well (Livingstone and Hubel 1982; Weber et al. 1983).

The same may be true of orientation-specific patchy connections, which appear to be the dominant type of intrinsic connection in cat visual cortex, and which may exist in the monkey too within the non-blob system. Columns representing different orientations undoubtedly share common (non-oriented) inputs, and they may share some outputs too (e.g., the poorly-oriented cortico-tectal projection cells of layer 5; Finlay et al. 1976). Thus there is ample reason to interlace different orientations rather than have separate areas for each orientation: the latter solution would allow shorter, non-patchy intrinsic connections only at the price of longer inter-areal connections.

One can account in this manner for the patchiness of the intrinsic projections, but there still remains the question of why the intrinsic projections exist at all. Here there are as many possibilities as there are response properties in visual cortex. Subfields, sidebands, and end-zones; orientation-, direction- and velocity-selectivity; ocular dominance and disparity tuning; non-classical receptive fields; arguments can be made to support any of these possibilities and more (Mitchison and Crick 1982; Rockland et al. 1982; Gilbert and Wiesel 1983; Martin 1984; Gilbert 1985; Matsubara et al. 1985).

In speculating about the function of the patchy projections, there seem to be three key considerations, based on the evidence discussed earlier. First, they are quite *local* in action. They probably interconnect cells with overlapping receptive fields, and few if any of them extend beyond the 'column image', at least in area 17. Second, they probably interconnect cells with at least partially matching response properties. Third, they probably mediate reciprocal excitation between groups of neurons, not specialized inhibitory functions.

These considerations lead to the view that the patchy intrinsic projections perform an ensemble averaging operation, an operation that would serve to enhance the detection of weak signals in the presence of noise. Thus the response parameter to which the patchy projections should most obviously contribute is contrast sensitivity. It is of interest in this respect that many neurons in cat area 17 exhibit adaptation to low-contrast stimuli; this adaptation has a time constant of about 6 sec, is local in operation, and is orientation-specific (Ohzawa et al. 1985). One could speculate that the functional effectiveness of the tangential intrinsic connections increases as contrast levels are reduced.

In making excitatory connections between cortical neurons there is likely to be a trade-off between sensitivity and selectivity, since no two cells will have identical receptive field positions and identical response properties. The loss of selectivity is minimized, however, by restricting the connections to groups of neurons with approximately similar receptive field locations, approximately similar preferred orientations, and so on. It is due to the specificity of these connections, one imagines, that neuronal tuning curves for orientation and other parameters broaden only slightly as contrast is reduced (Albrecht and Hamilton 1982; Sclar and Freeman 1982; Skottun et al. 1987).

To the extent that the receptive fields of the interconnected cells are not exactly superimposed, the tangential connections are likely to cause some increase in receptive-field size over that which is produced by the direct geniculate inputs, especially when field dimensions are assessed by summation tests rather than by the minimum response method. This increase may be of functional significance, for example in allowing cells to respond to interrupted or fragmentary contours (Von der Heydt et al. 1984), as suggested by Nelson and Frost (1985). The main role of the tangential connections, however, is probably that of organizing concerted, highly sensitive responses by populations of neurons with common properties.

If these general ideas are correct, the patchy intrinsic projections could arise during development in response to the rule that 'cells that fire together, wire together'. One would expect them to emerge from exuberant, non-patchy tangential projections by an activity-dependent elimination of synapses, such as occurs in the formation of ocular dominance stripes (LeVay et al. 1978; Stryker and Harris 1986). The intrinsic projections of areas 17 and 18 are indeed more extensive and continuous in young kittens than in adult cats, but they still show some patchiness even at the youngest ages examined (Luhmann et al. 1986; Price 1986). Presumably some activity patterns, sufficient to cause a degree of parcellation of connections, already exist in these young kittens, but as other systems develop (ocular dominance columns, for example, which begin to appear during the third postnatal week; LeVay et al. 1978) the intrinsic projections are dissected further.

Acknowledgements

This work was supported by NIH grant EY05551. I thank Sacha Nelson for useful discussions.

References

Albrecht, D.G. and Hamilton, D.B. (1982) Striate cortex of monkey and cat: contrast response function. *J. Neurophysiol.,* 48: 217 – 237.

Albus, K. and Meyer, G. (1981) Spiny stellates and cells of origin of association fibres from area 17 to area 18 in the cat's neocortex. *Brain Res.,* 210: 335 – 341.

Allman, J.M., Miezin, F. and McGuiness, E. (1985) Stimulus specific responses from beyond the classical receptive field: Neurophysiological mechanisms for local-global comparisons in visual neurons. *Annu. Rev. Neurosci.,* 8: 407 – 430.

Barlow, H. (1981) Critical limiting factors in the design of the eye and visual cortex. *Proc. R. Soc. Lond. (Biol.),* 212: 1 – 34.

Bullier, J., Kennedy, H. and Salinger, W. (1984) Branching and laminar origin of projections between visual cortical areas in the cat. *J. Comp. Neurol.,* 228: 329 – 341.

Casagrande, V.A. and Harting, J.K. (1975) Transneuronal transport of tritiated fucose and proline in the visual system of the tree shrew. *Brain Res.,* 96: 367 – 372.

Cohen, J.L., Robinson, F., May, J. and Glickstein, M. (1981) Corticopontine projections of the lateral suprasylvian cortex: de-emphasis of the central visual field. *Brain Res.,* 219: 239 – 248.

Colonnier, M. (1968) Synaptic patterns on different cell types in the different laminae of the cat visual cortex. An electron microscope study. *Brain Res.,* 9: 268 – 287.

Curcio, C.A. and Harting, J.K. (1978) Organization of pulvinar afferents to area 18 in the squirrel monkey: evidence for stripes. *Brain Res.,* 143: 155 – 161.

DeYoe, E.A. and Van Essen, D.C. (1985) Segregation of efferent connections and receptive field properties in visual area V2 of the macaque. *Nature,* 317: 58 – 61.

Eysel, U.T. and Wörgötter, F. (1986) Specific cortical lesions abolish direction selectivity of visual cortical cells in the cat. *Neurosci. Abstr.,* 12: 583.

Ferster, D. (1986) Orientation selectivity of synaptic potentials in neurons of cat primary visual cortex. *J. Neurosci.,* 6: 1284 – 1301.

Ferster, D. (1987) Origin of orientation-selective EPSPs in simple cells of cat visual cortex. *J. Neurosci.,* 7: 1780 – 1791.

Finlay, B.L., Schiller, P.H. and Volman, S.F. (1976) Quantitative studies of single-cell properties in monkey striate cortex. IV. Corticotectal cells. *J. Neurophysiol.,* 39: 1352 – 1360.

Florence, S.L. and Casagrande, V.A. (1978) A note on the evolution of ocular dominance columns in primates. *Invest. Ophthalmol. Vis. Sci.,* 17: 291 – 292.

Freund, T.F., Martin, K.A.C., Smith, A.D. and Somogyi, P. (1983) Glutamate decarboxylase-immunoreactive terminals of Golgi-impregnated axoaxonic cells and of presumed basket cells in synaptic contact with pyramidal neurons of the cat's visual cortex. *J. Comp. Neurol.,* 221: 263 – 278.

Gabbott, P.L.A., Martin, K.A.C. and Whitteridge, D. (1987) Connections between pyramidal neurons in layer 5 of cat visual cortex (area 17). *J. Comp. Neurol.,* 259: 364 – 381.

Gilbert, C.D. (1977) Laminar differences in receptive field properties of cells in cat primary visual cortex. *J. Physiol.,* 268: 391 – 421.

Gilbert, C.D. (1985) Horizontal integration in the neocortex. *Trends Neurosci.,* 8: 160 – 165.

Gilbert, C.D. and Kelly, J.P. (1975) The projections of cells in different layers of the cat's visual cortex. *J. Comp. Neurol.,* 163: 81 – 106.

Gilbert, C.D. and Wiesel, T.N. (1979) Morphology and intracortical projections of functionally characterized neurones in the cat visual cortex. *Nature,* 280: 120 – 125.

Gilbert, C.D. and Wiesel, T.N. (1981) Projection bands in visual cortex. *Soc. Neurosci. Abstr.,* 7: 356.

Gilbert, C.D. and Wiesel, T.N. (1983) Clustered intrinsic connections in cat visual cortex. *J. Neurosci.,* 3: 1116 – 1133.

Gilbert, C.D. and Wiesel, T.N. (1985) Intrinsic connectivity and receptive field properties in visual cortex. *Vision Res.,* 25: 375 – 374.

Gilbert, C.D. and Wiesel, T.N. (1987) Relationships between cortico-cortical projections, intrinsic cortical connections and orientation columns in rat primary visual cortex. *Soc. Neurosci. Abstr.,* 13: 4.

Goodwin, A.W., Henry, G.H. and Bishop, P.O. (1975) Direction selectivity of simple striate cells: properties and mechanism. *J. Neurophysiol.,* 38: 1500 – 1523.

Gray, E.G. (1959) Axosomatic and axo-dendritic synapse of the cerebral cortex: an electron microscope study. *J. Anat. (Lond.),* 93: 420–434.

Hendrickson, A.E., Hunt, S.P. and Wu, J.-Y. (1981) Immunocytochemical localization of glutamic acid decarboxylase in monkey striate cortex. *Nature,* 292: 605–607.

Horton, J.C. (1984) Cytochrome oxidase patches: a new cytoarchitectonic feature of monkey visual cortex. *Phil. Trans. R. Soc. Lond. (Biol.),* 304: 199–253.

Horton, J.C. and Hubel, D.H. (1981) Regular patchy distribution of cytochrome-oxidase staining in primary visual cortex of macaque monkey. *Nature,* 292: 762–764.

Hubel, D.H. and Livingstone, M.S. (1985) Complex-unoriented cells in a subregion of primate area 18. *Nature,* 315: 325–327.

Hubel, D.H. and Livingstone, M.S. (1987) Segregation of form, color and stereopsis in primate area 18. *J. Neurosci.,* in press.

Hubel, D.H. and Wiesel, T.N. (1968) Receptive fields and functional architecture of monkey striate cortex. *J. Physiol. (Lond.),* 195: 215–243.

Hubel, D.H. and Wiesel, T.N. (1969) Visual area of the lateral suprasylvian gyrus (Clare-Bishop area) of the cat. *J. Physiol. (Lond.),* 202: 251–260.

Hubel, D.H. and Wiesel, T.N. (1974) Uniformity of monkey striate cortex: a parallel relationship between field size, scatter, and magnification factor. *J. Comp. Neurol.,* 158: 295–306.

Hubel, D.H., Wiesel, T.N. and LeVay, S. (1975) Functional architecture of area 17 in normal and monocularly deprived macaque monkeys. *Cold Spring Harbor Symp. Quant. Biol.,* 15: 581–589.

Humphrey, A.L. and Hendrickson, A.E. (1980) Radial zones of high metabolic activity in squirrel monkey striate cortex. *Neurosci. Abstr.,* 6: 315.

Humphrey, A.L. and Hendrickson, A.E. (1983) Background and stimulus-induced patterns of high metabolic activity in the visual cortex (area 17) of the squirrel and macaque monkey. *J. Neurosci.,* 3: 345–358.

Humphrey, A.L. and Norton, T.T. (1980) Topographic organization of the orientation column system in the striate cortex of the tree shrew *(Tupaia glis).* I. Microelectrode recording. *J. Comp. Neurol.,* 192: 531–548.

Humphrey, A.L., Skeen, L.C. and Norton, T.T. (1980) Topographic organization of the orientation column system in the striate cortex of the tree shrew *(Tupaia glis).* II. Deoxyglucose mapping. *J. Comp. Neurol.,* 192: 549–566.

Kaas, J.H., Hall, W.C., Killackey, H. and Diamond, I.T. (1972) Visual cortex of the tree shrew *(Tupaia glis):* architectonic subdivisions and representations of the visual field. *Brain Res.,* 42: 491–496.

Kato, H., Bishop, P.O. and Orban, G.A. (1978) Hypercomplex and simple/complex cell classifications in cat striate cortex. *J. Neurophysiol.,* 41: 1071–1095.

Katz, L.C., Burkhalter, A. and Dreyer, W.J. (1984) Fluorescent latex microspheres as a retrograde neuronal marker for in vivo and in vitro studies of visual cortex. *Nature,* 310: 498–500.

Lavie, V. and Hendrickson, A. (1986) Comparison between pre- and postembedding EM immunocytochemistry using antisera to GABA and GAD. *Neurosci. Abstr.,* 12: 128.

LeVay, S. (1973) Synaptic patterns in the visual cortex of the cat and monkey. Electron microscopy of Golgi preparations. *J. Comp. Neurol.,* 150: 53–86.

LeVay, S. (1988) Patchy intrinsic projections in visual cortex, area 18, of the cat: morphological and immunocytochemical evidence for an excitatory function. *J. Comp. Neurol.,* 269: 265–274.

LeVay, S. and Sherk, H. (1981) The visual claustrum of the cat. 1. Structure and connections. *J. Neurosci.,* 1: 956–980.

LeVay, S. and Sherk, H. (1983) Retrograde transport of [3H]proline: a widespread phenomenon in the central nervous system. *Brain Res.,* 271: 131–134.

LeVay, S., Stryker, M.P. and Shatz, C.J. (1978) Ocular dominance columns and their development in layer IV of the cat's visual cortex: a quantitative study. *J. Comp. Neurol.,* 179: 223–244.

LeVay, S., Wiesel, T.N. and Hubel, D.H. (1980) The development of ocular dominance columns in normal and visually deprived monkeys. *J. Comp. Neurol.,* 191: 1–51.

Livingstone, M.S. and Hubel, D.H. (1982) Thalamic inputs to cytochrome oxidase-rich regions in monkey visual cortex. *Proc. Natl. Acad. Sci. USA,* 79: 6098–6101.

Livingstone, M.S. and Hubel, D.H. (1984a) Anatomy and physiology of a color system in the primate visual cortex. *J. Neurosci.,* 4: 309–356.

Livingstone, M.S. and Hubel, D.H. (1984b) Specificity of intrinsic connections in primate primary visual cortex. *J. Neurosci.,* 4: 2830–2835.

Luhmann, H.J., Millan, L.M. and Singer, W. (1986) Development of horizontal intrinsic connections in cat striate cortex. *Exp. Brain Res.,* 63: 443–448.

Lund, J.S. (1973) Organization of neurons in the visual cortex, area 17, of the monkey *(Macaca mulatta). J. Comp. Neurol.,* 147: 455–496.

Maffei, L. and Fiorentini, A. (1976) The unresponsive regions of visual cortical receptive fields. *Vision Res.,* 16: 1131–1139.

Marin-Padilla, M. (1969) Origin of the pericellular baskets of the pyramidal cells of the human motor cortex: a Golgi study. *Brain Res.,* 14: 633–646.

Martin, K.A.C. (1984) Neuronal circuits in cat striate cortex. In: Jones, E.G. and Peters, A. (Eds.), *Cerebral Cortex,* Plenum Press, New York, pp. 241–284.

Martin, K.A.C. and Whitteridge, D. (1984) Form, function and intracortical projections of spiny neurones in the striate visual cortex of the cat. *J. Physiol.,* 353: 463–504.

Matsubara, J., Cynader, M., Swindale, N.V. and Stryker,

M.P. (1985) Intrinsic projections within visual cortex: evidence for orientation-specific local connections. *Proc. Natl. Acad. Sci. USA,* 82: 935 – 939.

Matsubara, J.A., Cynader, M.S. and Swindale, N.V. (1987) Anatomical properties and physiological correlates of the intrinsic connections in cat area 18. *J. Neurosci.,* 7: 1428 – 1446.

Maunsell, J.H.R. and van Essen, D.C. (1983) The connections of the middle temporal visual area (MT) and their relationship to a cortical hierarchy in the macaque monkey. *J. Neurosci.,* 3: 2563 – 2586.

McConnell, S.K. and LeVay, S. (1986) Anatomical organization of the visual system of the mink, *Mustela vision. J. Comp. Neurol.,* 250: 109 – 132.

McGuire, B.A., Hornung, J.-P., Gilbert, C.D. and Wiesel, T.N. (1984) Patterns of synaptic input to layer 4 of cat striate cortex. *J. Neurosci.,* 4: 3021 – 3033.

McGuire, B.A., Gilbert, C.D. and Wiesel, T.N. (1985) Ultrastructural characterization of long-range clustered horizontal connections in monkey striate cortex. *Neurosci. Abstr.,* 11: 17.

McIlwain, J.T. (1976) Large receptive fields and spatial transformation in the visual system. *Int. Rev. Physiol.,* 10: 223 – 248.

Meyer, G. (1983) Axonal patterns and topography of short-axon neurons in visual areas 17, 18 and 19 of the cat. *J. Comp. Neurol.,* 220: 405 – 438.

Michael, C.R. (1986) Functional and morphological identification of double and single opponent color cells in layer IVCb of the monkey's striate cortex. *Neurosci. Abstr.,* 12: 1497.

Michalski, A., Gerstein, G.L., Czarkowska, J. and Tarnecki, R. (1983) Interactions between cat striate cortex neurons. *Exp. Brain Res.,* 51: 97 – 107.

Mitchison, G. and Crick, F. (1982) Long axons within the striate cortex: their distribution, orientation, and patterns of connection. *Proc. Natl. Acad. Sci. USA,* 79: 3661 – 3665.

Montero, V.M. (1981) Topography of the cortico-cortical connections from the striate cortex in the cat. *Brain Behav.,* 18: 194 – 218.

Nelson, J.I. and Frost, B.J. (1978) Orientation-selective inhibition from beyond the classic visual receptive field. *Brain Res.,* 139: 359 – 365.

Nelson, J.I. and Frost, B.J. (1985) Intracortical facilitation among co-oriented, co-axially aligned simple cells in cat striate cortex. *Exp. Brain Res.,* 61: 54 – 61.

O'Leary, J.L. (1941) Structure of area striata of the cat. *J. Comp. Neurol.,* 75: 131 – 161.

Ohzawa, I., Sclar, G. and Freeman, R.D. (1985) Contrast gain control in the cat's visual system. *J. Neurophysiol.,* 54: 651 – 667.

Orban, G.A., Kato, H. and Bishop, P.O. (1979) Dimensions and properties of end-zone inhibitory areas in receptive fields of hypercomplex cells in cat striate cortex. *J. Neurophysiol.,* 42: 833 – 849.

Payne, B.R., Berman, N. and Murphy, E.H. (1980) Organization of direction preferences in cat visual cortex. *Brain Res.,* 211: 445 – 450.

Peters, A. and Fairen, A. (1978) Smooth and sparsely-spined stellate cells in the visual cortex of the rat: a study using a combined Golgi-electron microscope technique. *J. Comp. Neurol.,* 181: 129 – 172.

Peters, A. and Kimerer, L.M. (1981) Bipolar neurons in rat visual cortex. A combined Golgi-electron microscopic study. *J. Neurocytol.,* 10: 921 – 946.

Peters, A. and Regidor, J. (1981) A reassessment of the forms of nonpyramidal neurons in area 17 of cat visual cortex. *J. Comp. Neurol.,* 203: 685 – 716.

Price, D.J. (1986) The postnatal development of clustered intrinsic connections in area 18 of the visual cortex in kittens. *Dev. Brain Res.,* 24: 31 – 38.

Ribak, C.E. (1978) Aspinous and sparsely-spinous stellate neurons in the visual cortex of rats contain glutamic acid decarboxylase. *J. Neurocytol.,* 7: 461 – 478.

Rockland, K.S. (1985a) A reticular pattern of intrinsic connections in primate area V2 (area 18). *J. Comp. Neurol.,* 235: 467 – 478.

Rockland, K.S. (1985b) Anatomical organization of primary visual cortex (area 17) in the ferret. *J. Comp. Neurol.,* 241: 225 – 236.

Rockland, K.S. and Lund, J.S. (1982) Widespread periodic intrinsic connections in the tree shrew visual cortex. *Science,* 215: 1532 – 1534.

Rockland, K.S. and Lund, J.S. (1983) Intrinsic laminar lattice connections in primate visual cortex. *J. Comp. Neurol.,* 216: 303 – 318.

Rockland, K.S., Lund, J.S. and Humphrey, A.L. (1982) Anatomical banding of intrinsic connections in striate cortex of tree shrews *(Tupaia glis). J. Comp. Neurol.,* 209: 41 – 58.

Rockland, K.S. and Pandya, D.N. (1979) Laminar origins and terminations of cortical connections of the occipital lobe in rhesus monkey. *Brain Res.,* 179: 3 – 20.

Saint Marie, R.L. and Peters, A. (1985) The morphology and synaptic connections of spiny stellate neurons in monkey visual cortex (area 17): a Golgi-electron microscopy study. *J. Comp. Neurol.,* 233: 213 – 235.

Sclar, G. and Freeman, R.D. (1982) Orientation selectivity in the cat's striate cortex is invariant with stimulus contrast. *Exp. Brain Res.,* 46: 457 – 461.

Sesma, M.A., Casagrande, V.A. and Kaas, J.H. (1984) Cortical connections of area 17 in tree shrews. *J. Comp. Neurol.,* 230: 337 – 351.

Shatz, C.J. (1977) Anatomy of interhemispheric connections in the visual system of Boston Siamese and ordinary cats. *J. Comp. Neurol.,* 173: 497 – 518.

Shatz, C.J., Lindstrom, S. and Wiesel, T.N. (1977) The distribution of afferents representing the right and left eyes in the cat's visual cortex. *Brain Res.,* 131: 103 – 116.

Shatz, C.J. and Stryker, M.P. (1978) Ocular dominance in layer

IV of the cat's visual cortex and the effects of monocular deprivation. *J. Physiol. (Lond.),* 281: 267 – 283.

Sherk, H. (1986) Coincidence of patchy inputs from the lateral geniculate complex and area 17 to the cat's Clare-Bishop area. *J. Comp. Neurol.,* 253: 105 – 120.

Shipp, S. and Zeki, S. (1985) Segregation of pathways leading from area V2 to areas V4 and V5 of macaque monkey visual cortex. *Nature,* 315: 322 – 325.

Sillito, A.M. (1979) Inhibitory mechanisms influencing complex cell orientation selectivity and their modification at high resting discharge levels. *J. Physiol. (Lond.),* 289: 33 – 53.

Sillito, A.M., Kemp, J.A., Milson, J.A. and Bernardi, N. (1980) A re-evaluation of the mechanisms underlying simple cell orientation selectivity. *Brain Res.,* 194: 517 – 520.

Skottun, B.C., Bradley, A., Sclar, G., Ohzawa, I. and Freeman, R.D. (1987) The effects of contrast on visual orientation and spatial frequency discrimination: a comparison of single cells and behavior. *J. Neurophysiol.,* 57: 773 – 786.

Somogyi, P. (1977) A specific 'axo-axonal' interneuron in the visual cortex of the rat. *Brain Res.,* 136: 345 – 350.

Somogyi, P., Freund, T.F., Wu, J.-Y. and Smith, A.D. (1983a) The section-Golgi procedure. 2. Immunocytochemical demonstration of glutamate decarboxylase in Golgi-impregnated neurons and in their afferent synaptic boutons in the visual cortex of the cat. *Neuroscience,* 9: 475 – 490.

Somogyi, P., Kisvarday, Z.F., Martin, K.A.C. and Whitteridge, D. (1983b) Synaptic connections of morphologically identified and physiologically characterised large basket cells of the striate cortex of cat. *Neuroscience,* 10: 261 – 294.

Somogyi, P. and Hodgson, A.J. (1985) Antiserum to gamma-aminobutyric acid: III. Demonstration of GABA in Golgi-impregnated neurons and in conventional electron microscopic sections of cat striate cortex. *J. Histochem. Cytochem.,* 33: 249 – 257.

Spear, P.D. and Baumann, T.P. (1975) Receptive-field characteristics of single neurons in lateral suprasylvian visual area of the cat. *J. Neurophysiol.,* 38: 1403 – 1420.

Stryker, M.P. and Harris, W.A. (1986) Binocular impulse blockade prevents the formation of ocular dominance columns in cat visual cortex. *J. Neurosci.,* 6: 2117 – 2133.

Swindale, N.V., Matsubara, J.A. and Cynader, M.S. (1987) Surface organization of orientation and direction selectivity in cat area 18. *J. Neurosci.,* 7: 1414 – 1427.

Symonds, L.L. and Rosenquist, A.C. (1984) Corticocortical connections among visual areas in the cat. *J. Comp. Neurol.,* 229: 1 – 38.

Tanaka, K., Hikosaka, K., Saito, H., Yukie, M., Fukada, Y. and Iwai, E. (1986) Analysis of local and wide-field movements in the superior temporal visual areas of the macaque monkey. *J. Neurosci.,* 6: 134 – 144.

Tigges, J. and Tigges, M. (1979) Ocular dominance columns in the striate cortex of chimpanzee *(Pan troglodytes). Brain Res.,* 166: 386 – 390.

Tigges, J., Tigges, M., Anschel, S., Cross, N.A., Letbetter, W.D. and McBride, R.L. (1981) Areal and laminar distribution of neurons interconnecting the central visual cortical areas 17, 18, 19, and MT in squirrel monkey *(Saimiri). J. Comp. Neurol.,* 202: 539 – 560.

Tootell, R.B.H., Silverman, M.S., DeValois, R.L. and Jacobs, G.H. (1983) Functional organization of the second visual area in primates. *Science,* 220: 737 – 739.

Ts'o, D.Y., Gilbert, C.D. and Wiesel, T.N. (1986a) Relationships between horizontal interactions and functional architecture in cat striate cortex as revealed by cross-correlation analysis. *J. Neurosci.,* 6: 1160 – 1170.

Ts'o, D.Y., Gilbert, C.D. and Wiesel, T.N. (1986b) Relationships between color-specific cells in cytochrome oxidase-rich patches of monkey striate cortex. *Neurosci. Abstr.,* 12: 1497.

Tusa, R.J., Palmer, L.A. and Rosenquist, A.C. (1978) The retinotopic organization of area 17 (striate cortex) in the cat. *J. Comp. Neurol.,* 177: 213 – 236.

Van Essen, D.C., Newsome, W.T., Maunsell, J.H.R. and Bixby, J.L. (1986) The projections from striate cortex (V1) to areas V2 and V3 in the macaque monkey: asymmetries, areal boundaries, and patchy connections. *J. Comp. Neurol.,* 244: 451 – 480.

Vidyasagar, T.R. and Heide, W. (1986) The role of gabaergic inhibition in the response properties of neurones in cat visual area 18. *Neuroscience,* 17: 49 – 55.

Von der Heydt, R., Peterhans, E. and Baumgartner, G. (1984) Illusory contours and cortical neuron responses. *Science,* 224: 1260 – 1262.

Weber, J.T., Huerta, M.F., Kaas, J.H. and Harting, J.K. (1983) The projections of the lateral geniculate nucleus of the squirrel monkey: studies of the interlaminar zones and the S layers. *J. Comp. Neurol.,* 213: 135 – 145.

Wiesel, T.N., Hubel, D.H. and Lam, D.M.K. (1974) Autoradiographic demonstration of ocular-dominance columns in the monkey striate cortex by means of transneuronal transport. *Brain Res.,* 79: 273 – 279.

Wong-Riley, M.T.T. and Carroll, E.W. (1984) Quantitative light and electron microscopic analysis of cytochrome oxidase-rich zones in V-II prestriate cortex of the squirrel monkey. *J. Comp. Neurol.,* 222: 18 – 37.

Zeki, S.M. (1974) Functional organization of a visual area in the posterior bank of the superior temporal sulcus of the rhesus monkey. *J. Physiol.,* 236: 549 – 573.

Zeki, S. (1980) The representation of colours in the cerebral cortex. *Nature,* 284: 412 – 418.

T.P. Hicks and G. Benedek (Eds.)
Progress in Brain Research, Vol. 75
© 1988 Elsevier Science Publishers B.V. (Biomedical Division)

CHAPTER 15

Local, horizontal connections within area 18 of the cat

Joanne A. Matsubara

Department of Anatomy, Dalhousie University, Halifax, Nova Scotia B3H 4H7, Canada

Introduction

An intriguing feature of the neural circuitry in visual cortex is that many of the local connections are made among *groups* of neurons. This feature is clearly visible after making microinjections of tracers such as wheat germ agglutinin conjugated to horseradish peroxidase (WGA-HRP) or succinyl-concanavalin A (Con A). Such injections produce retrogradely labeled cells which are not uniformly distributed, but rather clustered into distinct 'patches' in the normal animal. The horizontal extent of the patchy connections is best seen when sections of tissue are cut in the tangential plane, roughly parallel to the cortical surface. Under these conditions, one can readily see that the patches occupy zones anterior, posterior, medial and lateral to the injection site. Most of the patches are located within 1.4 mm of the center of the injection, with an occasional patch positioned as far away as 3.4 mm. Even more intriguing is the finding that the patches are distributed periodically, exhibiting an interpatch spacing of about 1 mm. Since we know of at least 2 functional properties in visual cortex (preferred orientation of a line stimulus and ocular dominance), which are also organized periodically, each with a repeat spacing of about 1 mm, it was of interest to determine if the 'patchy' networks of interconnections correlate with particular aspects of cortical functional organization as revealed by electrophysiological recordings.

This paper reviews the anatomical properties and functional correlates of the horizontal connections in area 18 of the normal adult cat. Previous studies revealed that the preferred orientation of the majority of recording sites within the injected and labeled areas were different and, most frequently, orthogonal to each other (Cynader et al. 1987; Matsubara et al. 1987). This paper also reports findings from recent experiments in which WGA-HRP and γ-aminobutyric acid (GABA) were identified in the same neuron within the intrinsic patches. Although double-labeled cells were relatively rare among the population of HRP labeled neurons, their presence indicates that cross-column inhibition between areas in the different preferred orientations exists and may enhance orientation selectivity. Other circuits which may serve to sharpen orientation selectivity in visual cortex are also discussed.

Materials and methods

WGA-HRP and Con A injections

Microinjections of tracers were made into area 18 of normal adult cats. Two sensitive tracers were used in this study: wheat germ agglutinin conjugated to horseradish peroxidase (WGA-HRP, 1% or 0.5% in sterile saline) and succinyl-concanavalin A (Con A, 1% in sterile saline). We tried other tracers, such as rhodamine latex microspheres, but found them far less sensitive, resulting in fewer and weaker labeled neurons. In some cases, cortical maps of physiological response properties were first obtained before injec-

164

tions were made (see Materials and Methods in Matsubara et al. 1987). The total volume of the solution injected into the cortex was between 10 and 20 nl, as measured by observing the meniscus level of the micropipette before and after the injection. Following a survival time under anesthesia of 24 h, the animals were deeply anesthetized and perfused with phosphate buffer (0.1 M, pH 7.2 with 0.5% sodium nitrite), followed by 4% buffered paraformaldehyde and 0.1% glutaraldehyde and finally by 10% buffered sucrose. Blocks of tissue were cut in the horizontal plane, tangential to the surface of area 18.

Sections were processed for WGA-HRP using the standard tetramethylbenzidine (TMB) method (Mesulam 1978). Other sections were processed immunohistochemically to detect the Con A injection site and labeled neurons: after rinsing 3 times in phosphate-buffered saline (PBS, pH 7.3), the sections were incubated in a primary antibody made in rabbit against Con A (Sigma) for 18 – 24 h at room temperature. The optimal dilution of the antiserum was 1 : 40 000. The primary antiserum was tagged sequentially with biotinylated goat anti-rabbit antibody and aviden DH biotinylated HRP solution (VectaStain). The peroxidase label was then visualized with a red chromogen (carbazole) which was easily distinguishable from the black TMB reaction product.

Combined HRP and GABA immunohistochemistry

Sections processed for TMB were subsequently stabilized using the method of Horn and Hoffmann (1987). Briefly, sections were incubated in an ice-cooled solution of 5% ammonium heptamolybdate for 20 min and then further stabilized using the method of Rye et al. (1984). Next, sections were rinsed and placed into a solution of the primary antiserum made in rabbit against GABA (Immunonuclear Co.) for 18 – 24 h at room temperature. The optimal dilution of the antiserum was 1 : 1000. All incubation solutions contained 1% Triton X-100 and 1% normal goat serum. After incubation in the primary antibody against GABA, sections were processed as above using the Vecta-

Stain reagents (see immunohistochemistry for Con A). The peroxidase label was usually visualized with a diaminobenzidine (DAB) chromogen. Sections were incubated in a pre-soak solution containing 50 mg DAB, 200 mg dextrose and 40 mg ammonium chloride dissolved in 100 ml of phosphate buffer. After 20 min, 50 μl of a 1.2% glucose oxidase solution was added to every 0.5 ml of the pre-soak solution. The reaction was stopped by transferring the sections into phosphate buffer. Sections were then mounted onto gelatinized glass slides and air dried overnight. They were then dehydrated and coverslipped with DPX mounting medium. Using this method, HRP-labeled cells were identified by the presence of black granules in the cytoplasm, while the GABA-immunoreactive neurons were light brown in color. Double labeled neurons contained both black granules (HRP) as well as an opaque, light brown cytoplasmic stain (GABA).

Results

The intrinsic patches

Microinjections of WGA-HRP and Con A produced similar patterns of labeling consisting of retrogradely-filled cell bodies surrounded by a granular reaction product characteristic of anterograde and/or collateral transport (Fig. 1). The labeled cells were distinctly clustered into punctate patches in the normal animal. The majority of the patches were quasi-circular in outline, with a diameter of roughly 350 μm. The number of patches arising from a single injection ranged between 2 and 10 (mean 5.7, SD 2, $n = 15$). The mean value of 5.7 patches per injection site should be considered a minimal estimate of the number of intrinsic patches connected to a given cortical locus because the extent of labeling was, to some degree, dependent on the quality of the perfusion and subsequent histochemical reactions. Distant patches were more susceptible to fading than the ones closer to the injection site probably because there was less HRP or Con A in these cells.

Most of the patches were within 1.4 mm of the injection site center, with an occasional patch oc-

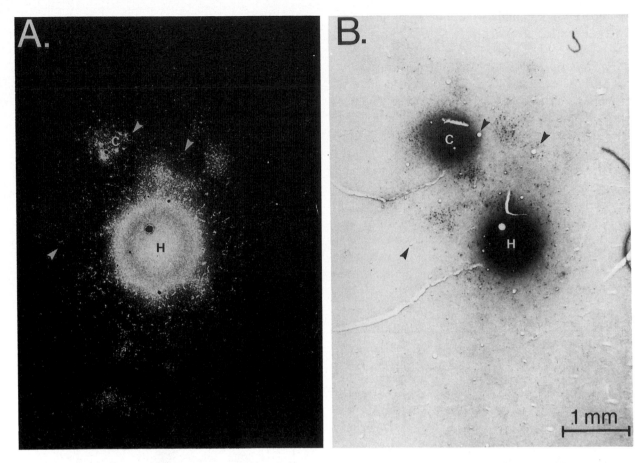

Fig. 1. Two photomicrographs illustrate the pattern of labeling resulting from the WGA-HRP (A, in dark-field) and Con A (B, in bright field) injection sites. The section on the right was reacted for both HRP and Con A in order to identify both injection sites (H, WGA-HRP; C, Con A) for alignment purposes. Cross-sections of selected blood vessels are marked for alignment purposes as well (arrowheads). Patches of Con A (in B) or WGA-HRP (in A) labeled neurons can be seen. The spacing between patches is about 1 mm.

curring as far away as 3.4 mm (Fig. 2). The patches were periodically distributed with an interpatch spacing of about 1 mm. The extent of labeling was greater along the anterior-posterior (AP) rather than the medial-lateral (ML) cortical axis. Moreover, along this axis, the labeling was usually more extensive in the posterior than the anterior direction. Sections of tissue cut in the coronal plane revealed labeled cells in vertical columns running through all 6 cortical layers. The patches appear as vertical strips of label. The width of the patches varied slightly from lamina to lamina, but on average, measured about 350 μm. Within each

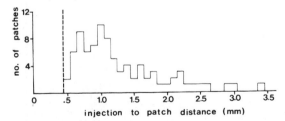

Fig. 2. Histogram illustrating the distance between the center of the injection site and each labeled patch from 11 injections. The dashed line at the far left indicates the zone in which we were unable to identify labeled neurons because of the intense reaction product within the core and halo of the injection site itself. Although most of the intrinsic patches occur within 1.4 mm of the injection site, there are rare patches as far away as 3.4 mm from the injection site.

patch, both pyramidal and non-pyramidal cells were labeled (Fig. 3).

Functional properties of the intrinsic patches

In those experiments in which cortical maps of functional properties were made prior to the injection of the tracers, we compared the pattern and positions of the intrinsic patches to the surface organization of the following receptive field properties: eye preference, receptive field location and preferred orientation. We were unable to detect any relationship between the eye preference of the injected and labeled cell regions. Injections into areas predominantly driven by the contralateral eye resulted in labeled regions exhibiting varied eye preference distributions. In some animals they were like the injection site and in others there were equal numbers of contralateral and ipsilateral eye-dominated regions. The overall distribution of the patches around the injection site was elongated along the A-P cortical axis and since the cortical magnification factor is greatest along this same axis, it appears that the elongation in the distribution of the patches effectively compensates for the functional asymmetry in the magnification factor, so that a population of connected cells represents a roughly circular region of visual space.

Unlike eye preference, we did find a significant relationship between the preferred orientation of the injected and labeled regions. The preferred orientations of most, but not all, of the recording sites within the injected and labeled areas were dif-

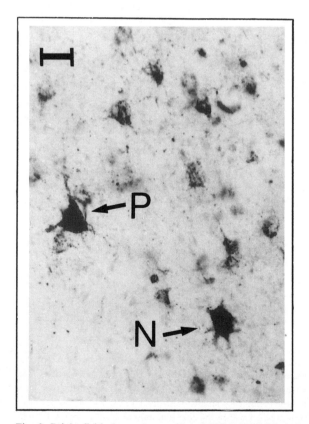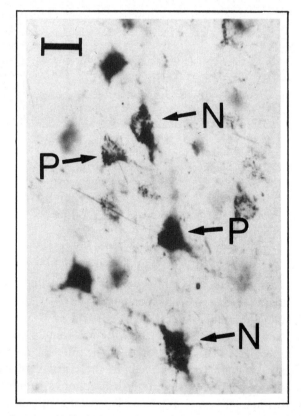

Fig. 3. Bright-field photomicrographs of WGA-HRP labeled neurons from two intrinsic patches in area 18. Coronal sections were processed using the TMB method and were not counterstained. Pyramidal cells (P) and non-pyramidal forms (N) were seen in the patches. Scale bars indicate 15 μm.

ferent and, most frequently, orthogonal to each other. This was a highly specific projection, since regions with orientation values like those of the injection site were 'within range', yet not labeled. The orientation values of the injection site, labeled areas and surrounding nonlabeled areas are shown in the circular polar graphs in Fig. 4. They illustrate that most of the preferred orientations within the labeled areas are different from those of the injection site. This result is also evident from the histograms below the circular graph. The angular difference between the mean of the injection sample ($|\bar{\gamma}_{inj}|$) and the individual preferred orientations within the injection site ($|\bar{\gamma}_{inj} - \gamma|$) are shown on the far left. The normalized difference represents the degree of spread in the preferred orientation values within the injection zone. Notice that the overall spread of the injection site does not exceed ± 27 degrees. The middle histogram illustrates the angular difference between the mean orientation value of the injected area and the individual preferred orientations of the labeled regions ($|\bar{\gamma}_{inj} - \beta|$). This histogram clearly illustrates that the preferred orientations of the labeled areas are not only different from those of the injection site but tend to encompass those orientations representing the larger difference values as well. The angular difference between the mean preferred orientation of the injected and labeled region in 43SPC is 63 degrees.

The specificity of the connections in 43SPC is apparent upon analysis of the preferred orientations within the control area (i.e., a circular area surrounding and exclusive of the injection site, whose radius is defined as the maximum distance between the center of the injection and the most distant patch of labeling). The circular polar graph on the far right ('control' in Fig. 4) shows that all preferred orientations, including ones like those in the injection site, were present in the control region. This fact is, again, evident in the histogram below the polar graph, which identifies the normalized difference angles between the mean orientation of the injection site and the individual preferred orientation within the control area

($|\bar{\gamma}_{inj} - \alpha|$). The control histogram indicates that regions with orientations like those found in the injection site were 'within range' of the injection site. In spite of this, however, we found very few

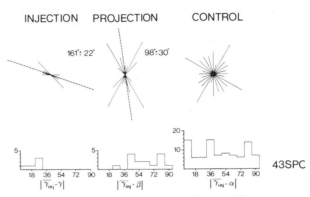

Fig. 4. Individual orientation values of the injection site, labeled areas (projection) and surrounding nonlabeled areas (control) are shown in polar coordinates. The mean preferred orientation of the injected area was 161° ($\pm 22°$) and is indicated by the dashed line. The mean orientation value of the labeled regions was 98° ($\pm 30°$). Note that most of the preferred orientations within the labeled regions are different from those in the injection site. The specificity of this connection is evident from the polar graph on the far right, which illustrates the preferred orientations within the surrounding control areas. The control area is defined as a circular area (surrounding and exclusive of the injection site) whose radius is the distance between the center of the injection and the most distant patch of labeling. Note all orientations, including ones like those in the injected areas, were present and 'within range' of the injection site. The normalized angular difference values are shown below the circular polar graphs. These histograms indicate the difference between the mean preferred orientation of the injected areas ($|\bar{\gamma}_{inj} = 161°|$) and the individual orientations of the injected ($|\bar{\gamma}_{inj} - \gamma|$), labeled ($|\bar{\gamma}_{inj} - \beta|$), and control ($|\bar{\gamma}_{inj} - \alpha|$) regions. The histogram of the normalized angular difference of the orientations in the injection site represents the degree of spread in the preferred orientation values within the injection zone. Note that the overall spread of the injection does not exceed $\pm 27°$. The middle histogram illustrates the normalized angular difference between the injected and labeled regions. This histogram clearly indicates that the preferred orientation of the labeled areas are not only different from those of the injection site, but tend to encompass those orientations representing the larger difference values. The difference between the mean of the injected and the mean of the labeled regions is 63°. The histogram on the far right indicates that all orientations, including ones like those in the injected area (i.e., with difference values near 0) were present and 'within range' of the injection site.

regions with 'like' orientation preference labeled.

These results lead us to speculate that inhibition between areas with different preferred orientations, might sharpen orientation selectivity by narrowing the range of stimulus orientations that excite a given cortical cell. Results from experiments in which sections of tissue were cut in the coronal plane (see Fig. 3) indicated that some of the labeled neurons comprising the intrinsic patches were non-pyramidal, and thus, possible candidates for GABAergic, inhibitory interneurons. Direct proof of the existence of inhibitory neurons within the intrinsic patches is presented in the next section.

Double-labeled neurons within the intrinsic patches

Combining HRP histochemistry with GABA-immunocytochemistry allowed us to answer, directly, the question of how many, if any, of the cells within the intrinsic patches were GABA-immunoreactive. Preliminary results in which both HRP and GABA have been localized to individual neurons within the intrinsic patches in area 18 are shown in Fig. 5. The edge of an WGA-HRP injection site can be seen in the top corner of panels A and B. Curved arrows point to double-labeled neurons, each containing black granules (HRP reaction product) and an opaque, brown cytoplasmic stain (GABA reaction product). The curved arrow with asterisk in panels C and D points to the same double labeled cell photographed at different focal planes. The straight, single arrows point to GABA-positive neurons while the double arrows point to four neurons which contained only black granules indicative of HRP labeling. Thus, these results indicate that GABA-positive (hence, presumably, inhibitory) neurons participate in the patchy, local connections in area 18. Our data suggest that the number of these presumed basket cells, is, however, relatively low in comparison to the pyramidal neurons which are found in abundance within the patches.

Discussion

Results from combined electrophysiological mapping and tracing studies indicate that the majority of the interconnections in area 18 are between regions of different preferred orientations. Our studies also revealed that, in addition, a small subset of the interconnections are between regions with similar preferred orientations. This can be seen in the cumulative histogram in Fig. 6 which shows the normalized difference angles between the mean orientation of the injection site and the individual orientation values of the injected, labeled and control regions from 7 injections. Notice that there is a small degree of overlap between the orientation range of the injected areas and the normalized difference angle between the injected and labeled regions. It is difficult to know at this time whether this subset of our data represents a connection between cells with similar preferred orientations or merely reflects a smearing in the results due perhaps to connections between broadly tuned neurons or to an effective injection site that has a larger spread than the one observed histologically. However, the vast majority of the interconnected regions exhibit different preferred orientations. Circuitry of this type may serve to enhance orientation selectivity if the overall effect of such a circuit is one of inhibition between cells with different preferred orientation biases and overlapping orientation ranges.

Perhaps the best evidence in favor of such a circuit comes from neuropharmacological studies in which local administration of bicuculline, a GABA antagonist, at the recording site causes a reversible loss of orientation selectivity (Sillito 1975; Tsumoto et al. 1979; Sillito et al. 1980). Recent, preliminary studies in which GABA, itself, is administered iontophoretically also suggest that orientation selectivity is enhanced by cross-column inhibition. In these studies, the administration of GABA at a locus lateral to the recording site caused a reduction in the orientation tuning of neurons at that recording site (Worgotter and Eysel 1987). These results indicated that orientation selectivity was affected only when GABA was injected approx. 500 μm to 1 mm from the recording electrode. There was less of an effect in the orientation

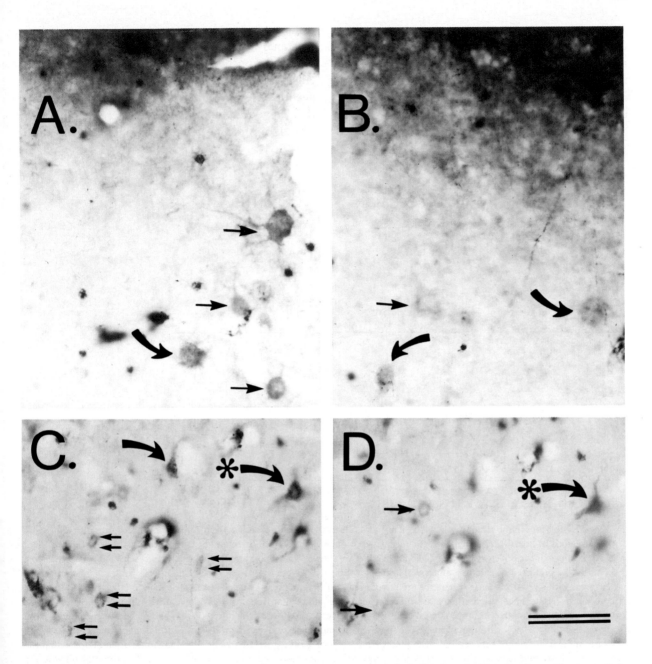

Fig. 5. Photomicrographs of horizontal sections processed for WGA-HRP and GABA immunohistochemistry. Portions of the WGA-HRP injection site are visible in the top corner of panels A and B. GABA-immunoreactive neurons were identified by the light, opaque brown cytoplasmic stain (single arrows in A, B and D). WGA-HRP labeled neurons were distinguished by the presence of black granules in the cytoplasm (double arrows in C). Double labeled neurons possess both an opaque light brown stain (GABA) and black granules (WGA-HRP). Three double labeled neurons are illustrated in A and B (curved arrows). Panels C and D were taken at different focal planes through the same section of tissue and illustrate a single patch of labeled cells approx. 1 mm from the injectoin site center. The curved arrow with asterisk points to the same double labeled cell. Scale bar indicates 100 μm.

tuning of neurons at the recording site when GABA was delivered at distances of 1 mm or more, suggesting that individual patches at varying distances from a given locus may play different roles in cortical processing. Nearest patches or cortical zones may enhance orientation tuning while more distant patches may mediate changes in other response properties. These possibilities await further analysis.

Other approaches have been taken towards elucidating the functional role of the patchy connections. Recent fine structural studies have shown that the pyramidal cells with clustered axonal collaterals primarily make synaptic contact onto

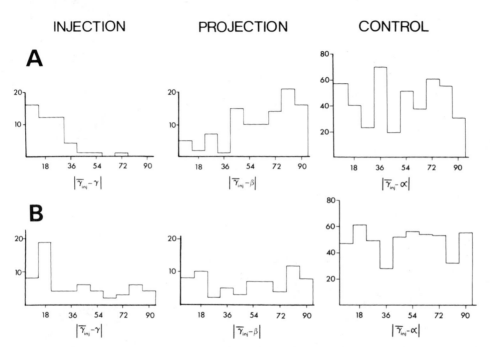

Fig. 6. (A) Histograms in the same format as those in Fig. 4, illustrating results obtained from 7 injections placed into physiologically identified regions of area 18. The angular difference between the mean preferred orientation of the injection site and the individual orientation values of the injected, labeled, and control areas are shown. The histogram on the far left (injection) indicates the degree of spread in the preferred orientation values within the injection zone. Note that, as in Fig. 4, the injection sites were confined to cortical areas with a relatively narrow range of preferred orientation values (i.e., ±30°). The middle histogram illustrates the angular difference between the mean orientation value of the injected area and the individual orientation values of the labeled regions. Most of the preferred orientations within the labeled areas were different from those of the injected areas and tended to encompass those values representing the large difference values. The specificity of the connection is evident from the histogram on the far right, which shows the angular difference between the mean preferred orientation of the injected area and the individual orientations within the control areas. Note that regions 'within range' of the injection site possessed preferred orientation values like those of the injected areas (i.e., with difference values near 0°). Yet relatively few areas exhibiting orientations like those of the injection site were labeled. (B) Cumulative histograms obtained from 5 injections placed into regions possessing a wide range of preferred orientation values. As in A, the cumulative angular difference between the mean preferred orientation of each injected region and the individual orientation value of the injected, labeled, and control areas are presented. The normalized difference angles of the injected regions are distributed more uniformly than in A, indicating that the range of preferred orientation values in the injected zone was broad. The middle histogram illustrates the normalized angular difference between the injected and labeled regions. In contrast to A, this histogram indicates that more preferred orientation values representing the smaller difference angles were labeled after injections. Presumably the connections were to areas with different preferred orientations, but because the injected zone includes a more complete range of orientations, the labeled areas also include a relatively complete range of values.

spines of other pyramidal cells and only rarely make contact with the dendritic shafts of GABA-immunoreactive neurons (Kisvarday et al. 1986; LeVay 1987). Thus, these fine structural studies indicate that the patchy connections are made predominantly by pyramidal cells onto other pyramidal cells. Results of Kisvarday et al. (1986) and LeVay (1987) at first glance appear inconsistent with our findings reviewed here. If connections between regions with different preferred orientations are made exclusively by pyramidal cells (hence, presumably excitatory) onto other pyramidal cells, then orientation selectivity should be broadened and not sharpened. How can we reconcile these differences? It is more than likely that cross-column inhibition between regions with different preferred orientations occurs by a multisynaptic network. Thus, long-range pyramidal cells, perhaps due to developmental biases, may project preferentially to other pyramidal cells which, in turn, may synapse upon inhibitory interneurons which then sharpen orientation tuning of nearby neurons within their own cortical column. Under such conditions, one might expect to find within a given vertical, orientation column, a small population of cells (i.e., the inhibitory interneurons and some pyramidal cells) which are tuned to non-optimal orientations. Lee et al. (1977) and more recently Murphy and Sillito (1986) have reported such findings. Recordings made from perpendicular penetrations in area 17 of the cat showed that a small population of cells, encountered occasionally in all cortical laminae, exhibited orientation preferences that differed markedly from the basic columnar unit.

Finally, as was shown in this study and in others (Martin et al. 1983), GABA-positive neurons with horizontally-directed axons (presumptive basket cells) are also present in the intrinsic patches and likely mediate cross-columnar, monosynaptic inhibition between regions with different preferred orientations. Fine structural studies by Kisvarday et al. (1986) indicate that basket cells make synaptic contact primarily with the apical dendrites of nearby pyramidal cells. Furthermore, each basket cell influences several hundred neurons and there is a convergence of 10–30 basket cells onto a postsynaptic target. Together, these studies suggest that basket cells are strategically positioned to inhibit all excitatory inputs (including those from cells in the same intrinsic patch as the basket cell) which converge onto apical dendrites of pyramidal cells.

References

Cynader, M.S., Swindale, N.V. and Matsubara, J.A. (1987) Functional topography in cat area 18. *J. Neurosci.,* 7: 1401–1413.

Horn, A.K.E. and Hoffmann, K.P. (1987) Combined GABA-immunocytochemistry and TMB-HRP histochemistry of pretectal nuclei projecting to the inferior olive in rats, cats and monkeys. *Brain Res.,* 409: 133–138.

Kisvarday, Z.F., Martin, K.A.C., Freund, T.F., Magloczky, Z.S., Whitteridge, D. and Somogyi, P. (1986) Synaptic targets of HRP-filled layer III pyramidal cells in the cat striate cortex. *Exp. Brain Res.,* 64: 541–552.

Lee, B.B., Albus, K., Heggelund, P., Holme, M.J. and Creutzfeldt, O.D. (1977) The depth distribution of optimal stimulus orientations for neurons in cat area 17. *Exp. Brain Res.,* 27: 301–314.

LeVay, S. (1987) Fine structure of patchy intrinsic projections of cat area 18. *Abstract Extrageniculo-striate Visual Mechanisms Symposium of IBRO.*

Martin, K.A.C., Somogyi, P. and Whitteridge, D. (1983) Physiological and morphological properties of identified basket cells in the cat's visual cortex. *Exp. Brain Res.,* 50: 193–200.

Matsubara, J.A., Cynader, M.S. and Swindale, N.V. (1987) Anatomical properties and physiological correlates of the intrinsic connections in cat area 18. *J. Neurosci.,* 7: 1428–1446.

Mesulam, M.M. (1978) Tetramethylbenzidine for horseradish peroxidase neurochemistry. *J. Histochem. Cytochem.,* 26: 106–117.

Murphy, P.C. and Sillito, A.M. (1986) Continuity of orientation columns between superficial and deep laminae of the cat primary visual cortex. *J. Physiol.,* 381: 95–110.

Rye, D.B., Saper, C.B. and Wainer, B.H. (1984) Stabilizing of the tetramethylbenzidine (TMB) reaction product: application for retrograde and anterograde, tracing and combination with immunocytochemistry. *J. Histochem. Cytochem.,* 32: 1145–1153.

Sillito, A.M. (1975) The contribution of inhibitory mechanisms to the receptive field properties of neurons in the striate cortex of the cat. *J. Physiol. (Lond.),* 250: 305–329.

172

Sillito, A.M., Kemp, J.A., Milson, J.A. and Berardi, M. (1980) A re-evaluation of the mechanisms underlying simple cell orientation selectivity. *Brain Res.,* 194: 517 – 520.

Tsumoto, T., Eckart, W. and Creutzfeldt, O.D. (1979) Modification of orientation sensitivity of cat visual cortex neurons by removal of GABA-mediated inhibition. *Exp.* *Brain Res.,* 34: 351 – 363.

Wortgotter, F. and Eysel, U.T. (1987) Changes in direction and orientation tuning of visual cortical cells determined by fast fourier analysis: a zone model of inhibitory convergence. *IBRO abstract* #1308.

T.P. Hicks and G. Benedek (Eds.)
Progress in Brain Research, Vol. 75
© 1988 Elsevier Science Publishers B.V. (Biomedical Division)

CHAPTER 16

Role of visual areas 17 and 18 of the cat in pattern vision

S. Bisti

Istituto di Neurofisiologia del C.N.R., Pisa, Italy

During the past two decades the performance of the visual system in analyzing spatial patterns has been widely studied in both man and other mammals. A convenient way used to describe the spatial characteristics of the visual system was to determine its contrast sensitivity function.

It is now widely accepted that every visual scene observed in good light with the resting eye is seen through a spatial frequency window. However, vision is a dynamic process resulting from a continuous interaction between spatial and temporal characteristics of a visual scene and, whenever the objects or the eyes move, the visual band pass is altered. It was reported that, in both man and other animals, the detectability of gratings at low spatial frequencies is enhanced by movement or temporal modulation of the visual stimulus (Kulikowski and Tolhurst 1973; Tolhurst 1973; Blake and Camisa 1977).

However, recent results (Burr and Ross 1982) have shown that the perceptual effect of image motion is more complex: contrast sensitivity functions measured either with stationary gratings or with gratings drifted at different speeds have the same peak sensitivity and bandwidth. What changes with drift speed is the position of the curves on the spatial frequency axis. The higher the velocity, the lower the spatial frequency at which the curves peak (Fig. 1).

In this paper, I will discuss the possible neurophysiological correlate in the cat of these psychophysical results. Recent results obtained by recording single units at the level of cortical areas 17 and 18 (Bisti et al. 1985) support the hypothesis according to which area 17 processes patterns in stationary or quasi-stationary situations while area 18 processes patterns moving at high velocities. In addition, I will present evidence of the possible role of the Y system in the perception of patterns during movement.

Spatio-temporal properties of neurones of area 17

The neurones of area 17 are very selective for different parameters of the visual stimulus such as orientation, direction of movement (Hubel and Wiesel 1962) and spatial frequency (see for reference, Maffei 1978). When stimulated with sinusoidal drifting or alternating gratings, each neurone responds to a narrow range of frequencies and this selectivity is little affected by changing the temporal frequency of the stimulus (Tolhurst and Movshon 1975; Bisti et al. 1985). As shown in Fig. 2 for 3 simple and 3 complex cells, the spatial frequency tuning curves remain rather similar when either the temporal frequency (the number of cycles of the grating which pass any point of the screen in a given time) (Fig. 2A,B) or the velocity

Correspondence to: Dr. Silvia Bisti, Istituto di Neurofisiologia del C.N.R., Via S. Zeno, 51, 56100 Pisa, Italy.

(Fig. 2C,D) or the rate of alternation (Fig. 2E,F) is increased. The only detectable effect is on the responsiveness of the cell.

Therefore it seems possible to conclude that, when the temporal properties of the stimulus are changed, the spatial tuning curves of striate neurones remain largely invariant showing only a shift along the amplitude axis.

Spatio-temporal properties of neurones of area 18

Neurones of area 18 respond selectively to a narrow range of spatial frequencies (Movshon et al. 1978; Berardi et al. 1982). At variance with the properties of neurones of area 17 their spatial frequency tuning curves are changed dramatically when the temporal characteristics of the drifting grating are changed (Bisti et al. 1985). It is easily

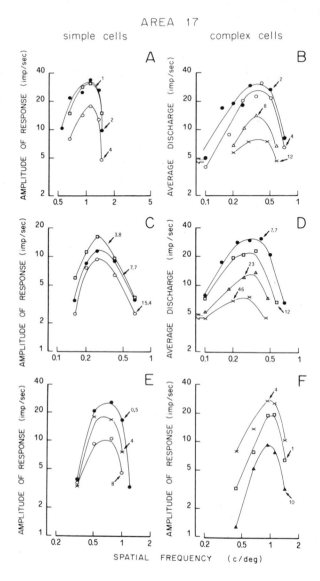

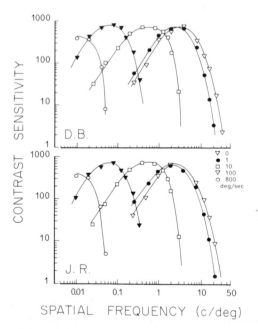

Fig. 1. Contrast sensitivity curves for 2 observers for sinusoidal gratings drifting at various speeds. On the abscissa is reported the spatial frequency of the gratings and on the ordinate the contrast sensitivity. Different symbols indicate different drift speeds. Note that at all drift speeds, the curve has the same height, width and general shape. (Redrawn from Burr and Ross 1982.)

Fig. 2. Spatial frequency tuning curves for 3 simple and 3 complex cells of area 17 for drifting and alternating gratings. When the stimulus was a drifting grating, amplitude of modulation (peak-to-trough) for simple cells and average discharge for complex cells were reported as a function of spatial frequency. A and B, stimulus: grating drifting at constant temporal frequency. Temporal frequency: □, 1 Hz; ●, 2 Hz; ○, 4 Hz; △, 8 Hz; ×, 12 Hz. Contrast 0.1 (A), 0.25 (B). C and D, stimulus: grating drifting at constant velocity. Velocity: □, 3.8 deg/sec; ●, 7.7 deg/sec; □, 12 deg/sec; ○, 15.4 deg/sec; △, 23 deg/sec; ×, 46 deg/sec. Contrast 0.1 (C), 0.25 (D). E and F, the contrast of the grating was sinusoidally modulated in time at constant temporal frequency. For simple cells amplitude of the modula-

noted that the complex cell in Fig. 3 becomes responsive to a different range of spatial frequencies upon changing of the velocity of the drifting gratings. The spatial selectivity of this neurone moves towards lower spatial frequencies when the stimulus velocity is increased. All neurones of area 18 show a similar behaviour.

An interesting point is that the shift of the tuning curves along the spatial frequency axis is strictly related to the motion of the visual stimulus. If the same temporal variations as those obtained with a drifting grating are produced by alternating a stationary grating in phase, no shift in the spatial frequency tuning curve is observed and the cell behaves very much like a neurone recorded from

area 17. As shown in Fig. 4, different drift velocities cause a shift of the spatial frequency tuning curve of a complex cell along the x-axis (Fig. 4A), whereas three different rates of grating alternation simply cause a reduction in the amplitude of

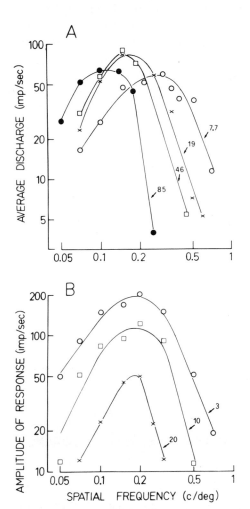

Fig. 4. Spatial frequency tuning curves of a complex cell of area 18. Each curve in (A) is obtained with drifting gratings of constant velocity. Numbers in the figure indicate the velocities in deg/sec. Velocity: ○, 7.7 deg/sec; ×, 1,9 deg/sec; □, 46 deg/sec; ●, 85 deg/sec. Spontaneous firing rate 0.2 impulses/sec. Each curve in (B) is obtained with square-wave gratings alternated at constant temporal frequency. The second harmonic of the cell discharge is reported as a function of the spatial frequency. Numbers in the Figure indicate the temporal frequencies in Hz. Temporal frequency: ○, 3 Hz; □, 10 Hz; ×, 20 Hz. Contrast, 0.17. Mean luminance, 7 cd/m². (Redrawn from Bisti et al. 1984b, 1985.)

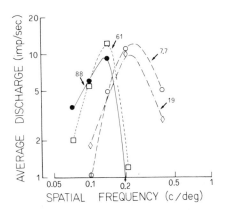

Fig. 3. Spatial-frequency tuning curves of a complex cell of area 18. Each curve is obtained with drifting gratings of constant velocity. Numbers in the Figure indicate the velocities in deg/sec. Velocity: ○, 7.7 deg/sec; ◇, 19 deg/sec; □, 61 deg/sec; ●, 88 deg/sec. Spontaneous firing rate, 0.2 impulses/sec. Contrast, 0.4. Mean luminance, 7 cd/m² (Redrawn from Bisti et al. 1985).

(Fig. 2, continued)

tion and for complex cells amplitude of the second harmonic component were reported as a function of spatial frequency. Temporal frequency: ●, 0.5 Hz; □, 1 Hz; ×, 4 Hz; ○, 8 Hz; ▲, 10 Hz. Contrast 0.1 (E), 0.1 (F). Mean luminance in all cases 7 cd/m². In B and D the arrows on the ordinate axis indicate the spontaneous firing rate of the cells. (From Bisti et al. 1985.)

the response (Fig. 4B). This peculiar characteristic of area 18 neurones in their response to visual stimuli is not only made evident by using periodic stimuli such as sinusoidal gratings, but it holds true even with aperiodic stimuli such as bars (Bisti et al. 1984a). Single neurones respond to a large variety of bar widths, and for each size the response is obtained only in a limited range of drifting velocities. The larger the bar, the higher the drift velocity has to be in order to elicit an optimal response from the cell (Fig. 5).

Taken together, these results seem to indicate that the spatial properties of area 18 neurones are strongly dependent upon the velocity of the visual stimulus, whereas for area 17 neurones the spatial properties are independent from either the velocity or the temporal characteristics of the visual stimulus. Several authors (for reference, see Orban 1984) have already suggested a dichotomy of function between visual areas 17 and 18. Area 17 would

be involved in pattern detection and area 18 in movement detection. Bisti et al. (1985) suggested a complementary role for the two visual areas in pattern analysis. Both area 17 and 18 would be involved in pattern analysis, the former in a stationary or semi-stationary situation and the latter during motion. Area 18 neurones would simply take over the task of area 17 neurones for high velocities of pattern movement, when area 17 neurones are no longer able to respond. The shift of the spatial frequency characteristics with velocity could be a way by which a given number of neurones cope with a large variety of stimuli at different velocities.

Responses of area 17 and 18 neurones to the harmonics of a complex stimulus

Several years ago Maffei et al. (1979) reported that simple cells of area 17 can detect the harmonics of a luminance gradient rather than the luminance

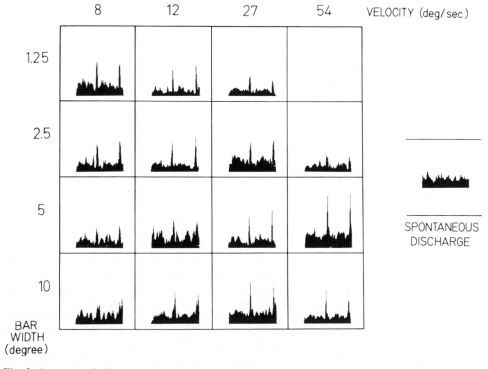

Fig. 5. Average peristimulus time histogram of the response of a complex cell to bars of different width drifting at different velocities. Records in each row are responses to bars of the same width drifted at different velocities. Records in each column are responses to bars of different width drifted at the same velocity. (Bisti, Galli, Maffei, unpublished data.)

difference in the gradient. As shown in Fig. 6, the response of the cell is very similar whether the stimulus is a sinusoidal or a square wave grating of the same contrast. However, when the visual stimulus consists of a grating in which the fundamental is missing (square wave grating minus the fundamental) the cell does not fire even if the stimulus has, to the human observer, contours. This is true provided that the stimulus does not contain the fundamental harmonic component to which the cell is tuned.

We tested the question of whether or not area 18 neurones are more sensitive to the harmonics of the stimulus rather than to contours. The results of the experiment are reported in Fig. 7 (Bisti, Galli, and Maffei, unpublished data). We first determined two spatial frequency tuning curves of a simple-like cell for two different drift velocities. Then we chose as a stimulus a square wave grating of spatial frequency (0.05 cycles/deg) near to the peak of sensitivity for a drifting velocity of 77 deg/sec; the third harmonic of such a grating (0.15 cycles/deg) is near to the peak of sensitivity for a drifting velocity of 26 deg/sec. The contrast of the stimulus was set to keep the third harmonic (the amplitude of which is 3 times lower than that of the fundamental) supra-threshold. The grating was then drifted at 77 deg/sec, at which velocity the cell responded mainly to the fundamental component of the stimulus. As soon as the velocity of the grating was decreased the cell response showed an increase in the third harmonic component with a decrease of the fundamental (compare Fig. 7D and E). At a lower velocity the cell became tuned to high spatial frequencies (Fig. 7A), making possible its response to the third harmonic.

Projections to area 18 and effects of monocular deprivation

Area 18 of the cat receives robust projections from multiple sources (Wilson 1968; Kawamura 1973; Abramson and Chalupa 1985; Freund et al. 1985a,b; Humphrey et al. 1985) and the interaction of all these inputs could account for the spatio-temporal properties of area 18 neurones. An input to cortical neurones which deserves a special interest is represented by the direct projections from Y cells of the dorsal lateral geniculate. The terminal axons of Y cells in area 18 arborize for several millimeters and often terminate in two to three separate clumps (Humphrey et al. 1985) indicating that each neuron of area 18 may receive converging inputs from a relatively wide retino-

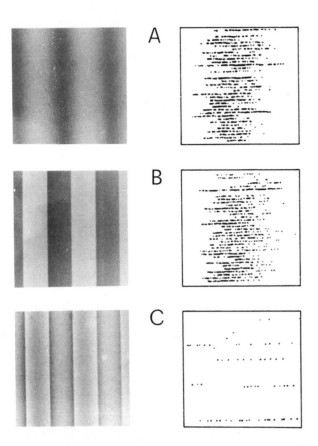

Fig. 6. Responses of a simple cell to drifting gratings of different profile but of the same periodicity. The periodicity of the grating was that for which the cell gave maximal responses: 0.5 cycle/deg with a velocity of 2.7 deg/sec, contrast 0.15 for the sinusoidal grating and 0.118 for the square-wave grating and average luminance 5 cd/m². On the left, visual stimuli are illustrated: sinusoidal, square-wave and missing fundamental gratings. The missing-fundamental grating (C) is obtained by subtraction of the fundamental harmonic (in A) from the square-wave grating (in B). Each dot in the responses reported on the right is a nervous impulse. Each row of dots is the response to a period of the grating. (From Maffei et al. 1979.)

topic region of the LGN. Different velocities of the visual stimulus may activate different populations of Y cells and this could subserve the mechanism of the shift of the tuning curves as a function of the drifting velocity.

Monocular deprivation in kittens is known to alter the pattern of cortical arborizations of Y cells in area 18 from both the normal and the deprived laminae of the LGN (Friedlander et al. 1986). While there is a shrinkage in the axonal arborizations of the deprived Y cells, there is an expansion of axonal arborization of the normal neurones. If the Y input is involved in the mechanism of the shift of tuning curves at varying velocities, an alteration of such a mechanism may be expected in neurones recorded in a cat which had one eye sutured during the critical period of postnatal development. Experiments are now in progress to test this hypothesis. Preliminary results (Bisti and Trimarchi, unpublished results) show that in monocularly deprived cats the spatial frequency tuning curves do not shift along the spatial frequency axis with increases of the velocity of the visual stimulus and this is true for neurones driven from either the deprived or the normal eye.

Behavioural experiments in monocularly deprived cats are under way to check if and to what extent the perception of moving objects is altered.

Acknowledgments

I wish to thank Prof. L. Maffei and Dr. L. Galli for helpful discussions and critical reading of the manuscript.

References

Abramson, B.P. and Chalupa, L.M. (1985) The laminar distribution of cortical connections with the tecto- and cortico-recipient zones in the cat's lateral posterior nucleus. *Neuroscience*, 15: 81 – 95.

Berardi, N., Bisti, S., Cattaneo, A., Fiorentini, A. and Maffei, L. (1982) Correlation between the preferred orientation and spatial frequency of neurons in visual areas 17 and 18 of the cat. *J. Physiol.*, 323: 603 – 618.

Bisti, S., Galli, L. and Maffei, L. (1984a) Interaction between size and velocity in the response of area 18 neurons of the cat. *Perception*, 13: A22.

Bisti, S., Carmignoto, G., Galli, L. and Maffei, L. (1984b) Spatial response characteristics of neurones of cat area 18 at different speeds of the visual stimulus. *J. Physiol.*, 349: 23P.

Bisti, S., Carmignoto, G., Galli, L. and Maffei, L. (1985) Spatial frequency characteristics of neurones of area 18 in the cat: dependence on the velocity of the visual stimulus. *J. Physiol.*, 359: 259 – 268.

Blake, R. and Camisa, J.M. (1977) Temporal aspects of spatial vision in the cat. *Exp. Brain Res.*, 28: 325 – 333.

Burr, D.C. and Ross, J. (1982) Contrast sensitivity at high velocities. *Vision Res.*, 22: 479 – 484.

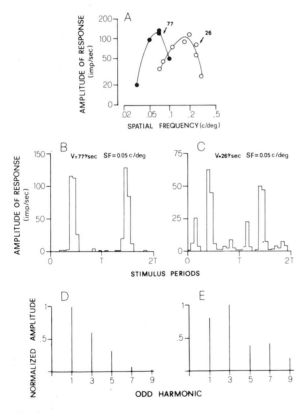

Fig. 7. (A) Spatial-frequency tuning curves of a simple-like cell of area 18. Each curve is obtained with gratings drifting at constant velocities. Velocity: ○, 26 deg/sec; ●, 77 deg/sec. Contrast, 0.15. (B) and (C) Peristimulus time histogram of the responses to a square-wave grating of spatial frequency 0.05 cycles/deg drifted at 77 deg/sec (B), at 26 deg/sec (C). Contrast, 0.25. (D) and (E) Normalized odd Fourier components of the response reported in (B) and (C), respectively. (Bisti, Galli, Maffei, unpublished data.)

Freund, T.F., Martin, K.A.C. and Whitteridge, D. (1985a) Innervation of cat visual areas 17 and 18 by physiologically identified X- and Y-type thalamic afferents. I. Arborization patterns and quantitative distribution of postsynaptic elements. *J. Comp. Neurol.*, 242: 263 – 274.

Freund, T.F., Martin, K.A.C., Somogyi, P. and Whitteridge, D. (1985b) Innervation of cat visual areas 17 and 18 by physiologically identified X- and Y-type thalamic afferents. II. Identification of postsynaptic targets by GABA immunocytochemistry and Golgi impregnation. *J. Comp. Neurol.*, 242: 275 – 291.

Friedlander, M.J., Martin, K.A.C. and Alones, V. (1986) The effect of monocular deprivation on the ultrastructure of functionally identified geniculocortical circuitry in the cat. *Soc. Neurosci. Abstr.*, 16: 786.

Hubel, D.H. and Wiesel, T.N. (1962) Receptive fields, binocular interaction and functional architecture in the cat's visual cortex. *J. Physiol.*, 160: 106 – 154.

Humphrey, A.L., Sur, M., Ulrich, D.J. and Sherman, S.M. (1985) Termination patterns of X- and Y-cell axons in the visual cortex of the cat: Projections to area 18, to the 17/18 border region, and to both area 17 and 18. *J. Comp. Neurol.*, 233: 190 – 212.

Kawamura, K. (1973) Cortical fiber connections of the cat cerebrum. III. The occipital region. *Brain Res.*, 51: 41 – 60.

Kulikowski, J.J. and Tolhurst, D.J. (1973) Psychophysical evidence for sustained and transient detectors in human vision. *J. Physiol.*, 232: 149 – 162.

Maffei, L. (1978) Spatial frequency channels: neural mechanisms. In: *Handbook of Sensory Physiology, vol. VIII*, Springer-Verlag, Berlin.

Maffei, L., Morrone, M.C., Pirchio, M. and Sandini, G. (1979) Responses of visual cortical cells to periodic and nonperiodic stimuli. *J. Physiol.*, 296: 27 – 47.

Movshon, J.A., Thompson, I.D. and Tolhurst, D.J. (1978) Spatial and temporal contrast sensitivity of neurones in area 17 and 18 of the cat's visual cortex. *J. Physiol.*, 283: 101 – 120.

Orban, G.A. (1984) Neuronal operations in the visual cortex. In: *Studies of Brain Function*, Springer-Verlag, Berlin.

Tolhurst, D.J. (1973) Separate channels for the analysis of the shape and the movement of a moving visual stimulus. *J. Physiol.*, 231: 385 – 402.

Tolhurst, D.J. and Movshon, J.A. (1975) Spatial and temporal contrast sensitivity of striate cortical neurones. *Nature*, 257: 674 – 675.

Wilson, M.E. (1968) Cortico-cortical connections of the cat visual areas. *J. Anat.*, 102: 357 – 386.

T.P. Hicks and G. Benedek (Eds.)
Progress in Brain Research, Vol. 75
© 1988 Elsevier Science Publishers B.V. (Biomedical Division)

CHAPTER 17

The transfer of visual information across the corpus callosum in cats, monkeys and humans: spatial and temporal properties

N. Berardi, S. Bisti, A. Fiorentini and L. Maffei

Istituto di Neurofisiologia del C.N.R., Via S. Zeno 51, 56100 Pisa, Italy

In mammals, retino-cortical connections are such that each half of the visual field projects only to the contralateral hemisphere. The role of callosal connections is generally associated with the task of binding together the two halves of the visual field in order to grant perceptual continuity across the vertical meridian and/or to subserve binocular functions such as depth perception.

It is known that neurones projecting across the corpus callosum can belong to any class of cortical cells (simple, complex and hypercomplex) and that most of them are binocular (Berlucchi et al. 1967; Hubel and Wiesel 1967; Shatz 1977a; Harvey 1980; Innocenti 1980). The site of origin of callosal connections is also known (Shatz 1977b; Harvey 1980; Innocenti 1980; Symonds 1982). What is not known, is what type of visual information is transmitted across the corpus callosum.

To provide a quantitative description of the visual spatial and temporal characteristics of the information transmitted by the corpus callosum is the aim of our experiments.

For this purpose, split-chiasm animals are an ideal preparation for separating callosal and geniculo-cortical inputs to the visual cortex. In-

deed, the section of the crossed optic fibers at the chiasm level makes the visual cortex of each side connected directly (i.e., by the geniculo-cortical pathway) only by way of the ipsilateral eye. It is therefore possible, for example, to record binocular single units in one hemisphere of a split-chiasm animal and to compare ipsilateral visual stimulation with stimulation through the contralateral eye, which evokes activity reaching the binocular unit through callosal connections.

It will be shown at the electrophysiological, behavioural and psychophysical levels that the callosal transfer characteristics are similar to those of a low pass filter. In addition, the responsiveness of the callosal pathway to contrast is dramatically reduced with respect to that of the direct geniculo-cortical pathway.

1. Transfer of visual information across the corpus callosum in the cat

Berardi et al. (1987) have recently shown, by means of visual evoked potentials (VEPs) and single unit recordings at the level of the 17/18 border of the visual cortex of the cat, that the contrast gain of the callosal pathway is considerably lower than the gain of the direct, geniculo-cortical system, with ratios of signal amplitude as low as 0.1 for the same stimulus contrast. In addition,

Correspondence to: Dr. Lamberto Maffei, Istituto di Neurofisiologia del C.N.R., Via S. Zeno, 51, 56100 Pisa, Italy.

high spatial and temporal frequencies are strongly attenuated in the process of callosal transfer. Within our sample of neurones in split-chiasm cats, the difference in signal amplitude between the callosal and the direct input is much stronger for area 17 than for area 18 cells.

The relevance of the finding that the callosal pathway has lower contrast gain and spatial resolution is emphasized by the results obtained in an alert split-chiasm cat, which show that the differences between the callosal and the direct pathway are not the consequence of a higher susceptibility of the former to anaesthetics, but rather reflect the different properties of the two pathways.

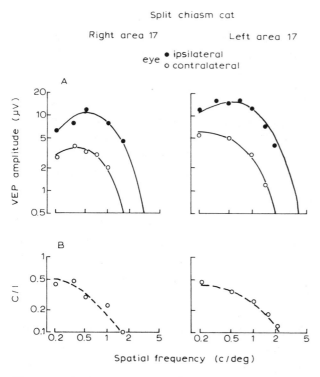

Fig. 1. (A). VEPS in area 17 of a split-chiasm cat. The VEP amplitude is shown as a function of the spatial frequency of the visual stimuli, which are sinusoidal gratings alternating in phase at 5 Hz. Results from the right (left side) and left (right side) area 17 are shown. Filled circles, data obtained for the ipsilateral eye. Open symbols, data obtained for the contralateral eye. The contrast of the gratings was 27%. (B). Ratio between the values for the contralateral (C) and the ipsilateral (I) eye of (A) plotted as a function of the spatial frequency.

In Fig. 1A, the spatial transfer characteristics (VEPs) for the direct (upper curve, filled symbols) and callosal (lower curve, open symbols) pathways are compared for both areas 17 of a split-chiasm cat. The ratio between the contralateral (C) and ipsilateral (I) eye responses is reported in Fig. 1B. The resulting curve (dashed line) can be interpreted as describing the filtering properties of the callosal connections in the spatial frequency domain.

2. Transfer of visual information across the corpus callosum in the monkey

Recently, experiments comparable to those reported above for the cat have been performed in 2 split-chiasm monkeys (long tail macaques).

Electrophysiological recordings were performed at the V1/V2 border in response to gratings of various spatial and temporal frequencies and contrasts. Qualitatively, the results are very similar to those reported for the cat. When the responses are elicited by the eye contralateral with respect to hemisphere from which the recordings are made, high spatial and temporal frequencies are very much attenuated. The sensitivity to contrast is also dramatically reduced. An example of the transfer characteristics obtained with VEPs in the spatial domain is reported in Fig. 2. Filled symbols are the results for the direct ipsilateral input, while open circles are the results for the indirect callosal pathway (contralateral eye).

3. Interhemispheric transfer of learning for pattern discrimination in behaving split-chiasm cats

The existence of a constraint for the activation of the callosal input at the 17/18 border, namely the need for visual stimuli of high contrasts and/or low spatial frequencies, has important implications for the physiological role of the corpus callosum.

A consequence of it would be, indeed, a lack of 'cross talk' between the hemispheres, at least at the 17/18 border, when the patterns inspected are of low contrast and high spatial frequency. In view of

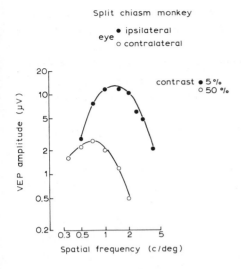

Fig. 2. VEPs at the V1/V2 border of a split-chiasm monkey. Modulation transfer function in the spatial domain. Filled circles, data obtained for the ipsilateral eye; open symbols, data obtained for the contralateral eye. The contrast of the stimulus is indicated in the figure. The temporal frequency of alternation was 5 Hz.

this fact, and of the possibility that the modulation transfer function for the callosal input to other visual areas (for instance, those possibly involved in the transfer of learning) also could have similar properties of attenuation to those of area 17, it was imperative to study whether a constraint for the interhemispheric transfer of visual information was present in the performance of a behaving, split-chiasm cat.

For this purpose, our cats were trained (three split-chiasm and one normal cat) to discriminate between two gratings of equal contrast and spatial frequency but of different orientation, with a forced-choice paradigm and under conditions of monocular vision. Once the learning process was completed with one eye, each animal was tested on the same task with the other eye. For split-chiasm cats, retention of the performance level attained with the trained eye (interocular transfer) is considered an indication of interhemispheric transfer (see Berlucchi and Sprague 1981; Berlucchi and Marzi 1982).

The normal cat showed complete interocular

transfer at all spatial frequencies tested (3.2, 1.6 and 0.8 cycles/deg, contrast 10 – 15%). The results for the split-chiasm cats are exemplified in Fig. 3. At medium-low spatial frequencies (0.6 cycles/deg) a moderate contrast (17%) is sufficient to allow complete interocular (interhemispheric) transfer of learning effects. For a higher spatial frequency (1.1. cycles/deg) there was no interocular transfer, even if the contrast of the gratings was increased to 30%. Similar results were obtained for cat 3 and cat 1. Complete interocular transfer of learning effects with gratings of moderate contrast was found only when the gratings were of medium-low spatial frequency. In order to obtain an interocular transfer for the higher spatial frequencies, the contrast had to be increased to much higher values.

We do not know from our experimental paradigm if the transfer of learning effects involves mainly visual areas higher in the cortical hierarchy than areas 17 and 18 or if the transfer of visual information at the 17/18 border is also important. Therefore, we cannot say whether the impairment in contrast gain demonstrated by our experiment is at the level of callosal connections at the 17/18 border or at the level of callosal connections between other visual areas.

However, it is clear that there is a limitation in the interhemispheric transfer of visual information subserved by the corpus callosum, which clearly

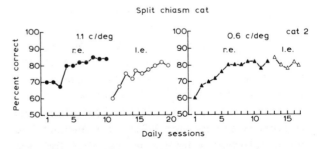

Fig. 3. Learning curves of a split-chiasm cat for the monocular forced-choice discrimination of sinusoidal gratings of different orientation. Each point is the percentage of correct responses in a daily session of 40 trials. Left side: spatial frequency 1.1 cycles/deg, contrast 30%, right side: spatial frequency 0.6 cycles/deg, contrast 17%. R.E., right eye; L.E., left eye.

184

affects the interhemispheric transfer of learning in split-chiasm cats.

4. Interhemispheric transfer of visual information in humans

In humans, the interhemispheric transfer of visual information cannot be investigated with the same procedure as in animal split-chiasm preparations. To our knowledge, only one case of a human patient with a traumatic longitudinal transection of the chiasm has been reported in the literature (Blakemore 1970).

It is possible, however, to investigate the interhemispheric transfer psychophysically taking into account that stimuli presented laterally either in the left or right visual hemifields project separately to the two hemispheres. Previous experiments on interhemispheric transfer in humans were based on measurements of reaction times to stimuli presented laterally.

We have approached this problem in a different way (Berardi and Fiorentini, 1987), making use of a visual discrimination task that is subject to the phenomenon of perceptual learning. The discriminanda were periodic patterns (complex gratings) consisting both of the sum of two sinusoids of spatial frequency f and 3f, respectively and of contrast in the ratio 1: (1/3), but differing from each other for the relative spatial phase of the two harmonic components (Fig. 4). The discrimination of such gratings, when presented briefly according to a temporal two-alternative forced-choice procedure, may be very difficult to perform when first tested in inexperienced subjects. However, the percentage of correct responses increases progressively with repetition of trials, and reaches a stable level that is then maintained for a long time (Fiorentini and Berardi 1981). This phenomenon of perceptual learning is specific for the parameters of the stimulus (orientation and spatial frequency) and does not transfer from the upper to the lower visual field, although it transfers intraocularly.

All these properties put together may indicate that the effect of learning is restricted to populations of neurones selectively activated by the stimulus. Therefore, one would expect that the effect of learning in complex grating discrimination will not transfer from one hemisphere to the other, at least at a sufficiently long distance from the vertical meridian.

Our findings show that this is indeed the case, if the discrimination is tested for complex gratings of relatively low spatial frequency removed 5 deg from the vertical meridian. As shown in Fig. 4, the discrimination performance improves with increasing numbers of trials for the visual hemifield tested first (left field, open symbols) until a stable performance is reached. This effect of learning, however, is not retained when the stimuli are removed from the left to the right hemifield (filled symbols).

The results obtained closer to the vertical meridian are quite different. In this case the effects of

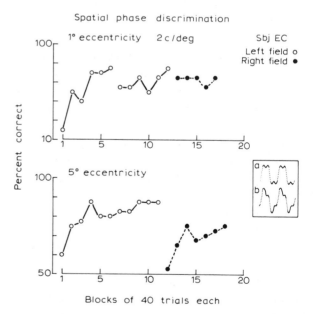

Fig. 4. Learning curves of a human subject for the forced-choice discrimination of two complex gratings having the luminance profiles shown in the insert. Each point is the percentage of correct responses in a block of 40 trials. The gratings' inner edge was removed laterally 5 deg (bottom) or 1 deg (top) from the fixation point either in the left (open symbols) or right (filled symbols) hemifield. Horizontal gratings of fundamental frequency 2 cycles/deg, contrast 10% (top), 15% (bottom) presented for 100 msec (top), 150 msec (bottom).

learning are transferred from one visual hemifield to the other, provided the fundamental spatial frequency of the gratings does not exceed 2 cycles/deg. For gratings of higher spatial frequency (4 cycles/deg) however, no transfer of learning effects occurs from one hemifield to the other, even if the stimuli are presented close to the vertical midline.

Control experiments have shown that the transfer of learning effects between two non-overlapping areas of the visual field (for gratings of fundamental frequency not exceeding 2 cycles/deg) is peculiar to areas on opposite sides of the vertical meridian. There is no transfer between two non-overlapping areas lying on the same side of the vertical meridian. In addition, it has been found that the interhemispheric transfer of learning is selective for the orientation of the stimuli to be discriminated and that it occurs intraocularly.

These findings are consistent with an interhemispheric transfer of information between regions symmetrical with respect to the vertical meridian and limited to a strip of a few degrees on either side of it. Within these regions, it seems to occur between structures which are not only orientation selective, but which are also tuned to the same stimulus orientation and which receive inputs from the two eyes. This is reminiscent of the properties of callosal connections between visual cortical areas, as described for the cat (Berlucchi and Rizzolatti 1968).

An alternative explanation of our findings, in terms of a bilateral cortical representation of a central vertical strip of the retinae, seems to be ruled out by the results of an experiment in which reaction times were measured for the discrimination of complex gratings presented laterally or various eccentricities (Berardi, Fiorentini and Gravina, in preparation).

If the interpretation in terms of callosal interhemispheric transfer is correct, then our psychophysical findings in humans are in very good agreement with the limitations of the callosal transfer of spatial frequency information demonstrated for the cat and the monkey.

Acknowledgements

We gratefully acknowledge the kind collaboration of the ENEA CNR Laboratorio animali da esperimento, Casaccia (Roma). N.B. is a Research Fellow of the Scuola Normale Superiore, Pisa.

References

Berardi, N. and Fiorentini, A. (1987) Interhemispheric transfer of visual information in humans: spatial characteristics. *J. Physiol.*, 384: 633 – 647.

Berardi, N., Bisti, S. and Maffei, L. (1987) The transfer of visual information across the corpus callosum: Spatial and temporal properties in the cat. *J. Physiol.*, 384: 619 – 632.

Berlucchi, G. and Marzi, C.A. (1982) Interocular and interhemispheric transfer of visual discrimination in the cat. In: Ingle, D.J., Goodale, M.A. and Mansfield, R.J.W. (Eds.), *Analysis of Visual Behaviour*, M.I.T. Press, Cambridge, MA, pp. 719 – 750.

Berlucchi, G. and Rizzolatti, G. (1968) Binocularly driven neurons in visual cortex of split chiasm cats. *Science*, 159: 308 – 310.

Berlucchi, G. and Sprague, J.M. (1981) The cerebral cortex in visual learning and memory, and in interhemispheric transfer in the cat. In: Schmitt, F.O., Wordern, F.G., Adelman, G. and Dennis, J.G. (Eds.), *The Organization of the Cerebral Cortex*, M.I.T. Press, Cambridge, MA.

Berlucchi, G., Gazzaniga, M.S. and Rizzolatti, G. (1967) Microelectrode analysis of transfer of visual information by the corpus callosum. *Arch. Ital. Biol.*, 105: 583 – 596.

Blakemore, C. (1970) Binocular depth perception and the optic chiasm. *Vision Res.*, 10: 43 – 47.

Fiorentini, A. and Berardi, N. (1981) Learning in grating waveform discrimination; specificity for orientation and spatial frequency. *Vision Res.*, 21: 1149 – 1158.

Harvey, A.R. (1980) A physiological analysis of subcortical and commissural projections of areas 17 and 18 of the cat. *J. Physiol.*, 30: 507 – 534.

Hubel, D.H. and Wiesel, T.N. (1967) Cortical and callosal connections concerned with the vertical meridian of visual fields in the cat. *J. Neurophysiol.*, 30: 1561 – 1573.

Innocenti, G.M. (1980) The primary visual pathway through the corpus callosum: morphological and functional aspects in the cat. *Arch. Ital. Biol.*, 118: 124 – 188.

Shatz, C. (1977a) Abnormal interhemispheric connections in the visual system of Boston siamese cats: a physiological study. *J. Comp. Neurol.*, 171: 229 – 246.

Shatz, C. (1977b) Anatomy of interhemispheric connections in the visual system of Boston siamese and ordinary cats. *J. Comp. Neurol.*, 173: 497 – 518.

Symonds, L.L. (1982) Connections among cortical visual areas in the cat. *Ph.D. Dissertation*, University of Pennsylvania, Philadelphia, PA.

CHAPTER 18

Cortico-cortical callosal connectivity: evidence derived from electrophysiological studies

Franco Leporé[1], Maurice Ptito[1], Louis Richter[1] and Jean-Paul Guillemot[2]

[1]Département de Psychologie, Group de Recherche en Neuropsychologie Expérimentale, et Centre de Recherche en Sciences Neurologiques, Université de Montréal, Montréal, Québec, [2]Département de Kinanthropologie, Université du Québec, Montréal, Québec, Canada

Introduction

One of the principal sources of cortico-cortical connections beyond the primary visual areas concerns the commissural system. In man, the major commissure, namely, the corpus callosum, is made up of some 200 million fibres (Blinkov and Glezer 1968). This may actually be a gross underestimation of the total number of fibres, since Innocenti (1986), using the electron microscope, has suggested that this figure may have to be at least quadrupled since the light microscope, from which these numbers were derived, does not reveal the fine callosal axons which constitute the majority of callosal fibres.

Many of the regions wherein callosal neurons originate (the callosal cell zone) and those on which they terminate (the callosal terminal zone) have been identified anatomically. These studies show that most visual areas in higher mammals receive from, and send axons through, the callosum. They demonstrate, moreover, that the callosal zones, both of origin and termination, are

smallest in the primary visual areas, being limited to the region of the vertical meridian representation; they are more widely distributed in the 'higher order' areas (Heath and Jones 1971; Sanides 1978, 1979; Van Essen et al. 1982). In the cat, the callosal organization follows this general pattern (see Fig. 1), the distribution being fairly narrow in area 17 and increasing thereafter, callosal neurons basically occupying the entire extents of the anterior ectosylvian (AEV) and lateral suprasylvian (LS) visual areas (Seagraves and Rosenquist 1982a,b; Miceli et al. 1986). This general organization has also been confirmed electrophysiologically (Hubel and Wiesel 1967; Berlucchi and Rizzolatti 1968; Harvey 1980; Berlucchi 1981; Leporé et al. 1981, 1986; Leporé and Guillemot 1982; Antonini et al. 1983; Berlucchi et al. 1986; Payne 1986; Ptito et al. 1987).

Our group has been interested in identifying the pattern of distribution of callosal neurons within these areas, defining their physiological properties and verifying with neurobehavioral studies the principal hypotheses concerning callosal function. In the studies we will be introducing in the present essay, we will limit our description to defining, using electrophysiological techniques, the pathways through which a cell in a particular visual area may be influenced by the other side. Parts of the studies

Correspondence to: Dr. F. Leporé, Dept. de Psychologie et Centre de Recherche en Sciences Neurologiques, Université de Montréal, C.P. 6128, Succ. A., Montréal, Québec, Canada H3C 3J7.

reported here may have appeared in abstract form or as portions of published papers (Leporé and Guillemot 1982; Antonini et al. 1983; Leporé et al. 1986; Ptito et al. 1987).

A number of anatomical descriptions of the callosal terminal and cell zones and the pattern of interhemispheric connections have been determined for the cat (see above). They generally show that all areas have reciprocal homotopic callosal connections as well as quite extensive heterotopic connections whereby 'higher order' areas also receive from, but do not send to, lower order areas. These anatomical connections are instrumental in determining some of the receptive field (RF) properties of the recipient cell.

Methods and procedures

The basic procedure for examining how the contralateral cortex affects the RFs in each of the visual areas, and also for carrying out the studies to be reported below, has been described in detail elsewhere (Leporé and Guillemot 1982). In summary, single cell activity was recorded in normal and chiasm-sectioned animals. The recording site was one of the known visual areas, such as 17, 18, 19, LS and AEV. In most experiments, the animal was first rendered quiescent with a light dose of ketamine, and then anaesthetized deeply with fluothane, nitrous oxide and oxygen and placed in the stereotaxic apparatus. After exposing the target cortex, fluothane was shut off and the ad-

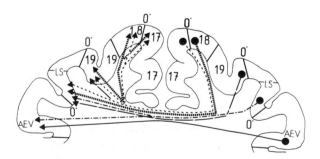

Fig. 1. Schematic organization of callosal projections to different visual areas as revealed by anatomical studies. (Adapted from Heath and Jones 1971.)

ministration of nitrous oxide and oxygen (70:30 ratio, respectively) was continued until the end of the experiment. Glass microelectrodes were used for most of the experiments, although tungsten electrodes were also occasionally employed. Transection of the chiasm was carried out at least 1 month prior to the electrophysiological recording. The transbuccal approach described by Myers (1956) was used to expose and section the chiasm. Histological verifications of completeness of lesion and of electrode placement were carried out on Kluver-Barrera (Kluver and Barrera 1953) stained sections. Only data obtained from animals which showed complete transection of the chiasm were retained for the analyses.

Results

Using the chiasm-sectioned preparation, any response evoked through the contralateral eye is presumed to pass through the callosum. Depending on the recording procedure and site, about one-third to one-half of all units which were visually responsive were found to be binocularly driven. RF properties of these callosally activated units were typical for the area under investigation: sizes were large for units in AEV and LS and small for those in areas 17, 18 and 19. Directional selectivity and orientation tuning were also very similar for callosally and thalamo-cortically determined fields for the same unit. Both complex and hypercomplex RFs, but no simple type RFs, were found. One consistent observation, which is important in specifying one of the putative functions of the callosum, was that the medial borders of the two RFs either touched or straddled the vertical meridian (Cynader et al. 1981, 1986; Leporé and Guillemot 1982; Antonini et al. 1983; Di Stefano et al. 1984; Leporé et al. 1986; Ptito et al. 1987). This is generally taken as indicating that the corpus callosum is involved in mid-line fusion (Berlucchi 1972, 1981; Leporé et al. 1986).

To confirm that the contralateral input to a particular cell is really coming through the callosum, one need only carry out a very simple procedure:

transect, in these chiasm-sectioned animals, the posterior third of the callosum before recording in the various visual areas. The effects of this procedure are quite dramatic: in all the visual areas examined so far (17, 18, 19, LS and AEV), the contralaterally determined RFs disappear. In a few cases, we were able to carry out this procedure while a cell was in the process of being recorded. The immediate disappearance of the contralateral RF, with minimal modification of the ipsilateral RF, confirmed without much doubt that the callosum was involved in specifying the RF of the contralateral eye (Antonini et al. 1983).

A second procedure for studying the nature of the callosal message is to record directly from callosal fibres. Whereas the method described above gives information about how callosal inputs affect the RF properties of the recipient cells in the callosal terminal zones, the latter procedure gives more precise indications about the output of the cells in the callosal cell zones. RFs of callosal axons have many features in common with those in the visual areas in general and the callosal terminal zones in particular: they have well-defined RFs, many are direction and/or orientation selective, etc. As was the case of callosally recipient cells, moreover, the medial borders of the RFs abutted or straddled the vertical meridian. They also show, however, some notable differences: simple type RFs were frequently encountered, the RF sizes were generally larger and the tuning to the various parameters tested was less tight (Leporé et al. 1986). These results may reflect a genuine difference between the properties of these fibres and those of the cells in the terminal zones. The results obtained by Maffei and collaborators (Maffei et al. 1986) may be cited in possible support of this interpretation. They used the split-chiasm preparation and recorded from the callosal terminal zone of area 17. They showed that the spatial frequency tuning of callosally recipient cells had a higher cutoff frequency when stimulated through the ipsilateral eye than through the contralateral eye (i.e., via the callosum). The results, when recording from callosal axons, may also reflect a sampling bias in favour of large fibres, which predominate in this structure, and/or a bias towards 'higher order' areas, such as LS and AEV, which have larger and less finely tuned RFs and also extensive callosal interconnections.

Both of these methods provide significant insights into the nature of the information coming from the other side and about how it affects the properties of the recipient cells. They say little, however, about where the information is originating, other than that it is coming from the opposite hemisphere. Given the large number of visual areas which send axons through the callosum and their extensive interconnections, it is not without interest, and quite in keeping with the theme of this symposium, to try and obtain some idea about the information flow beyond primary visual cortex. We have therefore combined the recording of callosal axonic activity or the response of cells in the callosal terminal zones of

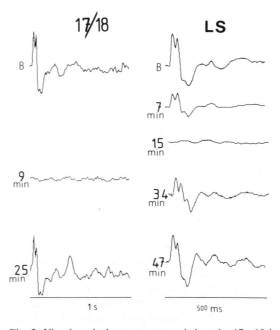

Fig. 2. Visual evoked response recorded at the 17–18 border and in LS to a flashed whole-field stimulus recorded before (B), during (17/18: 9 min, LS: 15 min) and after (17/18: 25 min, LS: 47 min) topical application of marcaine to the structure. Recuperation time: 17/18: 25 min, LS: 47 min; number of sweeps: 10; time base: 17/18: 1 sec; LS: 500 msec.

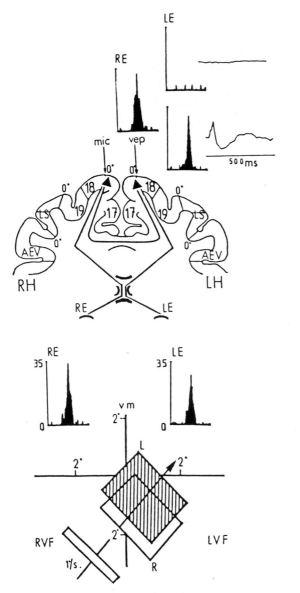

split-chiasm cats with selective inactivation of specific cortical areas.

Cortical inactivation was made possible with topical application of 5% marcaine. This was achieved by using a piece of gelfoam, generously infiltrated with this solution, cut to the appropriate dimensions and placed over the area to be inactivated. This local anaesthetic exerts its effects by blocking sodium channels along the axons so that the spike cannot travel to the terminals. Among its more desirable properties is that it blocks almost all activity in the neurons which it contacts, its principal effects are of relatively short duration and they are reversible. As a matter of fact, this reactivation of neuronal function can be accelerated, in the case of surface structures such as the cortex, by extensive washing with isotonic saline. The extent and chronology of the effects can be illustrated by looking at the visual evoked response recorded in the structure before, during and after anaesthetic blocking. This is illustrated in Fig. 2, which shows that the visual evoked response to a flashed whole-field stimulus virtually disappears during blockade and reappears following repeated washing with isotonic saline in about 20 min.

Some of the effects of contralateral blockade are predictable from the known anatomical organization of the callosal system. A binocular cell record-

Fig. 3. Effects of marcaine application to areas 17 – 18 of one hemisphere on the response of a cell situated in the callosal recipient zone of the other hemisphere in a split-chiasm cat. The schematic coronal section illustrates the principal visual areas and the fact that the chiasm section leaves intact only the ipsilateral visual pathways. Each post-stimulus histogram represents the response of the cell to five sweeps of the stimulus within the RF of one eye. The stimulus is a white bar moving at 1 deg/sec. The histograms next to the RF representations at the bottom of the figure illustrate the normal response of each eye before marcaine administration. In the cases where marcaine abolished the response for that eye, the resulting flat histogram (top of pair) as well as the one obtained following recuperation (bottom of pair) are shown. In cases where no effect was seen, only the histogram obtained during marcaine application is shown. The curves next to the histograms represent the visual evoked response to whole-field stimulation obtained in the area during and after marcaine blockade. Only the histograms obtained following marcaine application to areas 17 – 18 of the left hemisphere, where an effect was produced, are indicated. The schematic circuit diagram is the deduced pathway representing information flow between the hemispheres. Abbreviations: LVF: left visual field; RVF: right visual field; RE: right eye; LE: left eye; RH: right hemisphere; LH: left hemisphere; R: receptive field of right eye; L: receptive field of left eye; mic: microelectrode position; vep: visual evoked response electrode position; AEV: anterior ectosylvian visual area; LS: lateral suprasylvian visual area; vm: vertical meridian; s: seconds; ms: milliseconds; arrow: direction of sweep.

ed at the border region of areas 17 and 18 of a split-chiasm cat loses the response which can be evoked from the contralateral eye when the homotopic contralateral cortex is inactivated with marcaine. This is illustrated in Fig. 3, which shows the response of a cell at the border of areas 17 and 18 in a split-chiasm cat. The response evoked from stimulation of the ipsilateral eye is unaffected by marcaine application to the contralateral cortex whereas the response of the contralateral eye is completely abolished by the anaesthetic. These results indicate that the callosal input to the cell in the border regions of areas 17–18 originates in homotopic contralateral cortex.

Other pathways, however, are more difficult to predict. Take for example a cell recorded in LS of a split-chiasm cat. It could receive its callosal input from the homotopic contralateral area; however, it could also receive all or some of its input from a number of other areas. An idea of the circuitry can be derived from an examination of the results presented in Fig. 4. The electrode was positioned in the PMLS subdivision of LS of the right hemisphere (Clare-Bishop area of Hubel and Wiesel 1969; Palmer et al. 1978). The cell was binocularly driven and had a RF typical of this area. Blocking the contralateral, left areas 17–18 abolished the response which could be evoked through the left eye only. Neither eye was effective in driving the cell when the ipsilateral areas 17–18 or left LS cortex were blocked with the topical application of marcaine. By a process of elimination, it may be concluded that cells in areas 17–18 of the left side project to cells in homolateral regions of the right side, which in turn project to LS of the left side, after which the information is retransmitted to LS of the right side. This of course does not mean that each intervening step involves only one synapse or that intervening areas, such as area 19, are not also involved in the process. Rather, this schematic circuit constitutes an attempt to define a flow diagram for information transfer across the hemispheres, given the available data.

Another example is shown in Fig. 5. These results were obtained from an axon recorded in the

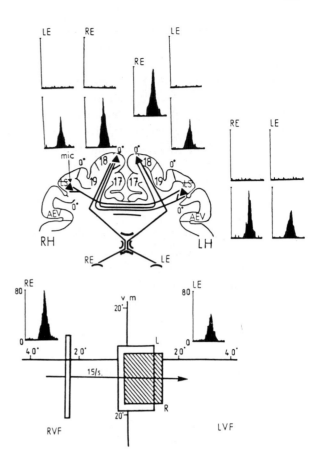

Fig. 4. Effects of marcaine application to different visual areas on the response of a cell situated in the LS callosal recipient zone of a split-chiasm cat. The schematic coronal section illustrates the principal visual areas and the fact that the chiasm section leaves intact only the ipsilateral visual pathways. Each post-stimulus histogram represents the response of the cell to 5 sweeps of the stimulus within the RF of one eye. The histograms next to the RF representations at the bottom of the figure illustrate the normal response of each eye before marcaine administration. The stimulus is a white bar traveling in the illustrated direction at 15 deg/sec. In the cases where marcaine abolished the response for that eye, the resulting flat histogram as well as the one obtained following recuperation are shown. In cases where no effect was obtained, only the histogram obtained during marcaine application is shown. Each sub-set of histograms is positioned next to the area to which marcaine was applied: in a clockwise fashion, starting from the left, are indicated histograms following marcaine application to areas 17–18 of the right hemisphere, to areas 17–18 and lateral suprasylvian of the left hemisphere, respectively. The schematic circuit diagram is the deduced pathway representing information flow between the hemispheres. Abbreviations, see Fig. 3.

corpus callosum of a normal cat. Here, application of the blocker to areas 17 – 18 of either side abolished the responses which could be evoked from the two eyes. Since the electrode is in the callosum, it is therefore difficult to know which is the primary hemisphere and which is the callosally activated hemisphere. However, given the organization of the RFs, which were mainly situated in the left hemifield, the most likely hypothesis is that the right hemisphere is the primary hemisphere which then projects through the callosum to homotopic contralateral areas 17 – 18. However, since the response to both eyes is eliminated by the application of marcaine to either cortex, it must be further hypothesized that the electrode is actually recording from a fibre which leaves areas 17 – 18 of the left hemisphere and projects to some unknown area in the right hemisphere. The results also indicate that LS of the left hemisphere is bypassed by the information flow since its inactivation had no effect on the response to stimulation of either eye.

It is clear from the result obtained using this technique that the callosal connectivity is more complex than that which can be derived from a simple inspection of the results of anatomical techniques. This scheme, moreover, certainly is oversimplified, since, as already indicated, some well-known visual areas, such as 19, which have quite extensive callosal projections and have been shown to be connected to both ipsilateral and contralateral LS, were not inactivated.

One complicating factor, which becomes evident from the above figure, was that the cat had normal visual pathways. To determine which was the primary hemisphere and which was the callosally recipient hemisphere, the primary site had to be deduced from the RF positions in visual space. Although the assumption that the hemifield which contains the largest portion of the RFs is the primary field is quite likely, it is not without risk. There is no a priori impediment for the callosally determined fields to be wider than those determined through the normal thalamo-cortical pathway. To circumvent this difficulty and possible source

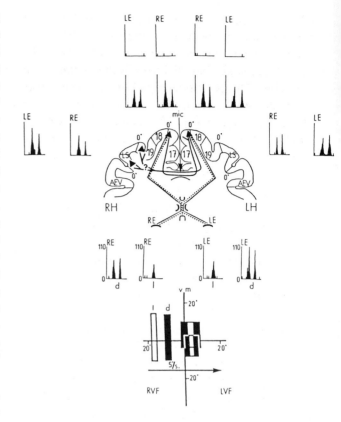

Fig. 5. Effects of marcaine application to different visual areas on the response of a cell situated in the splenium of the corpus callosum of a normal cat. The schematic coronal section illustrates the principal visual areas and the fact that the visual pathways are intact. Each post-stimulus histogram represents the response of the cell to five sweeps of the stimulus within the RF of one eye. The histograms next to the RF representations at the bottom of the figure illustrate the normal response of each eye before marcaine administration to a white (l) or a dark (d) bar. The stimulus used during blockade is a dark bar traveling in the illustrated direction at 5 deg/sec. In the cases where marcaine abolished the response for that eye, the resulting flat histogram as well as the one obtained following recuperation are shown. In cases where no effect was obtained, only the histogram obtained during marcaine application is shown. Each sub-set of histograms is positioned next to the area to which marcaine was applied: in a clockwise fashion, starting from the left, are indicated histograms following marcaine application to LS of the right hemisphere, to areas 17 – 18 of the right hemisphere, to areas 17 – 18 and lateral suprasylvian of the left hemisphere, respectively. The schematic circuit diagram is the deduced pathway representing information flow between the hemispheres. Abbreviations, see Fig. 3.

of error, therefore, additional recordings were carried out in callosal axons but of split-chiasm cats. The results are presented in Fig. 6. The fibre,

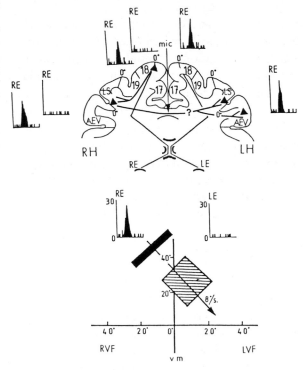

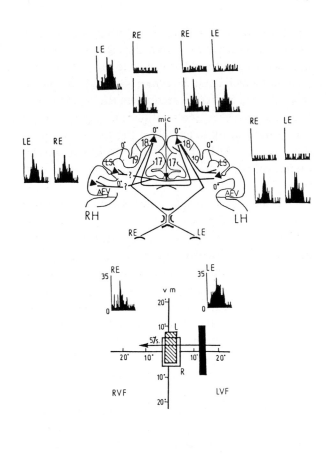

Fig. 6. Effects of marcaine application to different visual areas on the response of a cell situated in the splenium of the corpus callosum of a split-chiasm cat. The schematic coronal section illustrates the principal visual areas and the fact that the chiasm section leaves intact only the ipsilateral visual pathways. Each post-stimulus histogram represents the response of the cell to 5 sweeps of the stimulus within the RF of one eye. The histograms next to the RF representations at the bottom of the figure illustrate the normal response of each eye before marcaine administration. The stimulus used during blockade is a dark bar traveling in the illustrated direction at 8 deg/sec. In the cases where marcaine abolished the response for that eye, the resulting flat histogram as well as the one obtained following recuperation are shown. In cases where no effect was obtained, only the histogram obtained during marcaine application is shown. Each sub-set of histograms is positioned next to the area to which marcaine was applied: in a clockwise fashion, starting from the left, are indicated histograms following marcaine application to LS of the right hemisphere, to areas 17 – 18 of the right hemisphere, to areas 17 – 18 and lateral suprasylvian of the left hemisphere, respectively. The schematic circuit diagram is the deduced pathway representing information flow between the hemispheres. Abbreviations, see Fig. 3.

Fig. 7. Effects of marcaine application to different visual areas on the response of a cell situated in the splenium of the corpus callosum of a split-chiasm cat. The schematic coronal section illustrates the principal visual areas and the fact that the chiasm section leaves intact only the ipsilateral visual pathways. Each post-stimulus histogram represents the response of the cell to 5 sweeps of the stimulus within the RF of one eye. The histograms next to the RF representations at the bottom of the figure illustrate the normal response of each eye before marcaine administration. The stimulus used during blockade is a dark bar traveling in the illustrated direction at 5 deg/sec. In the cases where marcaine abolished the response for that eye, the resulting flat histogram as well as the one obtained following recuperation are shown. In cases where no effect was obtained, only the histogram obtained during marcaine application is shown. Each sub-set of histograms is positioned next to the area to which marcaine was applied: in a clockwise fashion, starting from the left, are indicated histograms following marcaine application to LS of the right hemisphere, to areas 17 – 18 of the right hemisphere, to areas 17 – 18 and lateral suprasylvian of the left hemisphere, respectively. The schematic circuit diagram is the deduced pathway representing information flow between the hemispheres. Abbreviations, see Fig. 3.

whose responses are shown in this example, was monocularly driven through the right eye. Applying marcaine to the left cortex had no effect on the response which could be evoked through the eye on this side; but it disappeared when the block was to the right cortex. A similar abolition of the response was produced by inactivating the right LS cortex but not the left. The circuit proposed above, therefore, is the one which is most consistent with these data.

One interesting result which seemed to emerge from two of the previous figures (Figs. 4 and 5) is that the callosal flow of information is not unidirectional but involves quite an extensive amount of reciprocally flowing activity. We tested this idea more specifically using the same preparation as above: we recorded axonal activity in the splenium of split-chiasm cats. If information flow proceeds only in one direction, then all fibres in these split-chiasm animals should be monocularly driven, as was the case for the fibre shown in Fig. 6; if, on the other hand, callosal activity is also bidirectional, then some fibres should respond to stimulation of either eye. More than one-third of the fibres recorded in the callosum of split-chiasm cats were in fact binocularly driven, showing that callosal crossover is not the exception but part of the rule. The results obtained with the fibre presented in Fig. 7 give some indication of the type of complexity one can expect in the system. The procedure and interpretation are similar to those presented above and will not be repeated. Again, however, the extrapolated flow diagram could not easily be predicted from purely anatomical considerations.

These studies are still in progress and not all the possible combinations and interrelations have been identified. Moreover, as indicated above, for purely technical and strategic reasons, a number of intervening or adjacent areas have not been inactivated. This leads to results which may be either partial or inconclusive. A definitive answer to the problems posed in this work will only be given when this procedure is applied to all the appropriate areas, a task which presents some additional difficulties, not the least of which is the increase in testing time which will be required for each unit.

Conclusion

In conclusion, therefore, it may be stated that the electrophysiological procedure, combined with localized inactivation, exposed in the present experiment, is a powerful tool for studying functional cortico-cortical callosal connections beyond the primary visual area. The results confirm the predictable functional relationships which exist between homotopic areas. They also show, however, that the circuitry for callosal function involves not only the more obvious interhemispheric connections but also extensive intrahemispheric relations and bidirectional information flow.

Acknowledgements

These experiments were made possible in part thanks to grants from the Natural Sciences and Engineering Research Council of Canada, and the Fond FCAR of the Ministry of Education of the Province of Québec to F.L., M.P. and J.-P.G., and from the Medical Research Council of Canada to F.L.

References

Antonini, A., Berlucchi, G. and Leporé, F. (1983) Physiological organization of callosal connections of a visual lateral suprasylvian cortical area in the cat, *J. Neurophysiol.*, 49: 902–921.

Berlucchi, G. (1981) Recent advances in the analysis of the neural substrates of interhemispheric communication. In: O. Pompeiano and C. Ajmone-Marsan (Eds.), *Brain Mechanisms of Perceptual Awareness and Purposeful Behavior*, Raven Press, New York, pp. 133–152.

Berlucchi, G. (1972) Anatomical and physiological aspects of visual function of corpus callosum, *Brain Res.*, 37: 371–392.

Berlucchi, G. and Rizzolatti, G. (1968) Binocular driven neurons in visual cortex of split-chiasm cats, *Science*, 159: 308–310.

Berlucchi, G., Tassinari, G. and Antonini, A. (1986) The organization of the callosal connections according to

Sperry's principle of supplemental complementarity. In: F. Leporé, M. Ptito and H.H. Jasper (Eds.), *Two Hemispheres, One Brain: Functions of the Corpus Callosum*, Alan Liss, New York, pp. 167 – 170.

Blinkov, S.M. and Glezer, I.I. (1968) *The Human Brain in Figures and Tables. A Quantitative Handbook*, Plenum Press, New York.

Cynader, M.S., Leporé, F. and Guillemot, J.-P. (1981) Interhemispheric competition during postnatal development, *Nature*, 290: 139 – 140.

Cynader, M.S., Gardner, J., Dobbins, A., Leporé, F. and Guillemot, J.-P. (1986) Interhemispheric communication and binocular vision: functional and developmental aspects. In: F. Leporé, M. Ptito and H.H. Jasper (Eds.), *Two Hemispheres, One Brain: Functions of the Corpus Callosum*, Alan Liss, New York, pp. 189 – 209.

DiStefano, M.R., Bedard, S., Marzi, C.A. and Leporé, F. (1984) Lack of binocular activation of cells in area 19 of the siamese cat, *Brain Res.*, 303: 391 – 395.

Harvey, A.R. (1980) A physiological analysis of subcortical and commissural projections of areas 17 and 18 of the cat, *J. Physiol. (Lond.)*, 302: 507 – 534.

Heath, C.J. and Jones, E.G. (1971) The anatomical organization of the suprasylvian gyrus of the cat, *Ergeb. Anat. Entwicklungsgesch.*, 45: 1 – 64.

Hubel, D.H. and Wiesel, T.N. (1967) Cortical and callosal connections concerned with the vertical meridian of visual fields in the cat. *J. Neurophysiol.*, 30: 1561 – 1573.

Hubel, D.H. and Wiesel, T.N. (1969) Visual area of the lateral suprasylvian gyrus (Clare-Bishop area) of the cat, *J. Physiol (Lond.)*, 202: 251 – 260.

Innocenti, G.M. (1986) What is so special about callosal connections. In: F. Leporé, M. Ptito and H.H. Jasper (Eds.), *Two Hemispheres, One Brain: Functions of the Corpus Callosum*, Alan Liss, New York, pp. 75 – 81.

Kluver, H. and Barrera, E. (1953) A method for the combined staining of cells and fibres in the nervous system, *J. Neuropathol. Exp. Neurol.*, 12: 400 – 403.

Leporé, F., Ptito, M., Samson, A. and Guillemot, J.-P. (1981) The influence of the contralateral hemisphere on the receptive field properties of cells in the visual cortex of the cat. *Rev. Canad. Biol.*, 40: 60 – 66.

Leporé, F. and Guillemot, J.P. (1982) Visual receptive field properties of cells innervated through the corpus callosum in the cat, *Exp. Brain Res.*, 46: 413 – 424.

Leporé, F., Ptito, M. and Guillemot, J.P. (1986) The role of the corpus callosum in midline fusion. In: F. Leporé, M. Ptito and H.H. Jasper (Eds.) *Two Hemispheres, One Brain: Functions of the Corpus Callosum*, Alan Liss, New York, pp. 211 – 230.

Maffei, L., Berardi, N. and Bisti, S. (1986) Interocular transfer of adaptation after effect in neurons of area 17 and 18 of split chiasm cats, *J. Neurophysiol.*, 55: 966 – 976.

Miceli, D., Leporé, F., Ward, R. and Ptito, M. (1986) Anatomical organization of interhemispheric connections of the anterior ectosylvian visual area in the cat. In: F. Leporé, M. Ptito and H.H. Jasper (Eds.) *Two Hemispheres, One Brain: Functions of the Corpus Callosum*, Alan Liss, New York, pp. 139 – 149.

Myers, R.E. (1956) Function of the corpus callosum in interocular transfer, *Brain*, 118: 358 – 373.

Palmer, L.A., Rosenquist, A.C. and Tusa, R.J. (1978) The retinotopic organization of the lateral suprasylvian areas in the cat, *J. Comp. Neurol.*, 177: 237 – 256.

Ptito, M., Tassinari, G. and Antonini, A. (1987) Electrophysiological evidence for interhemispheric connections in the anterior ectosylvian sulcus in the cat, *Exp. Brain Res.*, in press.

Payne, B.R. (1986) Role of callosal cells in the functional organization of cat striate cortex. In: F. Leporé, M. Ptito and H.H. Jasper (Eds.), *Two Hemispheres, One Brain: Functions of the Corpus Callosum*, Alan Liss, New York, pp. 231 – 254.

Sanides, D. (1978) The retinotopic distribution of visual callosal projections in the suprasylvian visual areas compared to the classical visual areas (17, 18, 19) in the cat, *Exp. Brain Res.*, 33: 435 – 443.

Sanides, D. (1979) Commissural connections of the visual cortex of the cat. In: I. Steele-Russell, M.W. van Hof and G. Berlucchi (Eds.), *Structure and Function of the Cerebral Commissures*, University Park Press, Baltimore, MD, pp. 236 – 244.

Seagraves, M.A. and Rosenquist, A.C. (1982a) The distribution of the cells of origin of callosal projections in cat visual cortex, *J. Neurosci.*, 2: 1079 – 1089.

Seagraves, M.A. and Rosenquist, A.C. (1982b) The afferent and efferent callosal connections of retinotopically defined areas in cat cortex, *J. Neurosci.*, 2: 1090 – 1107.

Van Essen, D.C., Newsome, W.T. and Bixby, J.L. (1982) The pattern of interhemispheric connections and its relationship to extrastriate visual areas in the macaque monkey, *J. Neurosci.*, 2: 265 – 283.

T.P. Hicks and G. Benedek (Eds.)
Progress in Brain Research, Vol. 75
© 1988 Elsevier Science Publishers B.V. (Biomedical Division)

CHAPTER 19

Influence of areas 17, 18, and 19 on receptive-field properties of neurons in the cat's posteromedial lateral suprasylvian visual cortex

Peter D. Spear

Department of Psychology and Neurosciences Training Program, University of Wisconsin, Madison, WI 53706, U.S.A.

Location and inputs of posteromedial lateral suprasylvian cortex

The cat's cortex contains a large number of visual areas in addition to striate cortex (area 17). Besides extrastriate areas 18 and 19, at least ten extrastriate visual cortical areas have been identified on the basis of pathway tracing and electrophysiological mapping studies (Fig. 1). The posteromedial lateral suprasylvian (PMLS) visual area is among the largest and best studied of these extrastriate visual cortical areas. The PMLS area was discovered in 1943 by Marshall et al. (1943) and later studied by Clare and Bishop (1954), after whom the area sometimes is named. More recent electrophysiological studies have shown that PMLS neurons have well-defined visual receptive fields and that the area is organized visuotopically (e.g., Hubel and Wiesel 1969; Wright 1969; Spear and Baumann 1975; Turlejski and Michalski 1975; Camarda and Rizzolatti 1976; Palmer et al. 1978).

One of the features of PMLS cortex that makes it extremely useful for understanding how visual information is integrated in the brain is that it is the target of several parallel visual pathways (see Rosenquist (1985) and Spear (1985) for reviews). One such pathway comes from the retina through the dorsal lateral geniculate body (dLGB) to PMLS cortex (a retinothalamic pathway). Within

the dLGB, projections to PMLS cortex arise from the geniculate wing (GW), the medial interlaminar nucleus (MIN), and the C layers. The A layers of the dLGB, which provide the major thalamic inputs to cortical areas 17 and 18, do not project to PMLS cortex. Physiological (Berson 1985; Rauschecker et al. 1987) and anatomical (reviewed by Rosenquist 1985; Spear 1985) studies suggest that the dLGB inputs to PMLS cortex arise from Y and W cells; few, if any, dLGB X cells appear to project to PMLS cortex. A second pathway to PMLS cortex arises from the superior colliculus and passes through the thalamus to PMLS cortex (a tectothalamic pathway). The thalamic nuclei involved in this pathway are the lateral posterior nucleus (LP), the posterior nucleus of Rioch (PN), and the C layers of the dLGB. A third pathway arises from the nucleus of the optic tract in the pretectum and passes through the pulvinar (PUL), the MIN, and the C layers of the dLGB to PMLS cortex (a pretectothalamic pathway). A fourth pathway involves direct corticocortical inputs to PMLS cortex (a corticocortical pathway). These corticocortical inputs arise from a variety of visual areas, including areas 17, 18, 19, 20a, 21a, 21b, anteromedial lateral suprasylvian (AMLS) cortex, and ventral lateral suprasylvian (VLS) cortex of both hemispheres.

My colleagues and I have long been interested in

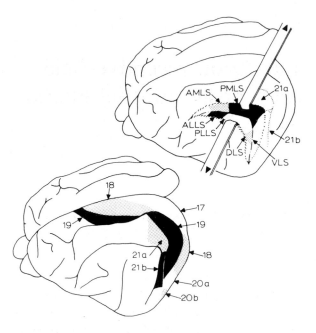

Fig. 1. Drawing of dorsolateral views of the cat brain to show the locations of 13 cortical visual areas that have been defined by pathway tracing and electrophysiological mapping studies. The visual areas are shown only for the left hemisphere; dorsal is up and anterior is to the left. In the uppermost drawing, the suprasylvian sulcus is shown opened by retractors so that the two banks of the sulcus can be seen. The drawings are based on the work of Tusa et al. (1981), and the visual areas are labeled according to their terminology. The six visual areas on the banks of the suprasylvian sulcus are the anteromedial (AMLS), anterolateral (ALLS), posteromedial (PMLS), posterolateral (PLLS), dorsal (DLS), and ventral (VLS) lateral suprasylvian visual areas. The remaining areas are numbered. Several additional cortical visual areas in the cat also have been described (see Rosenquist (1985) for review) but are not shown in the figure. (This figure is adapted from one kindly provided by A.C. Rosenquist.)

knowing how these various input pathways influence the visual response properties of neurons in PMLS cortex. One reason for this interest is a desire to understand how visual information is processed by the brain — how multiple inputs are combined and integrated to produce the spatial and temporal receptive-field properties of neurons in a target area. A second reason stems from a

desire to understand the neural plasticity, or compensation, that can occur in a target area after the influences of one or more inputs have been removed (Spear 1979, 1985; Tong 1988). To study plasticity of neural input-processing and integration, it is necessary to understand neural input-processing in normal adult animals.

To address these questions, my colleagues and I have sought to determine the effects of removing inputs from areas 17, 18, and 19 on the response properties of PMLS neurons in adult cats. We have focused on areas 17, 18, and 19 because they are the major cortical targets of the geniculocortical pathway in cats, because they provide the major corticocortical inputs to PMLS cortex, and because they are the areas most commonly removed in studies of compensation after 'visual cortex' damage in cats and other species. All of the studies I will describe here have involved making aspiration lesions of various combinations of areas 17, 18, and 19 and then comparing the response properties of PMLS neurons with those in normal cats. In our earliest experiments, we attempted to study PMLS neurons after reversible cooling of areas 17, 18, and 19. These attempts met with failure; we saw no changes in the responses of PMLS neurons during cooling of areas 17, 18, and 19 (Spear and Baumann, unpublished data). Presumably, there was no effect because the receptive fields of PMLS cells are very large and encompass regions of visuotopic representation in areas 17, 18, and 19 that are buried in sulci and inaccessible to the cooling plate. When we made aspiration lesions, however, we saw very clear and rapid changes in PMLS response properties (Spear and Baumann 1979a). Two kinds of information can be obtained from studies of this kind. First, any changes that occur when a source of afferents is removed provide information about the influences of those afferents on the responses of target PMLS neurons. Second, any response properties that remain provide information about the contributions made by remaining afferents from thalamus and other cortical areas.

Receptive-field organization of PMLS neurons

We began by investigating the effects of removing various combinations of areas 17, 18, and 19 on the basic receptive-field organization of PMLS neurons. Before discussing these results, I will briefly summarize results from our laboratory on the receptive-field organization of PMLS cells in normal adult cats (Spear and Baumann 1975; Smith and Spear 1979; Spear et al. 1985; McCall et al. 1988).

Normal receptive-field organization

About 85% of PMLS neurons encountered in single-cell recordings respond to light. These cells can be divided into four classes on the basis of their receptive-field properties (Fig. 2A). The large majority (about 80%) of PMLS cells are direction selective. They respond better to moving than to stationary flashed stimuli (about half give no response to flashed stimuli), and the response is strongly dependent on the direction of stimulus movement (Fig. 3). Directions of movement deviating more than 45 – 90° to either side of a preferred direction generally result in no response. The remaining 20% of PMLS cells are about evenly divided among the other three receptive-field classes (Fig. 2A). Cells in the movement-sensitive class respond best to moving stimuli but are not sensitive to the direction of stimulus movement. Cells in the stationary class give a transient response to the onset and/or offset of a stationary flashed stimulus and this response is equal to or greater than that to a moving stimulus. Cells in the indefinite class have diffuse ill-defined receptive fields or give indefinite responses to light.

The receptive fields of PMLS neurons generally are circular or elliptical and are relatively large (average of about 280 deg^2). Most PMLS cells are sensitive to the size of a visual stimulus. This size-sensitivity is due in part to spatial summation — the response of the cell increases as the size of the stimulus is increased within the excitatory receptive-field center. In addition, about 40% of PMLS cells have an inhibitory surround that results in a decreased response as the size of the stimulus is increased beyond the receptive-field center. When an inhibitory surround is present, it nearly always completely encircles the excitatory receptive-field center. Although most PMLS cells prefer moving stimuli, there is little selectivity to stimulus veloci-

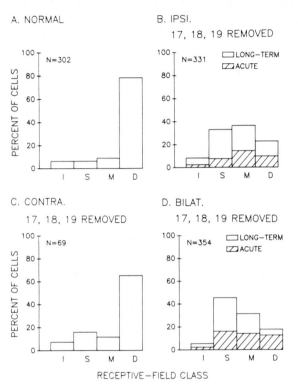

Fig. 2. Percentages of PMLS cells with different receptive-field properties in normal cats (A) and cats with ipsilateral (B), contralateral (C), or bilateral (D) removal of areas 17, 18, and 19. All cats were at least 6 months old at the time of the cortical lesion. Cross-hatched portions of each bar are results from cats studied within a day of the cortical lesion (acute lesion). Open portions of each bar are results from cats studied 2 weeks to more than a year after the lesion (long-term lesion). The height of each bar represents the sum of the open and cross-hatched portions. N is the number of cells studied in each condition. Receptive-field classes are: I, indefinite; S, stationary; M, movement sensitive; D, direction selective. Descriptions of the properties that characterize each class are given in the text. Data in A combined from Spear and Baumann (1975), Smith and Spear (1979), Spear et al. (1985), and McCall et al. (1988). Data in B combined from Spear and Baumann (1979a), Spear et al. (1980, 1988), and Tong et al. (1984). Data in C from Spear and Baumann (1979a). Data in D combined from Spear and Baumann (1979a,b) and Spear et al. (1988).

ty; good responses are obtained to stimuli moving from 5°/sec to over 200°/sec.

Influence of ipsilateral areas 17, 18, and 19

Removal of ipsilateral areas 17, 18, and 19 produces two main changes in the receptive-field properties of PMLS neurons (Spear and Baumann 1979a; Spear et al. 1980, 1988; Tong et al. 1984). First, there is a marked reduction in the percentage of direction-selective cells, from about 80% of the responsive cells in normal cats to about 20% in cats with ipsilateral areas 17, 18, and 19 removed

(Fig. 2B). Second, there is an increase in the percentage of cells that respond as well to stationary flashed stimuli as to stimulus movement. That is, the loss of direction-selective cells is not simply accompanied by an increase in the percentage of cells that are movement sensitive but not direction selective. Rather, a large proportion of the cells now give their optimal response to stationary flashing lights and are in the stationary receptive-field class.

As can be seen in Fig. 2B, these changes in PMLS receptive-field properties occur within

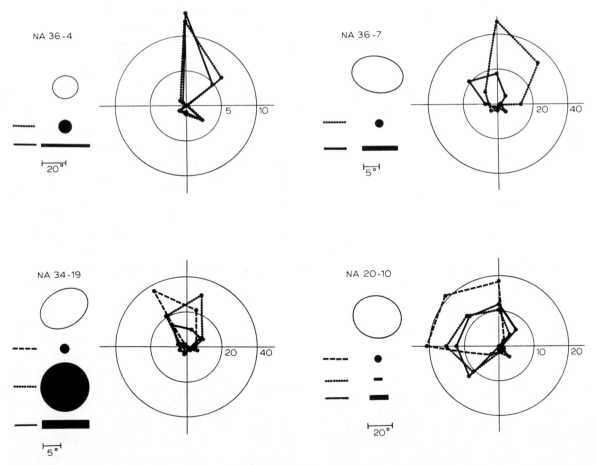

Fig. 3. Responses of four direction-selective cells in cat PMLS cortex to stimuli moving in different directions through the receptive field. Presentation of spot and slit stimuli were alternated for each of 8 directions of movement. Slits were oriented perpendicular to the movement direction. Polar diagrams show the mean response amplitude as a function of direction of the moving stimulus. Concentric circles indicate the number of spikes, as labeled. Receptive field (outline drawings) and stimulus (in black) sizes are given by the horizontal calibration bars. From Spear and Baumann (1975).

hours of removing inputs from ipsilateral areas 17, 18, and 19, and it seems safe to assume that the changes are immediate. Furthermore, at least in adult cats, no further alterations are observed during a period of more than a year after the lesion. Thus the effects are due to the removal of inputs from areas 17, 18, and 19 and not to secondary consequences of the lesion, such as retrograde degeneration in the thalamus or in PMLS cortex itself (which projects back to areas 17, 18, and 19).

One possible cause of these changes is that removal of areas 17, 18, and 19 simply silences PMLS cells with certain properties. Indeed, we do routinely find an increase in the percentage of cells that fail to respond to light in cats with cortical damage. However, the increase in nonresponsive cells is not sufficient to account for the loss of direction selective cells (Spear and Baumann 1979a). Furthermore, if a silencing of cells in one receptive-field class (e.g., direction selective) were the cause of an increase in percentages of cells in other classes, then the percentage of cells in all of the remaining receptive-field classes should increase equally. However, the percentage of cells in the indefinite class does not change at the same time that the percentages of cells in the movement-sensitive and stationary classes increase substantially (Fig. 2B). These considerations suggest that the changes in receptive-field properties that occur when inputs from areas 17, 18, and 19 are removed are due to the modification of specific properties of individual PMLS cells and not simply to a silencing of cells with certain properties.

Although there are changes in direction selectivity and responses to stationary flashed stimuli among PMLS neurons, other response properties appear to be normal following removal of ipsilateral areas 17, 18, and 19 (Spear and Baumann 1979a). The cells continue to respond to relatively small (1 – 2° or smaller) stimuli, most cells show spatial summation to increases in stimulus size within the receptive-field center, and about 35% of the cells have inhibitory surrounds — all properties that are similar to normal. Receptive-field size and the general features of visuotopic organization in

PMLS cortex also appear to be normal. Reponses of cells to different stimulus velocities also are unchanged.

Influence of contralateral areas 17, 18, and 19

The influence of inputs from contralateral areas 17, 18, and 19 have been assessed in two ways. First, recordings have been made from PMLS neurons contralateral to a unilateral lesion (Spear and Baumann 1979a). As shown in Fig. 2C, the percentages of direction-selective cells and cells in the other receptive-field classes are similar to normal in such animals. Second, recordings have been made in cats with a bilateral lesion of areas 17, 18, and 19 (Spear and Baumann 1979a,b; Spear et al. 1988) and compared with those ipsilateral to a unilateral lesion. Comparison of Figs. 2D and 2B shows that the effects are quite similar.

These results suggest that inputs from contralateral areas 17, 18, and 19 have little or no effect on the elaboration of receptive-field properties of PMLS neurons. However, three cautionary notes must be made. First, inputs from contralateral areas 17, 18, and 19 may well have small effects on direction selectivity and responses to stationary flashed stimuli that can only be detected with a much larger sample. That this may be the case is suggested by the observation that the percentage of direction-selective cells contralateral to a unilateral lesion is slightly lower than normal (compare Figs. 2C and 2A) and that the percentage of direction selective cells in cats with a bilateral lesion is slightly lower than in cats with a unilateral ipsilateral lesion (compare Figs. 2B and D). Second, receptive fields of neurons in areas 17, 18, and 19 are largely or entirely in the contralateral visual hemifield. However, PMLS cortex contains cells with receptive fields that extend 20 – 25° into the ipsilateral hemifield (Spear and Baumann 1975; Palmer et al. 1978), and these cells receive callosal input from the contralateral hemisphere (Rauschecker et al. 1987). Therefore, it is possible that inputs from contralateral areas 17, 18, and 19 influence the properties of those cells. Because the sample of such cells is very small, this possibility cannot be ruled out. Third, inputs from contralateral areas 17, 18, and 19 may well have effects on properties of PMLS cells that were not studied in these experiments.

Separate influences of areas 17, 18, and 19

To determine which inputs are responsible for receptive-field properties of PMLS neurons, experiments have been conducted in which areas 17, 18, and 19 were removed in various combinations (Spear and Baumann 1979a). In some cats, areas

18 and 19 were removed and most of area 17 was left intact. For each hemisphere, the portion of visuotopic representation that was removed in each cortical area was carefully reconstructed and related to the visual-field location of the receptive-field centers of PMLS cells that were recorded. We found that PMLS cells with inputs from areas 18 and 19 removed (and inputs from area 17 intact) have normal receptive-field organization (Fig. 4A, upper panel). In the same cats, PMLS cells with inputs from area 17 removed in addition to areas 18

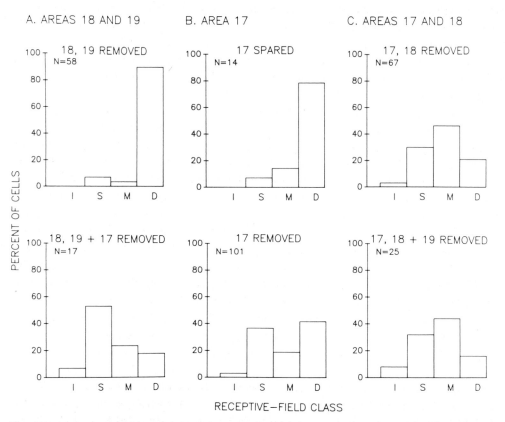

Fig. 4. Percentages of PMLS cells with different receptive-field properties in cats with lesions intended to include areas 18 and 19 (A), area 17 alone (B), or areas 17 and 18 (C). For each condition, data are presented with reference to detailed lesion reconstructions. In A, the upper panel (18, 19 removed) shows results for PMLS cells that had receptive-field locations corresponding to the region of visual-field representation that was damaged in areas 18 and 19, but not damaged in area 17, i.e., these results show effects of removing areas 18 and 19 alone. The lower panel (18, 19 + 17 removed) shows results for PMLS cells in the same cats but with receptive-field locations corresponding to the region of visual-field representation that was damaged in area 17 as well as areas 18 and 19. Similarly, in B, the results are divided into cells with receptive-field locations corresponding to the region of visual-field representation damaged (lower panel) or spared (upper panel) in area 17 (areas 18 and 19 were intact). In C, the results are divided into cells with receptive-field locations corresponding to the region of visual-field representation damaged only in areas 17 and 18 (upper panel) or in area 19 as well as in areas 17 and 18 (lower panel). Conventions as in Fig. 2. From Spear and Baumann (1979a).

and 19 show the typical effects associated with removal of areas 17, 18, and 19 (Fig. 4A, lower panel).

In other cats, cortical removal was limited to area 17. This lesion produces effects on PMLS neurons that are similar to those following removal of all three cortical areas (17, 18, and 19). However, the effects are of smaller magnitude (Fig. 4B, lower panel). For example, about 40% of the cells are direction selective, compared to about 20% when all three areas are removed. In some cases the damage to area 17 was incomplete, and cells with receptive-field locations that correspond to spared portions of area 17 have normal receptive-field properties (Fig. 4B, upper panel).

Finally, some cats had areas 17 and 18, but not area 19, removed. This lesion produces effects on PMLS receptive-field properties that are indistinguishable from the effects of removing all three areas (Fig. 4C, upper panel). Indeed, in the same animals, cells with inputs from area 19 inadvertently removed in addition to areas 17 and 18 are indistinguishable from cells with inputs only from areas 17 and 18 removed (compare upper and lower panels of Fig. 4C).

In a related study, Guedes et al. (1983) reported that transecting output fibers from areas 17 and 18 has no effect on the response properties of suprasylvian cortex neurons, a result that appears to be inconsistent with those just described. A possible reason for this difference is that the transections made by Guedes et al. (1983) may not have removed the outputs from both areas 17 and 18 that are in visuotopic correspondence with the suprasylvian cortex cells that were studied. A second possible reason for the difference is that Guedes et al. (1983) recorded from the VLS visual area after the transections whereas we recorded primarily from the PMLS area and to a lesser extent from the AMLS area (see Fig. 1). Thus Guedes et al. (1983) were studying a different extrastriate visual area of cortex.

Conclusions

Our results suggest that inputs from ipsilateral areas 17 and 18 have two main influences on the receptive-field organization of PMLS neurons. The first is to provide information for the elaboration of direction selectivity in PMLS cortex. It is not known whether the direction selectivity is transmitted from areas 17 and 18 and imposed on recipient PMLS neurons or whether the inputs from areas 17 and 18 provide a basis on which direction selectivity is elaborated by intrinsic PMLS cortex circuitry. The second influence of ipsilateral areas 17 and 18 is to inhibit responses of PMLS cells to stationary flashed stimuli. Presumably, removal of areas 17 and 18 removes the inhibition and thus increases the responses of many cells to stationary flashed stimuli.

About half of the PMLS cells appear to receive these functional influences from area 17 alone, and these cells change their response properties following removal of area 17 alone (Fig. 4B). Other PMLS cells appear to receive the functional information independently from both areas 17 and 18. For these cells it is necessary (and sufficient) to remove inputs from both cortical areas to produce a change in receptive-field organization. No PMLS cells seem to receive the functional information solely from area 18, because removal of area 18, even in combination with area 19, is not sufficient to produce a change in receptive-field organization (Fig. 4A). Apparently, the functional inputs from area 18 terminate only on PMLS cells that also receive the information independently from area 17. It is not clear what role is played by the known projections from area 19 to PMLS cortex.

There are a variety of pathways through which areas 17 and 18 could influence PMLS neurons. In addition to their direct projections to PMLS cortex, areas 17 and 18 provide indirect inputs via the superior colliculus, pretectum, and a number of thalamic nuclei (see Spear (1985) for review). It is known that removal of the corticotectal loop to PMLS cortex is not responsible for the loss of direction selectivity that occurs after removal of areas 17 and 18 (Smith and Spear 1979). However, it is not known whether the changes that occur in PMLS cortex are due to removal of one of the other indirect pathways or to removal of the direct corticocortical inputs.

It is important to stress that receptive-field properties such as receptive-field size, spatial summation, surround inhibition, and responses to different stimulus velocities, are unaffected by combined removal of areas 17, 18, and 19. Therefore these properties of PMLS neurons are elaborated on the basis of thalamic or other cortical inputs independent of areas 17, 18, and 19.

Spatial-frequency sensitivity of PMLS neurons

Like neurons elsewhere in the visual system, PMLS neurons respond selectively to different spatial frequencies in a visual stimulus (Gizzi et al. 1981; Shelepin 1983, 1984; DiStefano et al. 1985; Morrone et al. 1986; Zumbroich and Blakemore 1987). For example, when tested with drifting sine-wave gratings, individual PMLS neurons respond optimally to a relatively narrow range of spatial frequencies and fail to respond to spatial frequencies higher than a particular value − the spatial resolution, or visual acuity, of the neuron. The ranges of optimal spatial frequencies and spatial resolutions of PMLS neurons largely overlap those of neurons in areas 17 and 18 (see Orban (1984) for review). This raises the possibility that the spatial-frequency processing of PMLS neurons depends upon inputs from these cortical areas. Alternatively, PMLS neurons might process spatial-frequency information on the basis of thalamic inputs, independent of the corticocortical pathways. To test these possibilities, William Guido, Lillian Tong, and I have begun an investigation of the spatial-frequency sensitivity of PMLS neurons and the consequences of removing inputs from ipsilateral areas 17, 18, and 19.

Normal spatial-frequency sensitivity

To test spatial-frequency processing by PMLS neurons, we analyzed the responses to sine-wave gratings that drift across the receptive field in the preferred direction. In most cases, the grating covered 20° × 20° of visual field and extended beyond the receptive-field center. However, cells with inhibitory receptive-field surrounds often have their responses completely suppressed if the grating includes the surround region. Therefore, for these cells the grating was presented in a circular aperture the size of the excitatory receptive-field center. Each neuron was presented with a range of seven spatial frequencies at six different contrasts. On a given trial, one spatial frequency and contrast combination was presented for one second at a drift rate (temporal frequency) of 3 Hz. A run consisted of all 42 combinations of spatial frequencies and contrasts (presented in semi-random order) plus a blank 'stimulus' of the same mean luminance (30 cd/m^2) but with no grating. Ten such runs were presented to most cells that were studied. Thus each of the 42 stimuli (spatial frequency and contrast combinations) and the blank was presented 10 times.

Fig. 5A shows peristimulus time histograms of the ten responses of a PMLS neuron to one of the stimuli. The PSTH for each trial was subjected to Fourier analysis to determine the amplitude of the modulated discharge at the fundamental frequency of the stimulus (F1) and the mean discharge rate (F0) for that trial. Then the means and standard errors of the F0 and F1 responses for the ten trials were calculated. This analysis was carried out for the responses to each spatial frequency at each of six contrasts and for the maintained discharge during presentation of a blank screen. A response vs. contrast function for one spatial frequency is shown in Fig. 5B. From the response vs. contrast function, a contrast threshold was calculated for the spatial frequency (arrow in Fig. 5B). Contrast thresholds were determined in this way for all seven spatial frequencies and used to plot a contrast-sensitivity (inverse of contrast-threshold) function (Fig. 5C). From the contrast-sensitivity function, we determined the optimal spatial frequency, the spatial resolution (highest spatial frequency to which the cell gives a statistically significant response), and the maximal sensitivity of each neuron (arrows in Fig. 5C). We also measured maximal response strength for each neuron, which

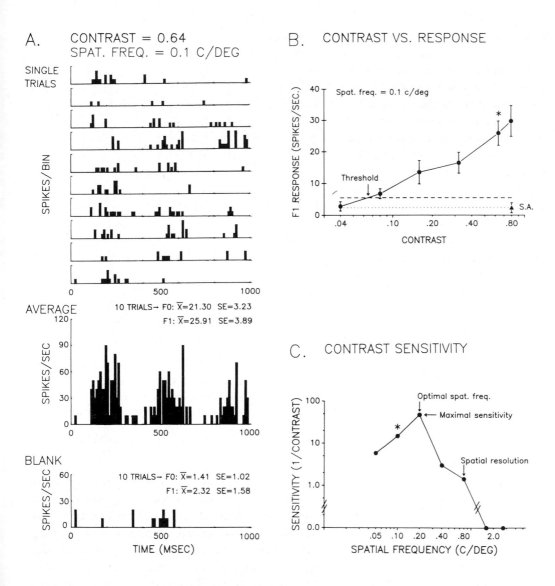

Fig. 5. (A) At the top are peristimulus time histrograms (PSTH) of the responses of a PMLS neuron to 10 presentations of a 0.1 cycles/deg sine-wave grating of 0.64 contrast. Each presentation lasted one second and included 3 cycles of the grating, which drifted across the receptive field in the preferred direction of the neuron. The average PSTH for all 10 trials is shown below. Also given are the means and standard errors (in spikes/sec) of the F0 and F1 responses for the 10 trials. At the bottom is the average PSTH for 10 presentations of a blank screen; this shows the neuron's maintained activity. The mean and standard errors of the mean discharge rate (F0) and the 3 Hz modulated discharge (F1) inherent in the neuron's maintained activity (analyzed as if a 3 Hz grating were present) also are given. (B) Means and standard errors of the F1 response to a 0.1 cycles/deg grating at each of six contrasts. The horizontal dotted line and triangle (labeled S.A.) shows the mean and standard error of the F1 activity during presentation of the blank screen; the horizontal dashed line is 2 standard errors above the mean. The point marked by the asterisk represents the results calculated from the PSTHs shown in A. The arrow indicates the contrast threshold for this spatial frequency. (C) Contrast-sensitivity (inverse of contrast-threshold) function of the same neuron to all seven spatial frequencies. The point marked by the asterisk comes from the contrast threshold determination shown in B. The vertical arrows indicate the optimal spatial frequency and the spatial resolution of this cell. The horizontal arrow indicates the maximal sensitivity. From Guido, Tong, and Spear (unpublished).

is the maximal discharge rate to any grating stimulus tested minus the discharge rate during presentation of the blank screen. So far we have obtained such data from 39 neurons in PMLS cortex of normal adult cats. One of the cells did not respond to drifting gratings even though it responded to spots of light on the tangent screen. The remaining cells gave both a modulated (F1) response and an overall increase in discharge rate (F0) to the grating stimuli (see Fig. 5A). In general, the results for the two response measures were very similar. Therefore, only the results for the fundamental response will be presented here.

In agreement with previous studies (Gizzi et al. 1981; Shelepin 1983, 1984; Morrone et al. 1986;

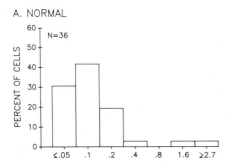

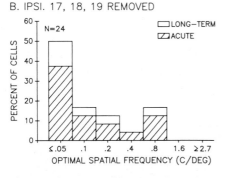

Fig. 6. Optimal spatial frequency for PMLS neurons in normal cats (A) and cats with ipsilateral areas 17, 18, and 19 removed (B). Results are based on the fundamental component of the Fourier-analyzed responses of each neuron. In B, cross-hatched portions of each bar are data from cats studied within a day of the cortical lesion. Open portions of each bar are data from cats studied more than 6 months after the lesion. The height of each bar represents the sum of the open and cross-hatched portions. N is the number of cells studied in each condition. From Guido, Tong, and Spear (unpublished).

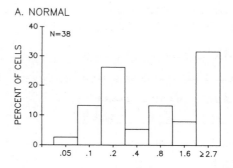

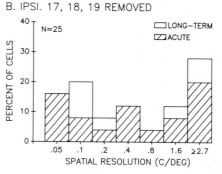

Fig. 7. Spatial resolution of PMLS neurons in normal cats (A) and cats with ipsilateral areas 17, 18, and 19 removed (B). Results are based on the fundamental component of the Fourier-analyzed responses of each neuron. Conventions as in Fig. 6. From Guido, Tong, and Spear (unpublished).

Zumbroich and Blakemore 1987), we found that PMLS cells are most sensitive to relatively low spatial frequencies (Fig. 6A). Although a few cells have an optimal spatial frequency of 1.6 cycles/deg or higher, the majority have an optimum between 0.05 and 0.2 cycles/deg. The spatial resolution of PMLS cells also tends to be low, although the range is relatively broad (Fig. 7A). About 70% of the cells have a spatial resolution between 0.05 and 1.6 cycles/deg. The highest spatial frequency tested was 2.7 cycles/deg, and about 30% of the cells gave a significant response to this stimulus. It is possible that these cells would have responded to even higher spatial frequencies had they been presented. However, the response to 2.7 cycles/deg was very weak for all but one of the cells. Therefore, it is likely that this spatial frequency is very close to the highest to which the cells respond. These results for the spatial resolution of normal

PMLS neurons are similar to those of other investigators (DiStefano et al. 1985; Zumbroich and Blakemore 1987).

Many PMLS cells in normal cats require relatively high grating contrasts for a significant response to occur. That is, contrast sensitivity tends to be relatively low. This is shown by Fig. 8A, which plots the maximal logarithmic sensitivity for each cell in the sample. The mean maximal logarithmic sensitivity for all cells is 1.87. Maximal response strength also tends to be low for normal PMLS neurons (Fig. 9A). Although maximal fundamental response rates as high as 45 spikes/sec are seen, the average maximal response strength for the sample is only 13.5 spikes/sec. Similar response rates are found for measures of mean discharge (the F0 response); the average maximal response strength for this measure is 19.1 spikes/sec.

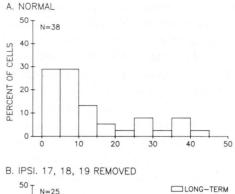

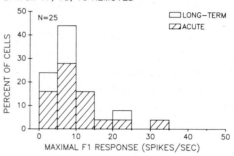

Fig. 9. Maximal strength of the fundamental response for PMLS neurons in normal cats (A) and cats with ipsilateral areas 17, 18, and 19 removed (B). Response strength was measured as the discharge rate to the grating stimulus minus the discharge rate during presentation of a blank screen. Conventions as in Fig. 6. From Guido, Tong, and Spear (unpublished).

Influence of ipsilateral areas 17, 18 and 19

So far we have investigated the spatial-frequency sensitivity of 20 PMLS cells in cats studied a day after removing ipsilateral areas 17, 18, and 19 and 10 PMLS cells in cats studied 6 months or more after the lesion. Among the 30 cells, only 20% (6 cells) were direction selective. Thus these cells showed the reduced direction selectivity that is typical of PMLS neurons with inputs from areas 17 and 18 removed. When tested with drifting gratings, two of the 30 cells gave no significant response even though they responded to spots of light on the tangent screen, and three cells had significant F0 responses but no significant F1 modulation to the gratings. For the responsive cells it was possible to generate spatial-frequency sensitivity functions using the same methods that were used in normal cats (Fig. 5).

Removal of areas 17, 18, and 19 produces a

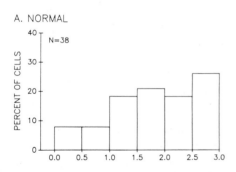

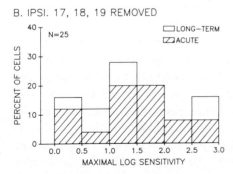

Fig. 8. Maximal logarithmic sensitivity of PMLS neurons in normal cats (A) and cats with ipsilateral areas 17, 18, and 19 removed (B). Results are based on the fundamental component of the Fourier-analyzed responses of each neuron. Conventions as in Fig. 6. From Guido, Tong, and Spear (unpublished).

slight reduction in maximal responsiveness and sensitivity among PMLS neurons. The average maximal fundamental response rate is 9.1 spikes/sec for PMLS cells with inputs from areas 17, 18, and 19 removed, which is significantly lower than normal ($t = 1.88$, $df = 61$, $p < 0.05$, one-tailed). As can be seen in Fig. 9 (compare Fig. 9B and 9A), this difference is due to a decrease in PMLS cells with the highest response rates (> 25 spikes/sec) after removal of areas 17, 18, and 19. The mean maximal logarithmic sensitivity for all cells is 1.48, about one-third of a log unit lower than normal ($t = 1.77$, $df = 61$, $p < 0.05$, one-tailed). This decrease is due to a reduced percentage of cells with the highest sensitivities rather than an overall reduction (leftward shift) in the distribution of sensitivities (compare Figs. 8B and 8A).

Despite these changes in maximal responsiveness and sensitivity, removal of inputs from areas 17, 18, and 19 has little or no effect on the optimal spatial frequency or spatial resolution of PMLS cells. As shown in Fig. 6B, the range of optimal spatial frequencies is 0.05 – 0.8 cycles/deg after removal of areas 17, 18, and 19. Although the percentage of cells with an optimum of 0.05 cycles/deg is somewhat higher than in normal cats, the two distributions overlap substantially (compare Figs. 6B and 6A) and are not significantly different. Similarly, there is no significant difference between the distributions of spatial resolutions for normal PMLS cells and PMLS cells with inputs from areas 17, 18, and 19 removed (compare Figs. 7A and B).

Conclusions

In reaching conclusions from these results, it is important to bear in mind several cautions. Our results on spatial-frequency sensitivity of PMLS neurons are based on relatively small samples of neurons both in normal cats and in cats with ipsilateral areas 17, 18, and 19 removed. Until additional neurons have been studied, any conclusions must be regarded as tentative. Furthermore, so far we have analyzed results only for spatial-frequency

sensitivity to drifting sine-wave gratings. We also have tested many of the same neurons with counterphased sine-wave gratings to assess the linearity of spatial summation and the spatial-frequency sensitivity of any nonlinear (second harmonic) responses to the gratings. Temporal-frequency sensitivity of responses to the optimal spatial frequency also has been tested for many PMLS cells. Until the results for these properties have been analyzed fully, our conclusions remain limited to spatial-frequency sensitivity to moving gratings.

With these cautions in mind, we suggest that inputs from ipsilateral areas 17, 18, and 19 have little influence on spatial frequency processing by neurons in PMLS cortex. Removing areas 17, 18, and 19 reduces the incidence of PMLS cells with the highest response rates and sensitivities; however, it has no significant effect on spatial resolution and optimal spatial frequency. Thus, while afferents from areas 17, 18, and 19 may enhance the responsiveness and sensitivity of some PMLS cells, they appear to have little influence on the selectivity of responses to spatial parameters of the stimuli. Unlike direction selectivity and relative responses to moving and stationary flashed stimuli, spatial resolution and optimal spatial frequency appear to depend more on inputs from other cortical areas or the thalamus than on areas 17, 18, and 19.

One important input for spatial-frequency processing may be the C layers of the dLGB. The spatial-frequency sensitivity of C-layer neurons is similar in many respects to those of cells in PMLS cortex. For instance, both the Y and W cells in the C layers have relatively low spatial frequency optima and low spatial resolutions. Furthermore, W cells in the C layers are noted for their poor contrast sensitivity and relatively weak responses (see Sherman (1985) for review). These comparisons suggest that the spatial-frequency processing by PMLS neurons may depend on afferents from Y and especially W cells in the C layers of the dLGB and that this processing occurs in parallel with that in areas 17, 18, and 19.

References

Berson, D.M. (1985) Cat lateral suprasylvian cortex: Y-cell inputs and corticotectal projection. *J. Neurophysiol.*, 53: 544–556.

Camarda, R. and Rizzolatti, G. (1976) Visual receptive fields in the lateral suprasylvian area (Clare-Bishop area) of the cat. *Brain Res.*, 101: 427–443.

Clare, M.H. and Bishop, G.H. (1954) Responses from an association area secondarily activated from optic cortex. *J. Neurophysiol.*, 17: 271–277.

DiStefano, M., Morrone, M.C. and Burr, D.C. (1985) Visual acuity of neurones in the cat lateral suprasylvian cortex. *Brain Res.*, 331: 382–385.

Gizzi, M.S., Katz, E. and Movshon, J.A. (1981) Spatial properties of neurons in the cat's lateral suprasylvian visual cortex. *Soc. Neurosci. Abstr.*, 7: 831.

Guedes, R., Watanabe, S. and Creutzfeldt, O.D. (1983) Functional role of association fibres for a visual association area: The posterior suprasylvian sulcus of the cat. *Exp. Brain Res.*, 49: 13–27.

Hubel, D.H. and Wiesel, T.N. (1969) Visual area of the lateral suprasylvian gyrus (Clare-Bishop area) of the cat. *J. Physiol. (Lond.)*, 202: 251–260.

Marshall, W.H., Talbot, S.A. and Ades, H.W. (1943) Cortical response of the anesthetized cat to gross photic and electrical afferent stimulation. *J. Neurophysiol.*, 6: 1–15.

McCall, M.A., Tong, L. and Spear, P.D. (1988) Development of neuronal responses in cat posteromedial lateral suprasylvian visual cortex, *Brain Res.*, 447: 67–78.

Morrone, M.C., DiStefano, M. and Burr, D.C. (1986) Spatial and temporal properties of neurons of the lateral suprasylvian cortex of the cat. *J. Neurophysiol.*, 56: 969–986.

Orban, G.A. (1984) *Neuronal Operations in the Visual Cortex*, Springer-Verlag, Berlin, 367 pp.

Palmer, L.A., Rosenquist, A.C. and Tusa, R.J. (1978) The retinotopic organization of lateral suprasylvian visual areas in the cat. *J. Comp. Neurol.*, 177: 237–256.

Rauschecker, J.P., von Grünau, M.W. and Poulin, C. (1987) Thalamo-cortical connections and their correlation with receptive field properties in the cat's lateral suprasylvian visual cortex. *Exp. Brain Res.*, 67: 100–112.

Rosenquist, A.C. (1985) Connections of visual cortical areas in the cat. In: A. Peters and E.G. Jones (Eds.), *Cerebral Cortex*, Plenum Press, New York, pp. 81–117.

Shelepin, Y.E. (1983) Spatial frequency characteristics of receptive fields of neurons in the lateral suprasylvian area of the cat cortex. *Neurophysiol.*, 14: 443–447.

Shelepin, Y.E. (1984) Comparison of topographic and spatial-frequency characteristics of the lateral suprasylvian and striate cortex in cats. *Neurophysiol.*, 16: 29–34.

Sherman, S.M. (1985) Functional organization of the W-, X-, and Y-cell pathways in the cat: a review and hypothesis. In: J.M. Sprague and A.N. Epstein (Eds.), *Progress in Psychobiology and Physiological Psychology*, Academic Press, Orlando, FL, pp. 234–314.

Smith, D.C. and Spear, P.D. (1979) Effects of superior colliculus removal on receptive field properties of neurons in lateral suprasylvian visual area of the cat. *J. Neurophysiol.*, 42: 57–75.

Spear, P.D. (1979) Behavioral and neurophysiological consequences of visual cortex damage: Mechanisms of recovery. In: J.M. Sprague and A.N. Epstein (Eds.), *Progress in Psychobiology and Physiological Psychology*, Academic Press, New York, pp. 45–90.

Spear, P.D. (1985) Neural mechanisms of compensation following neonatal visual cortex damage. In: C.W. Cotman (Ed.), *Synaptic Plasticity and Remodeling*, Guilford Press, New York, pp. 111–167.

Spear, P.D. and Baumann, T.P. (1975) Receptive-field characteristics of single neurons in lateral suprasylvian visual area of the cat. *J. Neurophysiol.*, 38: 1403–1420.

Spear, P.D. and Baumann, T.P. (1979a) Effects of visual cortex removal on receptive-field properties of neurons in lateral suprasylvian visual area of the cat. *J. Neurophysiol.*, 42: 31–56.

Spear, P.D. and Baumann, T.P. (1979b) Neurophysiological mechanisms of recovery from visual cortex damage in cats: properties of lateral suprasylvian visual area neurons following behavioral recovery. *Exp. Brain Res.*, 35: 161–176.

Spear, P.D., Kalil, R.E. and Tong, L. (1980) Functional compensation in lateral suprasylvian visual area following neonatal visual cortex removal in cats. *J. Neurophysiol.*, 43: 851–869.

Spear, P.D., Tong, L., McCall, M.A. and Pasternak, T. (1985) Developmentally induced loss of direction-selective neurons in the cat's lateral suprasylvian visual cortex. *Dev. Brain Res.*, 20: 281–285.

Spear, P.D., Tong, L. and McCall, M.A. (1988) Functional influence of areas 17, 18, and 19 on lateral suprasylvian cortex in kittens and adult cats: implications for compensation following early visual cortex damage, *Brain Res.*, 447: 79–91.

Tong, L. (1988) Mechanisms of functional compensation in the posteromedial lateral suprasylvian visual cortex (PMLS) of cats with an early visual cortex lesion (areas 17, 18, and 19). In: K-F. So (Ed.), *Vision – Structure and Function*, World Scientific Publ., Singapore, in press.

Tong, L., Kalil, R.E. and Spear, P.D. (1984) Critical periods for functional and anatomical compensation in lateral suprasylvian visual area following removal of visual cortex in cats. *J. Neurophysiol.*, 52: 941–960.

Turlejski, K. and Michalski, A. (1975) Clare-Bishop area in the cat: Location and retinotopical projection. *Acta Neurobiol. Exp.*, 35: 179–188.

Tusa, R.J., Palmer, L.A. and Rosenquist, A.C. (1981) Multiple cortical visual areas: visual field topography in the cat. In: C.N. Woolsey (Ed.), *Cortical Sensory Organization*, Humana Press, Clifton, NJ, pp. 1 – 31.

Wright, M.J. (1969) Visual receptive fields of cells in a cortical area remote from the striate cortex in the cat. *Nature*, 223: 973 – 975.

Zumbroich, T.J. and Blakemore, C. (1987) Spatial and temporal selectivity in the suprasylvian visual cortex of the cat. *J. Neurosci.*, 7: 482 – 500.

T.P. Hicks and G. Benedek (Eds.)
Progress in Brain Research, Vol. 75
© 1988 Elsevier Science Publishers B.V. (Biomedical Division)

CHAPTER 20

Stimulus selectivity and its postnatal development in the cat's suprasylvian visual cortex

Thomas J. Zumbroich*, Colin Blakemore and David J. Price**

University Laboratory of Physiology, Parks Road, Oxford OX1 3PT, U.K.

Our view of the processing of visual information in the cerebral cortex has changed radically over the past 20 years or so. According to classical ideas, signals from the eyes entered the striate cortex, which projected to one or two other specific visual areas in the peristriate belt, whence the visual messages disappeared into a huge tract of 'association cortex' stretching forward into the parietal and temporal regions. Two main discoveries have utterly changed our picture of cortical processing beyond area 17. First there is the finding that the posterior 'association cortex', at least in cats and primates, is in fact occupied by a remarkable patchwork of additional visual areas, each with its own representation of all or part of the visual field. These multiple visual zones may constitute an analytical cascade, in which at least some of the areas are functionally specialized for analysis of particular aspects of the visual stimulus. The other, related observation is that these extrastriate visual areas receive their own complex sets of afferent inputs from various parts of the posterior thalamus, in addition to the indirect cortico-cortical projections originating in area 17.

In the cat, the lateral suprasylvian cortex around

the suprasylvian sulcus is visually responsive and was subdivided by Palmer et al. (1978) into six regions on the basis of their topographical organization. The areas in the medial (PMLS) and lateral banks (PLLS) of the middle suprasylvian sulcus display a complicated pattern of afferent connectivity. They receive input from other visual cortical areas, including areas 17, 18, 19 and 20 (e.g., Symonds and Rosenquist 1984; Sherk 1986) and have thalamic afferents that originate not only from the C-laminae of the lateral geniculate nucleus (LGN) and the medial interlaminar nucleus (MIN), but to an even larger extent from the pulvinar/lateralis posterior complex (e.g., Tong et al. 1982; Raczkowski and Rosenquist 1980, 1983). Thus inputs from the geniculo-cortical, the cortico-thalamocortical, and the tecto-thalamocortical visual pathways converge on the cortex of the middle suprasylvian sulcus.

Neurons in the lateral suprasylvian cortex respond well to moving stimuli and are usually direction selective (Hubel and Wiesel 1969; Wright 1969). Their properties have led many authors to propose that this region is specialized for the analysis of image motion (e.g., Spear and Baumann 1975; Toyama and Kozasa 1982; Toyama et al. 1985; Blakemore and Zumbroich 1987).

Grating stimuli (regular patterns of light and dark bars) have been used extensively and to great effect in the analysis of the spatial structure and selective properties of the receptive fields of

---

* *Present address:* Department of Biology, B-022, University of California at San Diego, La Jolla, CA 92093, U.S.A.
** *Present address:* Department of Zoology, University of California, Berkeley, CA 94720, U.S.A.

neurons in other parts of the visual system, from the retina to areas 17 and 18. We have used drifting and contrast-modulated gratings, as well as conventional projected stimuli, to examine the selectivity of cells in both PMLS and PLLS of adult cats and also to study the postnatal development of PMLS.

Stimulus selectivity in the suprasylvian visual areas of the adult cat

Spatial selectivity

For areas 17 and 18 grating stimuli have proven powerful tools for the quantitative study of the selectivity of neurons for the spatial dimensions of stimuli, the structure of their receptive fields and the nature of spatial summation (e.g., Movshon et al. 1978a,b). The spatial properties of neurons in the suprasylvian cortex have received comparatively little attention (Blakemore and Zumbroich 1985; Di Stefano et al. 1985; Morrone et al. 1986; Zumbroich and Blakemore 1987). It is well known that at any position in the visual field the receptive fields of neurons in PMLS and PLLS are considerably larger, on average, than those of cells in area 17 (e.g., Spear and Baumann 1975; Zumbroich et al. 1986). This raises the possibility that neurons in the suprasylvian visual cortex are performing a fine spatial analysis of the image generalized over areas of the visual field larger than the receptive fields of striate neurons. Alternatively their preferred spatial dimensions might be large, in direct correspondence to their big receptive fields.

We recorded from isolated single units in areas PMLS and PLLS of adult cats, paralysed by an intravenous infusion of Flaxedil and anaesthetized by hyperventilation with 80% nitrous oxide supplemented when necessary with adjuvant intravenous anaesthetic. The corneae were protected by means of contact lenses with 3 mm artificial pupils, and the refractive state of the eyes was corrected with additional spherical lenses. We have described our methods in detail elsewhere (Blakemore and Zumbroich 1987). Each unit was initially assessed qualitatively and the receptive field was plotted by means of projected spots and bars. To measure spatial frequency selectivity an oscilloscope display screen was then centred on the receptive field and high-contrast gratings of sinusoidal luminance profile, of optimal orientation, direction of drift and temporal frequency, but different spatial frequencies, were presented under computer control in a pseudo-randomly interleaved series. The computer prepared averaged histograms of responses to each spatial frequency and to a blank trial with no grating present on the screen. Fourier analysis was then applied to decompose the response into its various temporal components.

Fig. 1 illustrates responses to drifting gratings for a unit recorded in PMLS. We have plotted the mean spike rate (f_0 Fourier component: filled squares) and the amplitude of modulation of the discharge at the temporal frequency of drift of the grating (fundamental, f_1, component: open circles). The spike histograms (Fig. 1B) show that the cell's discharge was weakly modulated at all spatial frequencies to which it responded, but the plot of the f_0 and f_1 components of the response versus spatial frequency suggests that the overall elevation of spike rate provides the more reliable description of the spatial selectivity of the neuron and gives a higher value of cut-off spatial frequency ('acuity').

The temporal pattern of response to moving sinusoidal gratings was quantitatively analysed for all cells to calculate the degree to which the response was composed of modulated and unmodulated components. Like the individual example of Fig. 1, the responses of the majority of cells in PMLS and PLLS were dominated by an unmodulated elevation of discharge, although some modulation occurred at the temporal frequency of drift, especially at low spatial frequencies (Zumbroich and Blakemore 1987). These properties are similar to those of *complex* cells in the striate cortex (Movshon et al. 1978b). In general, then, we based our assessment of neuronal responses to drifting gratings on measurement of the mean discharge (f_0) component. From spatial frequency tuning curves, like that in Fig. 1, we determined the *cut-off spatial frequency* (acuity), defined as the spatial frequency at which the response fell to a threshold level equal to the spontaneous activity plus 2 standard errors (SE) of the mean. The highest acuity we found for neurons in this part of the posterolateral suprasylvian cortex, bordering the middle suprasylvian sulcus, was 2.1 cycles per degree of visual angle (cycles/deg), which is considerably lower than the best values reported for cells in cat area 17 (e.g., Movshon et al. 1978c: 7

cycles/deg), but is roughly comparable to the maximum resolution in area 18 (e.g., Movshon et al. 1978c: less than 1.5 cycles/deg) and the superior colliculus (Bisti and Sireteanu 1976: 2.2 cycles/deg).

Fig. 2 shows the relationship between the eccentricity of the receptive field and the acuity for PMLS (A) and PLLS (B). For PMLS there was a significant negative linear correlation between the logarithm of the cut-off spatial frequency and eccentricity. A similar decline of spatial resolution with distance of the receptive field from the area

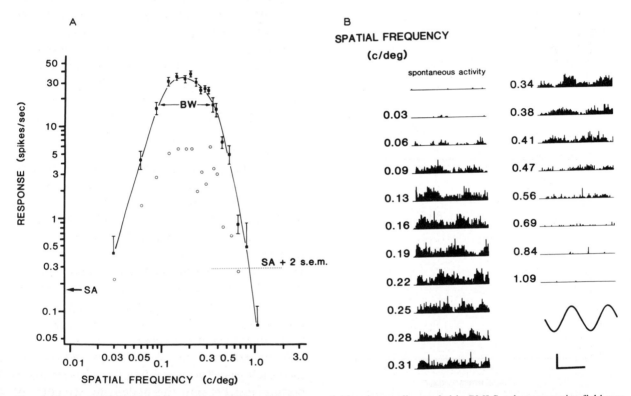

Fig. 1. This is a typical spatial-frequency tuning function for a spatial bandpass cell recorded in PMLS, whose receptive field was centred at an eccentricity of 5 deg. (A) Response, on a log scale, is plotted against the spatial frequency of a grating drifting across the receptive field in the optimal direction. Each data point represents the mean value of discharge (spikes/sec) for ten presentations of 2 cycles of a grating moving at a temporal frequency of 0.75 Hz. The filled squares ($\pm$ 1 SE) plot the overall elevation of discharge (f_0 Fourier component) and the unfilled circles indicate the component of the response modulated at the temporal frequency of the drifting grating (f_1). The arrow, marked SA, on the ordinate shows the mean level of spontaneous activity and the interrupted line is a suprathreshold level, defined as the spontaneous activity plus 2 SE, above which an f_0 response was considered to be significantly higher than background. The bandwidth (BW) at half-amplitude is shown. (B) These are the spike histograms for each of the spatial frequencies presented to this cell. The duration of each histogram represents two temporal periods of the grating and each is the average of ten presentations. The bin width was 12 msec. Vertical calibration: 100 spikes/sec. Horizontal calibration: 1.0 sec. (Data from Zumbroich and Blakemore 1987.)

centralis is evident at the level of the retina (e.g., Cleland et al. 1979), the LGN (e.g., Ikeda and Wright 1976) and striate cortex (e.g., Eggers and Blakemore 1978). For our limited sample from PLLS there was no clear relationship, the lowest acuity in the sample being at 18 deg and the second highest (still only about 1 cycle/deg) at 70 deg eccentricity. The part of PLLS that we investigated seems, then, to lack any obvious central specializa-

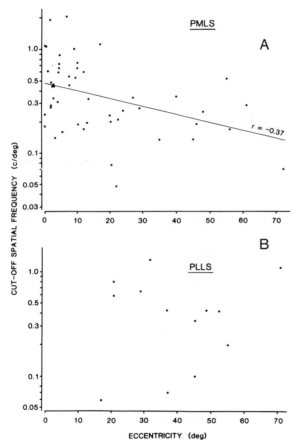

Fig. 2. The spatial 'acuity' or cut-off spatial frequency, defined as the highest spatial frequency for which the cell gave a response, was determined by finding the point at which the spatial-frequency tuning curve intersected the threshold criterion, 2 SE above the spontaneous activity (see Fig. 1A). Here, the acuity of units in (A) PMLS ($n = 49$) and (B) PLLS ($n = 13$) is plotted against eccentricity (radial distance of the response field centre from the area centralis). A linear regression equation was calculated for the data from PMLS (correlation coefficient, $r = -0.37$; $P < 0.01$ in a t-test). (Data from Zumbroich and Blakemore 1987.)

tion, with a concentration of cells with relatively higher resolution representing the area centralis.

A number of neurons (17.5% overall, but relatively more common in PLLS than in PMLS) showed very little or no attenuation of response at low spatial frequencies, and we classified them as *spatial low-pass* cells. Such cells, which respond well to large, rapidly moving patterns and even to overall changes in retinal illumination, are rare in area 18 and have never been described in area 17. For all the other *spatial bandpass* units, with a clear peak in the spatial frequency tuning function, we determined the optimal spatial frequency. Values of best spatial frequency for our sample ranged from 0.04 to 0.37 cycles/deg. The average optimal spatial frequency of neurons in the suprasylvian cortex (about 0.16 cycles/deg) was considerably lower than the value reported for area 17 (0.77 cycles/deg for a mostly central sample; Movshon et al. 1978c), but roughly comparable to that for area 18 (0.22 cycles/deg for a central sample; Movshon et al. 1978c).

From the spatial frequency tuning curves of bandpass units we also measured the narrowness of tuning for spatial frequency. The average full bandwidth at half-amplitude (see Fig. 1A) was 2.2 octaves (in both PMLS and PLLS) with a range from 0.5 to 4.7 octaves, whereas for areas 17 and 18 the mean value of bandwidth is about 1.5 octaves. Thus the suprasylvian visual cortex differs from areas 17 and 18 in its relatively high proportion of low-pass cells and the larger average bandwidth of the bandpass cells.

A comparison of the sizes of receptive fields and their preference for spatial frequency has led to important insights into the underlying structure of receptive fields for cells in the cat's striate cortex (Movshon et al. 1978a,b). We pursued a similar strategy; for each individual cell in PMLS and PLLS we multiplied the optimum spatial frequency (in cycles/deg) by the width of the receptive field (in deg), measured along the axis of motion used to determine spatial frequency preference. This product, the *spatial index*, describes how many cycles (each cycle consisting of one dark and one light bar) of a grating of optimum spatial frequency will fit across the width of the receptive field.

The receptive field was plotted as a 'response field' (Barlow et al. 1967), i.e. the region within which a moving spot or bar generated a response. The width of such a plot for a simple cell in the striate cortex (Hubel and Wiesel 1962) would correspond to the 'discharge centre', which in turn approximates to the central region within which spatial summation occurs (Movshon et al. 1978a). The spatial index would thus be expected to be 0.5 cycles for simple cells (the discharge centre being equal in width to an individual bar of the grating), but should have a higher value for complex cells. Fig. 3A shows the broad distribution of spatial index, ranging from one cell with a value just below 0.5, up to 5.4 cycles. The mean value for PMLS is 1.68 cycles and for PLLS 2.36 cycles. Thus, most of the cells had an optimal spatial frequency such that several bars of an optimal grating would be required to fill the width of the receptive field.

This point is further illustrated in Fig. 3B, in which we have plotted *preferred bar width* (i.e., half the optimal spatial period, where spatial period is the inverse of spatial frequency) versus the width of the receptive field. For a cell (such as a striate simple cell) whose spatial frequency preference is simply determined by summation across a spatial unit equal to the measured width of its response field, we would expect a slope of 1 in such a plot. As Fig. 3B illustrates, for all but one unit the response field diameter was larger than half of the preferred spatial period, just as Movshon et al. (1978a,b) found for complex cells in striate cortex.

Tests of linearity of spatial summation (see Zumbroich and Blakemore 1987, for details) provided further evidence that cells in the suprasylvian visual cortex share many features of their summation properties with complex cells in areas 17 and 18 (Movshon et al. 1978b) and also with Y-cells and non-linear W-cells in the LGN (Shapley and Hochstein 1975; Sur and Sherman 1982).

In conclusion, it seems most unlikely that the suprasylvian visual cortex continues a process started in striate cortex by extending a fine spatial analysis of the image over a wider region of space. The basic structure of the receptive fields of cells in PMLS and PLLS may be quite similar to that of non-linear striate complex cells, but the subunits that are presumed to make up each receptive field must be larger and therefore tuned to lower spatial frequencies, much like those of complex cells in area 18. Indeed those subunits may be provided by cortico-cortical input from area 18 or by direct afferent input from W-cells in the LGN or from neurons in other parts of the posterior thalamus.

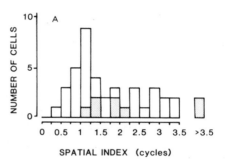

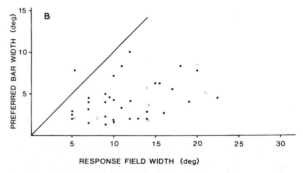

Fig. 3. (A) A histogram plotting the *spatial index* (the product of peak spatial frequency and response field width) for 33 neurons in PMLS (unfilled blocks) and 8 neurons in PLLS (stippled blocks). (B) Plot of half the value of the preferred spatial period (i.e. the optimal bar width) versus the receptive field width for 33 neurons in PMLS (filled dots) and 8 neurons in PLLS (open circles). The line with a slope of 1 is the expected relationship for neurons whose receptive field width is the same as the size of the summating unit determining selectivity for spatial frequency. (Data from Zumbroich and Blakemore 1987.)

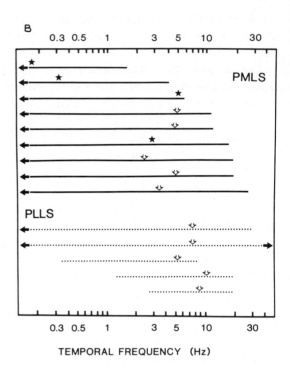

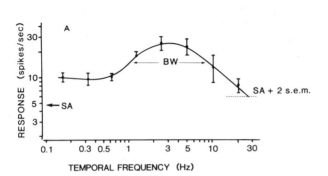

Fig. 4. (A) A temporal-frequency tuning curve for a neuron in PMLS, measured with drifting gratings of optimum spatial frequency (0.125 cycles/deg). Response (elevation of mean discharge, in spikes/sec) is plotted against temporal frequency (in cycles/sec). The arrow shows the mean level of spontaneous activity (SA) and the interrupted line is the level of maintained discharge plus 2 SE of the mean, above which a response was considered to be significantly higher than the background. The full temporal bandwidth at half-amplitude (BW) is indicated. (B) A diagram showing the full range of temporal frequencies over which each of the tested units gave a significant response to drifting gratings of the optimal spatial frequency. Solid lines indicate cells from PMLS, dotted lines those from PLLS. The lowest temporal frequency tested was 0.175 Hz: the solid arrows at the left indicate cells (mainly in PMLS) that still responded significantly at this frequency. One cell in PLLS (solid arrow at right) still responded at the highest temporal frequency tested (41 Hz). The open arrows point to the optimal temporal frequency for all cells in which a bandwidth could be measured. The stars indicate the point of greatest response, just before the high-frequency roll-off, for *temporal low-pass* neurons. (Data from Zumbroich and Blakemore 1987.)

Temporal selectivity

It is well established that cells in both PMLS (e.g., Spear and Baumann 1975; Camarda and Rizzolatti 1976; Blakemore and Zumbroich 1987) and PLLS (Blakemore and Zumbroich 1987; von Grünau et al. 1987) respond well to moving stimuli, a high proportion of them being selective for the direction of motion. This suggests that this part of the visual cortex could have a role in the perception of movement (e.g., Toyama and Kozasa 1982; Toyama et al. 1985). A knowledge of the preferences of neurons in the suprasylvian visual cortex for tem-

poral as well as spatial frequency is essential for an understanding of their motion selectivity. We therefore studied temporal selectivity in some detail, by measuring the responses to a grating of optimal spatial frequency moving in the best direction at various temporal frequencies of drift.

Fig. 4A gives an example of a temporal frequency tuning curve. This cell, located in PMLS, responded best between 1 and 10 Hz with a full-width at half-amplitude of 3.1 octaves. In Fig. 4B we have plotted, for each individual cell tested, the whole range of temporal frequencies to which the cell gave a response significantly elevated above the spontaneous level. All of the cells recorded in PMLS still responded above threshold even at the lowest temporal frequency presented (0.175 Hz). Four of them showed so little low temporal-frequency attenuation that their responses had not even fallen to half-amplitude at the lowest temporal frequency tested, and we classified them as *temporal low-pass* cells. The optimum temporal frequencies lay between less than 2.5 Hz and 10 Hz for both PMLS and PLLS. However, in our small sample from PLLS there was a tendency for at-

tenuation at low temporal frequencies to be more pronounced and for optimum teporal frequencies to be higher. The bandwidth of the temporal frequency tuning functions (full-width at half-amplitude) varied between 0.63 octaves up to more than 4 octaves, with a mean of 2.8 octaves for PMLS and 2.5 octaves in PLLS.

Thus units in both PMLS and PLLS responded to a wide range of temporal frequencies. Whereas in PLLS there was a trend towards more pronounced low-frequency attenuation and higher

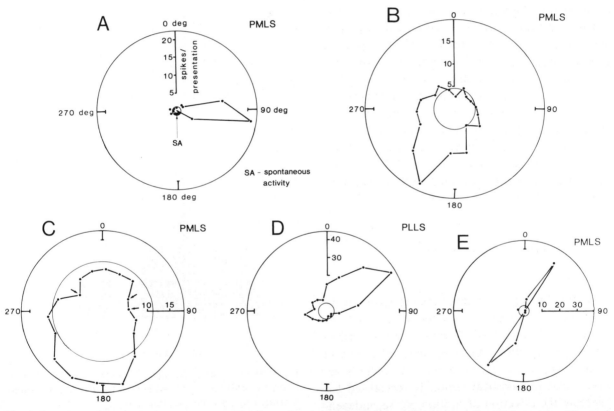

Fig. 5. Responses of representative neurons are plotted as a function of the direction of movement of a drifting grating. The angle on each polar plot shows the direction of motion while the radial dimension represents the response amplitude (spikes/presentation). The inner circle shows the mean level of spontaneous activity and the small arrows indicate directions at which the responses of the cells were significantly inhibited below the background level. (A) A sharply tuned uni-directional cell from PMLS (half-width = 18°; directionality = 1.0). (B) A uni-directional cell from PMLS that responded significantly over a total range of 140° (half-width = 21°; directionality = 0.96). (C) A broadly tuned uni-directional cell in PMLS that was inhibited by movement in directions roughly opposite to its preferred direction, the inhibition reaching statistical significance at about 120° clockwise and anticlockwise from the peak direction (half-width = 43°; directionality = 1.35). (D) A cell from PLLS that responded weakly but significantly to the direction opposite to the peak (half-width = 27°; directionality = 0.77). (E) A bi-directional cell in PMLS that was very narrowly tuned to the two opposite directions of motion (half-width = 13° and 12° for the two peak directions; directionality = 0.09). (Data from Blakemore and Zumbroich 1987.)

preferred temporal frequencies, units in PMLS showed little or no low temporal-frequency attenuation, like most units in area 17 and some in area 18 (Tolhurst and Movshon 1975; Movshon et al. 1978c).

Using the equation

velocity = temporal frequency/spatial frequency

we made a conservative estimate of the total range of angular velocities to which each cell would respond, corresponding to the range of temporal frequencies for which motion of a grating of *optimal spatial frequency* gave suprathreshold responses. We found that cells responded to the optimum spatial frequency over a wide range of velocities (typically from below 1 deg/sec to several hundred deg/sec), which was comparable to the range of effective velocities found with dot stimuli (Spear and Baumann 1975; Camarda and Rizzolatti 1976). Units in PLLS seem, on average, to prefer faster stimulus velocities than do units in PMLS, confirming findings with dot and line stimuli (von Grünau et al. 1987).

Direction and orientation selectivity

Although the first accounts of the properties of the receptive fields of cells in suprasylvian area (e.g., Hubel and Wiesel 1969; Wright 1969) described them as orientation selective, much like cells in areas 17 and 18, it has since become generally accepted that this cortical region is specialized for detecting the direction of motion per se, independent of the orientation of contours in the image. We have quantitatively studied the selectivity of cells in both PMLS and the adjacent area PLLS for gratings that either were made to drift in different directions (so as to measure directional tuning curves) or were held stationary at different orientations while their contrast was modulated (so as to provide a test for orientation selectivity in those cells that responded to such stimuli).

Direction selectivity

Fig. 5 illustrates a number of directional response curves from cells in PMLS and PLLS with different degrees of direction selectivity. As a quantitative measure of the degree of preference for one of the two alternative directions along the

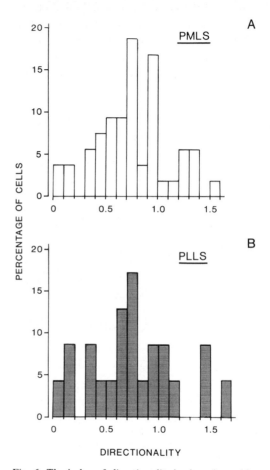

Fig. 6. The index of *directionality* is plotted as a histogram for cells from PMLS ($n = 53$, A) and PLLS ($n = 23$, B). Directionality was calculated according to:

$$\text{directionality} = 1 - (r_{opp}/r_{pd}),$$

where r_{pd} is the amplitude of response (minus spontaneous activity) for movement in the cell's principal preferred direction and r_{opp} is the response in the opposite direction. A value of zero indicates an equal response in the two directions; values up to 1 indicate increasing directional asymmetry; and values above 1 occur when the neuron is inhibited by stimuli moving in the direction opposite to its preferred. (Data from Blakemore and Zumbroich 1987.)

preferred axis we calculated an index of *directionality* from the cell's response (minus spontaneous activity) to a grating moving in the cell's preferred direction (r_{pd}) and its response above background to a grating moving in the opposite direction (r_{opp}):

$$\text{directionality} = 1 - (r_{opp}/r_{pd})$$

This measure gives positive values that increase from 0 to 1 as directional preference increases,

with values above 1 if the response is inhibited in the direction opposite to that of the peak. The distributions of the values of directionality for all cells analysed in PMLS and PLLS are plotted in Fig. 6. Seventy-nine percent of all cells in PMLS and 71% of all cells in PLLS showed strong direction preference (directionality > 0.5) and 26% of the sample from PMLS and 17% of that from PLLS were actually inhibited at the direction opposite to their best direction (directionality > 1.0). Comparison with similar studies in other regions

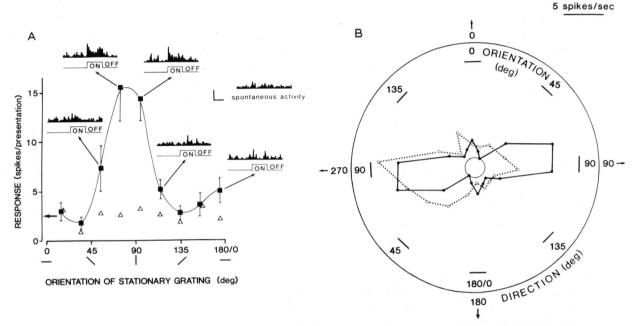

Fig. 7. (A) This tuning function plots the responses of a cell from PMLS to stationary gratings of optimum spatial frequency but different orientation, turned on and off without variation of mean luminance. The onset component (filled squares) and the offset component (open triangles) of the responses (spikes/presentation) are plotted separately. Each data point represents the mean response (± 1 SE) counted over the total 1.5 sec on or off period for ten stimulus presentations. The mean spontaneous activity measured during blank trials is indicated by a large filled arrow on the ordinate. Histograms (bin width, 12 sec; total sweep duration, 5.5 sec) collected during the stimulus presentations are shown adjacent to some of the data points. Calibration bars: vertical, 50 spikes/sec; horizontal, 1 sec. The cell gave clear onset responses to gratings at orientations near 90°, but no significant offset response for any orientation. (B) the onset responses to *stationary*, flashed gratings of different orientations for the cell illustrated in Fig. 7A are compared with the responses to gratings, also of optimum spatial frequency, *moving* in different directions. The angle on the polar plot represents direction or orientation, as indicated. The radial dimension plots the mean response (calibration bar, 5 spikes/sec). For both types of stimulus the duration of presentation was the same (1.5 sec). The mean level of spontaneous activity (1.6 spikes/sec) is shown by the inner circles. In the case of the flashed gratings (filled circles, continuous line) each data point appears twice, once on each half of the plot, in order to create a continuous function over the full range of 360°. Data points for the moving grating (open circles, dotted line) cover the full range of 360°. This allows direct comparison of the two response functions. The cell had a clear preference for vertical gratings whether stationary or moving, and when the grating was drifting the cell strongly preferred leftward motion. (Data from Blakemore and Zumbroich 1987.)

220

of the visual system confirms that the percentage of units with strong directional preference is indeed higher in the suprasylvian cortex than in any other cortical and subcortical visual structures so far investigated. In addition, cells were comparatively well tuned for the preferred direction of motion of a grating: on average the half-width at half-amplitude around the preferred direction was 23.2° for PMLS and 25.3° for PLLS, thus falling within the range found for complex cells in area 17 (e.g., Hammond and Andrews 1978).

The plot of the overall distribution of preferred directions of cells in the suprasylvian visual cortex revealed some anisotropies (Blakemore and Zumbroich 1987). Further analysis, taking into account the position of each cell's receptive field, showed a tendency for cells in PMLS to prefer centrifugal or centripetal motion, and in PLLS to prefer centrifugal motion, as had been reported earlier for PMLS (e.g., Spear and Baumann 1975).

Orientation selectivity

Following the initial suggestion that neurons in PMLS are orientation selective (Hubel and Wiesel 1969; Wright 1969), Spear and Baumann (1975) were the first specifically to address the problem of distinguishing orientation and direction selectivity. Their most definitive criterion involves testing with stationary, flashed stimuli "since, in the absence of moving stimuli, there is no possibility of confusing direction selectivity with orientation selectivity" (Smith and Spear 1979).

In our quantitative experiments, 27 cells out of a total of 60 units tested in PMLS and PLLS gave a sufficient response to stationary, contrast-modulated gratings of the optimum spatial frequency to permit their orientation selectivity to be assessed from spike counts and averaged histograms collected during the stimulus presentations. In Fig. 7A we illustrate the responses of a cell recorded in PMLS during the presentation (onset-response) and withdrawal (offset-response) of a grating, the contrast of which was instantaneously modulated between zero and 0.8 and back again, without change in mean luminance (square-wave modula-

tion; temporal period = 3 sec). The cell did not respond to the withdrawal of the grating at any orientation. It was, however, excited by the appearance of the grating stimulus when it was vertical (orientation = 90°), but not if it was rotated by more than about 45° in either direction. In Fig. 7B we have plotted the responses to both drifting and flashed gratings on the same polar coordinates. The cell was not only strongly direction selective but also showed a clear preference for a stationary grating flashed on at the orientation that was optimal for the response to a drifting grating.

Obviously, our determination of response as a function of orientation might have been contaminated by sensitivity to the spatial *position* of the luminance profile of the grating with respect to the centre of the receptive field. However, we are certain that spatial phase dependence *does not* account for our finding of orientation selectivity in the suprasylvian cortex. Firstly, our previous ex-

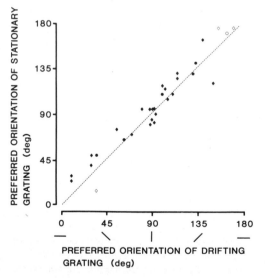

Fig. 8. The optimum orientation found with stationary gratings is plotted against the preferred orientation revealed with drifting gratings for 27 cells (PMLS, *n* = 22, diamonds; PLLS, *n* = 5, circles). Four units had distinct additional peaks in both response functions and data for these secondary peaks are plotted with open symbols. The interrupted line has a slope of +1, as expected for perfect agreement. (Data from Blakemore and Zumbroich 1987.)

periments (Zumbroich and Blakemore 1987) demonstrated that suprasylvian neurons behave highly non-linearly and never exhibit strong dependence on spatial phase, especially at spatial frequencies near the optimum, as used for our tests of orientation selectivity. Secondly, when we specifically investigated the effects of varying spatial position at different orientations, we never found evidence that the orientation selectivity was a spurious reflection of spatial phase dependence (Blakemore and Zumbroich 1987).

Finally, the most compelling evidence that orientation selectivity is a genuine property of those cells that respond to stationary gratings is the excellent correspondence between the independent estimates of preferred direction and orientation, illustrated in Fig. 8. This graph plots the preferred orientation of a stationary grating against the orientation of a grating moving in the optimum direction, for each cell tested. Four of the cells showed a clear bi-lobed orientation-tuning function, with a secondary preference for stationary gratings at about 90° to the orientation that gave rise to maximum response, and again there was good agreement with the presence of orthogonal accessory peaks in their directional tuning curves (open symbols in Fig. 8).

Although this kind of definitive test of orientation selectivity can obviously be applied only to cells that respond reliably to stationary stimuli, we have no reason to believe that inherent selectivity for orientation is restricted to the neurons that we were able to test in this way. Certainly those cells that did respond reliably to flashed stimuli were not distinctively different from the rest in a way that might set them aside as a special population.

Postnatal development of stimulus selectivity in PMLS

For a number of reasons it seems especially worthwhile to extend previous studies of the postnatal development of areas 17 and 18 (e.g., Hubel and Wiesel 1963; Blakemore and Van Sluyters 1975; Albus and Wolf 1984; Blakemore and Price

1987a,b) to that of the extrastriate area PMLS. Unlike areas 17 and 18, PMLS receives no direct thalamic input from the A-laminae of the LGN but only from the C-laminae, the MIN and pulvinar/lateral posterior complex (Tong et al. 1982; Raczkowski and Rosenquist 1980, 1983). Although there is a dense cortico-cortical projection from areas 17 and 18 (Symonds and Rosenquist 1984a,b), lesions of these more medial visual areas do not abolish visual responsiveness in the suprasylvian visual cortex (Spear and Baumann 1979) and some neurons even retain direction selectivity (Guedes et al. 1983). Therefore, PMLS is, in some respects, a parallel visual area, dominated by a pattern of afferent input very different from that of both areas 17 and 18. It seems to be specialized for the analysis of image motion, a function that might be especially important for the support of the simplest forms of visuomotor behaviour, which appear during the third week of life (Norton 1974, 1981).

We have recorded from single neurons in PMLS of kittens aged between 9 days and 8 weeks to study quantitatively their selectivity for a wide range of stimulus properties (Price et al. 1988; Zumbroich et al. 1988). We employed a sampling procedure aimed at exploring fairly uniformly through all layers of the cortex in regular steps of about 100 μm.

Onset of visual responsiveness

In the very young kittens, less than 12 days of age, much of PMLS appeared to be unresponsive to any of our stimuli and neurons were identified only by occasional spontaneous spikes or an injury discharge as the electrode was advanced. In the 9-day-old animal only one clearly responsive unit was isolated, in layer IV, during three long penetrations through PMLS. In the 10-day kitten we found several small clusters of responsive cells, separated by unresponsive zones, all located in the lower cortical layers (IV, V, VI). At 12 days of age a substantial fraction of neurons recorded were responsive, some of them located in the superficial layers; and by the end of the third week virtually every cell isolated could be visually excited.

Spatial selectivity

To investigate the change in spatial resolution of cells in PMLS with age we have plotted in Fig. 9 the *highest acuity* found amongst the sample of cells from each kitten, versus age. Such an analysis of the best cell recorded at each age provides an estimate of the contribution that PMLS might be able to make to the behavioural acuity at each particular age. The resulting graph (Fig. 9, filled squares) indicates that the highest acuity in PMLS rises sharply between 9 days and the end of the third week of life when it reaches the adult value of just over 2 cycles/deg. The rise in both the best values of acuity and the mean (Fig. 9, open triangles) was not accounted for by any progressive increase with age in the proportion of centrally placed receptive fields in the sample. In fact, the lack of correlation between acuity and eccentricity observed in kittens younger than 2 weeks makes it very unlikely that an increase in the highest acuity with age could simply be due to a bias in sampling. The same analysis performed for the *optimum* spatial frequency also demonstrated a considerable increase during the second and third week of life, after which values of around 0.5 cycles/deg were reached (Fig. 9, filled circles).

The proportion of visually responsive cells that were *selective* for spatial frequency (in the sense that they had spatial bandpass characteristics and could be assigned a bandwidth and a peak spatial frequency) increased with age from about 55% in the youngest kittens to about 80% in older kittens, close to the adult value of 85%. Over the same period of time there was a slight but significant *increase* in mean spatial bandwidth, most likely due to the recruitment into the population of bandpass

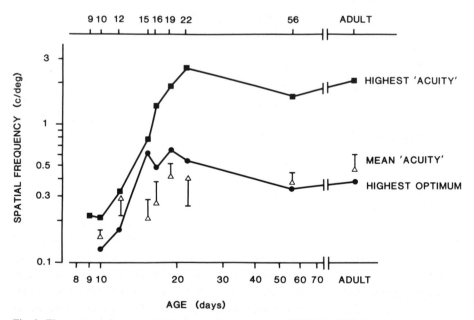

Fig. 9. The mean acuity (plus 1 SE) of responsive neurons in PMLS (unfilled triangles) is plotted versus age. The highest acuity (filled squares) and the highest optimum spatial frequency (filled circles) found amongst the entire sample at different ages are also plotted, to indicate our estimate of the upper limit of the performance of PMLS. There is a sharp rise between 10 and 20 days of age in all these indicators of spatial performance. There was no tendency for cells included from older kittens to have receptive field centres located closer to the area centralis than those from younger kittens. Note that the single visually responsive cell recorded in a 9-day-old animal was a spatial low-pass cell and therefore could not be included in this analysis of optimal spatial frequency. (Data from Zumbroich et al. 1988.)

cells of broadly tuned neurons that started out with low-pass characteristics.

As in adult PMLS, the widths of receptive fields in kittens were on average about twice the size of the preferred spatial period (4 times the preferred bar-width; see above). This and further tests with stationary contrast-modulated gratings presented at different spatial positions confirmed that *at all ages* responsive neurons in PMLS resemble striate complex cells with respect to the non-linearity of their responses and the spatial structure of their receptive fields.

Temporal selectivity

Despite the general sluggishness of cells in kitten PMLS, their responses were clearly dependent on the temporal frequency of a drifting grating. Inspection of individual temporal-frequency tuning functions of cells in very young animals showed that they responded best to temporal frequencies lower than those preferred in adults, and a quantitative analysis of this trend is shown in Fig. 10. Both the mean optimum temporal frequency and the mean high temporal-frequency cut-off of cell in PMLS increased over the first 3 weeks of life. The mean optimum temporal frequency continued to increase up to 8 weeks of age and even beyond, though none of the changes after 19 days of age reached clear statistical significance.

The proportion of temporal low-pass cells was substantially lower in kittens, even up to 2 months

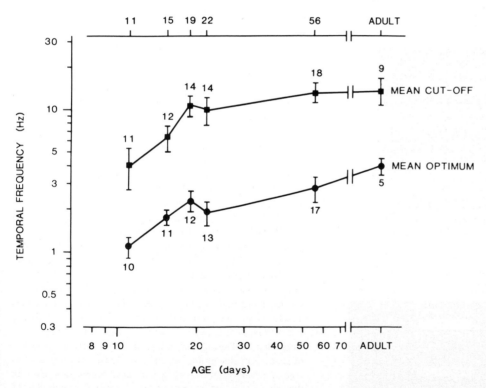

Fig. 10. The mean *high temporal-frequency cut-off* ($\pm$ SE, filled squares) and the mean *optimum temporal frequency* ($\pm$ SE, filled circles) of cells in PMLS are plotted for each age. The sample sizes are indicated above the error bars for the mean cut-offs and below them for the mean optimum temporal frequency. For cells with little or no obvious low temporal-frequency attenuation (low-pass cells) no optimum temporal frequency could be determined. For this graph, data from kittens aged between 10 and 12 days and between 15 and 16 days are pooled. Both functions increase up to 3 weeks of age: mean optimum temporal frequency continues to increase until 8 weeks and beyond, but note that the changes after 3 weeks of age do not reach statistical significance. (Data from Zumbroich et al. 1988.)

old, than in adults; immature neurons were unable to sustain responses to either very rapidly or very slowly modulated patterns. The gradual increase in high-frequency and low-frequency responsiveness led to a broadening, on average, of temporal bandwidth, which increased the absolute range of temporal frequencies to which the population of cells responded at older ages. Since little comparable work has been done on the development of temporal properties in other parts of the visual system, it is difficult to decide whether peripheral or central factors play the major role in the development of temporal selectivity in PMLS. It seems plausible, though, to speculate that the properties of retinal ganglion cells, which take about 16 weeks to achieve mature intensity-response functions and temporal resolution (Flynn et al. 1977), could be

responsible for the slow time-course of development of temporal properties in PMLS.

Direction selectivity

Because of the general sluggishness and strong habituation of many of the visually responsive cells recorded in very young kittens, we often found it more difficult to judge stimulus selectivity by ear than we had previously experienced in adult PMLS and we therefore decided to concentrate entirely on *quantitative* measurements of direction and orientation selectivity.

To summarize the overall change in the pattern of selectivity for motion with age, Fig. 11A shows the proportions of all quantitatively studied visually responsive cells that (1) had a significant direc-

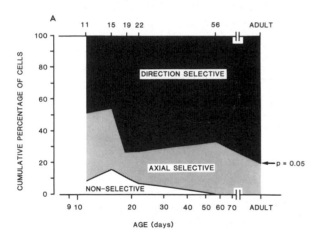

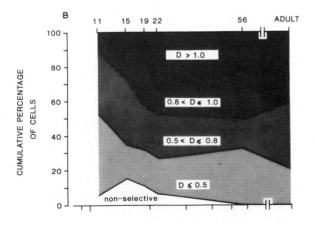

Fig. 11. (A) This graph shows the cumulative percentages of visually responsive cells that were *direction selective, axial selective* or *non-selective* at different ages. The height of each separate area in the graph represents the percentage of neurons of that type in the population of responsive units at the age shown on the abscissa. A statistical criterion was employed to distinguish between direction selectivity and axial selectivity: if the mean amplitude of response in one direction exceeded that in the opposite direction with significance at the $P < 0.05$ level, the cell was termed direction selective. A more conservative criterion for classifying cells as having a definite direction preference (e.g., $P = 0.01$) would shift the border up, increasing the fraction of axial selective units, while a laxer criterion (e.g., $P = 0.1$) would bring it down. Data from cats aged 10 and 12 days, and those from animals of 15 and 16 days, were pooled and plotted on the abscissa at 11 days and 15 days, respectively. The one visually responsive cell recorded at 9 days was axial selective and is not included in this graph. (B) An index of *directionality* was calculated for each cell's best direction (see legend to Fig. 6) and cells were divided into classes according to the strength of their direction preferences: directionality smaller than 0.5; between 0.5 and 0.8; between 0.8 and 1; and larger than 1. These classes are plotted with different densities of shading in this graph, which shows the cumulative percentage of cells in each of these groups at different ages. Even in the youngest animals (10 and 12 days, pooled, and plotted at 11 days on the abscissa) about half of the cells had directionality higher than 0.5, and at the end of the third week of postnatal life the distribution was very similar to that found in adult cats. The one cell assessed quantitatively in a 9-day-old animal was axial selective (directionality = 0.43) and is not included in this analysis. (Data from Price et al. 1988.)

tion preference (*direction selective*), (2) responded best to motion along one axis, but did not differ significantly in their responses to the two opposite directions (*axial selective*), and (3) gave a response over the whole range of directions and had no clear response peak (*non-selective*).

Even in the youngest animals, more than 90% of the visually responsive neurons were already selective for motion along a particular axis, by quantitative criteria, and half of them had a clear preference for one of the two directions along this axis.

To quantify further the strength of directional preference we classed all visually responsive cells at each age into groups according to their indices of directionality, as defined above (Fig. 11B). In the group of very young animals, aged 10 – 12 days, *no* cell was actually inhibited at the direction opposite to the preferred direction (directionality > 1), but about 50% had an index of directionality greater than 0.5. At about 3 weeks of age the distribution of directionality was already very similar to that found in adult PMLS.

With increasing age, not only did the proportion of direction selective cells and the strength of direction preference increase, but also those cells that were definitely direction selective or axial selective became more sharply tuned. At 10 – 12 days the mean half-width was 32.6°, but it decreased to the adult value (mean half-width 23.2°) by the end of the third postnatal week.

Orientation selectivity

In view of the great interest in the maturation of orientation selectivity in the striate cortex and area 18 (e.g., Hubel and Wiesel 1963; Blakemore and Van Sluyters 1975; Bonds 1979; Albus and Wolf 1984; Blakemore and Price 1987a,b) we thought it important to study this issue for PMLS (Price et al. 1988). Fortunately, even at only 10 – 12 days of age, almost 40% of responsive units recorded in PMLS responded reliably (by quantitative criteria) to stationary flashed gratings and we were therefore able to apply the same test that reveals orientation selectivity in most if not all cells in adult PMLS that respond to such stimuli (Blakemore and Zumbroich 1987).

Just as for neurons in the adult cat, we were able to compare the responses to stationary, contrast-modulated gratings of optimal spatial frequency, presented at different orientations, with the responses to gratings of the same spatial frequency drifting in different directions. At *all* ages, the vast majority of cells that responded reliably to the onset or withdrawal of a grating showed clear selectivity for its orientation (Price et al. 1988). Moreover, the preferred orientation determined quantitatively in this way was always very close to the independent determination, in the same cell, of the optimum orientation for a *drifting* grating (just as in Fig. 8).

In animals up to three weeks of age, a small proportion (about 10%) of visually responsive units were *non-selective* for the direction of motion of a grating. Some of these non-selective cells responded to stationary, flashed gratings and in every case they were also non-selective for the *orientation* of such a stimulus.

It must be emphasized that the orientation selectivity revealed with flashed gratings is quite subtle, even in the majority of cells from adult PMLS. In our experience and that of others (e.g., Spear and Baumann 1975), very few neurons appear to be distinctly orientation selective when tested by ear with single flashed bars. However, the close agreement between the preferred orientations for stationary and moving stimuli (see Fig. 8) is surely convincing evidence that the sensitivity of cells in PMLS to motion and its direction is constructed on a mechanism that is selective for the orientation of contours, as in the striate cortex and area 18. It is worth pointing out that even in area 17, many complex cells do not respond reliably to flashed bars. The subtle orientation selectivity of cells in PMLS is, then, another property that they share with striate complex neurons.

The overall picture that emerges from our studies of the postnatal development of PMLS (Price et al. 1988; Zumbroich et al. 1988) is, in some respects, very similar to that resulting from studies of area 17 and 18, but is, in some interesting ways, rather different.

The general time-course of maturation appears fairly similar in all three regions of cortex investigated. Cells begin to respond to visual stimuli at or just before the time of natural eye-opening. Neurons with some degree of stimulus selectivity are initially found in clusters lying in the deep layers of the cortex, in all three areas. The proportion of visually responsive units and the general degree of stimulus selectivity improve rapidly during the next 2–3 weeks in areas 17, 18 and PMLS. However, in certain important respects the maturation of PMLS seems surprisingly precocious compared with that of the other two areas. First, we find that, by only three weeks of age, cells in PMLS are virtually indistinguishable from those in the adult, except perhaps for their ability to respond to very high temporal frequencies and therefore high velocities – a property that may, in any case, be limited by retinal maturation (Zumbroich et al. 1988). The spatial tuning and spatial acuity of cells, the proportions that are direction selective and axial selective, the strengths of direction preference, the incidence of overtly orientation selective neurons and the angular tuning of cells for direction and orientation all seem fully developed at three weeks of age. Moreover, the huge majority of neurons in PMLS have clear selectivity for motion along one axis as soon as they begin to respond and more than half of them have a preference for one direction of motion (by statistical criteria) at around the time of eye-opening. By comparison, in the early stages of development of areas 17 and 18, there is a large fraction of cells with little or no stimulus selectivity, which gradually acquire selective properties during the first month of life (e.g., Blakemore and Van Sluyters 1975; Albus and Wolf 1984; Blakemore and Price 1987a).

Rather than there being an hierarchical progressive sequence of maturation of visual areas, areas 17, 18 and PMLS appear to develop in parallel, with, if anything, PMLS leading the more

'primary' visual areas in its maturation. This may imply that the postnatal development of PMLS is controlled by its own independent thalamic input.

It must be said, however, that McCall et al. (1988), who have also studied the postnatal development of PMLS, find a very much lower proportion of selective cells at young ages and report that maturation of stimulus selectivity is not complete until at least 8 weeks of age. They used qualitative methods and judged the properties of cells only by ear; such techniques would probably not reveal the statistically significant but subtle degrees of selectivity that we found for many cells in very young kittens. However, the disparity in results for older kittens is harder to explain because we found that at only 3 weeks of age, cells of PMLS are virtually indistinguishable from those in the adult in almost every respect. Further work will be needed to resolve this small difference in results.

Functional architecture

One of the most impressive aspects of the local organization of areas 17 and 18 is the 'columnar' representation of preferred orientation (e.g., Hubel and Wiesel 1962, 1965; Blakemore and Price 1987a). In both regions, cells lying in a radial group or column have very similar preferred orientations, but, if a microelectrode is driven obliquely or tangentially across the pattern of columns, orientation preferences shift from one group of cells to the next, usually in a steady progressive sequence. The scale of this 'functional architecture' is such that at least one column of neurons is available for any orientation that might appear at any position in the visual field.

In their first study of PMLS, Hubel and Wiesel (1969) noted that there was a tendency for cells recorded close together to have similar selective properties. We investigated this question in some detail in the adult cat and found clear evidence in many penetrations through PMLS that the preferences of cells change in a progressive sequence during oblique tracks but are very similar for cells recorded at different depths within a single radial column (Blakemore and Zumbroich 1987). There was a strong tendency for the preferred *directions* of cells to shift in small steps across the cortex of PMLS. However, there were sometimes *reversals* of preferred direction from one cell to the next and occasional differences of 180° in preferred direction between cells recorded at different depths within a single column. This led Blakemore and Zumbroich (1987) to the conclusion that the functional architecture of PMLS is based on a regular and sequential representation of the preferred *axis* of movement (or, indeed, of the equivalent preferred *orientation,* just as in area 17 and 18), rather than the preferred direction. Figure 12C shows a graphical reconstruction of a long, roughly tangential penetration through PMLS of an adult cat. The preferred axis of motion (left ordinate) or

preferred orientation (right ordinate) of the cells recorded is plotted as a function of the distance across the surface of the cortex from the point of entry. It is clear that there is a strong tendency for the preferred axis of motion (or orientation) to change smoothly and continuously across the cortex, at a maximum rate of about 360°/mm (much the same as in areas 17 and 18).

We used the same techniques to examine the development of functional architecture in young kittens and representative results are shown in Fig. 12A (for a 12-day-old animal) and Fig. 12B (for a 19-day-old animal). In the younger kitten, the responsive cells were found in small clusters in the deep layers of the cortex (layer IV and below). Nevertheless, there was a very clear tendency for closely neighbouring cells to have very similar

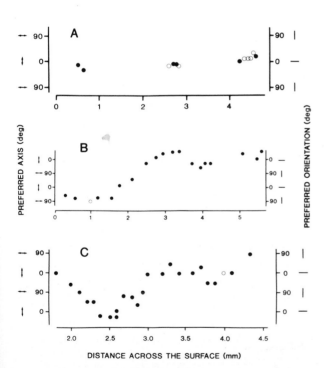

Fig. 12. These graphs show the results of an analysis of the distribution of stimulus selectivity from cell to cell, across the cortex of PMLS. The microelectrode was driven obliquely through the cortex and an attempt was made to isolate units in regular steps of 100 μm. The properties of cells were assessed quantitatively, by means of procedures described in the text, and each selective cell was assigned a preferred axis of motion.

Neurons that had a statistically significant preference for one of the two directions along this axis were classified as direction selective. The electrode penetration was subsequently reconstructed from examination of small electrolytic lesions placed at intervals along each track in Nissl-stained sections of the cortex (Blakemore and Zumbroich, 1987). The position of each recording site was then projected up to the surface of the cortex along the radial palisades of cell bodies, so that its locus could then be expressed as the equivalent distance across the cortical surface from the point of entry. The sequences of preferred *direction* in mature animals generally changed progressively from cell to cell along each penetration, but there were occasional reversals of direction preference from one cell to the next, which broke the regularity of the sequence. However, if the properties of cells were expressed in terms of their preferred *axis* of movement, regardless of which direction was preferred, these discontinuities were, of course, eliminated. The graphs here show such reconstructions for two young animals, aged 12 days (A) and 19 days (B) as well as for an adult animal (C). Direction selective cells are represented by filled circles, axial selective cells by unfilled. The left ordinate is the preferred axis of motion and the right ordinate is the equivalent preferred *orientation*, orthogonal to this axis. In the 12-day-old animal (A), responsive units were found in isolated groups in the lower layers of the cortex. Nevertheless, there was a clear tendency for neighbouring cells, lying in a single cluster, to have very similar preferred axes of motion. The result in the 19-day animal (B) was very similar to that in the adult (C): preferred axis (or orientation) tended to shift progressively across the cortex, at a rate up to 360°/mm, with occasional reversals of the whole sequence. (Data from Blakemore and Zumbroich (1987) and from Price et al. (1988).)

preferred axes of motion (and equivalent preferred orientations). By only 19 days of age (Fig. 12B), selective cells were encountered at almost all recording sites and the progressive sequence of preferred axes was just about as regular as that in the adult (Fig. 12C). Thus, in line with most of the other properties of PMLS, the columnar system seems to be virtually fully mature by the end of the third week.

Conclusions

Our results reinforce the prevalent view that the posterior lateral suprasylvian cortex has many properties that suit it for a role in the analysis of image motion. In particular, a very high proportion of neurons are direction selective. However, the inherent structure of the receptive fields of cells in this area is remarkably similar to that of neurons in the striate cortex and area 18. Virtually all cells that repond to stationary, flashed gratings are clearly orientation selective and their selectivity for motion (as for cells in areas 17 and 18) seems to be dependent on a mechanism that is sensitive to the orientation of contours. Even the columnar architecture of this cortical region appears to be built on a progressive representation of preferred axis of motion (or underlying preferred orientation) rather than preferred direction per se, just as in areas 17 and 18.

Spatial summation is highly non-linear for cells in the suprasylvian cortex, each receptive field appearing to consist of a number of sub-units, spatially summating across a region equal in size to about a quarter of the width of the whole receptive field. The spatial properties of cells in PMLS are shifted to lower spatial frequencies than those of striate neurons, implying that the subunits underlying the receptive fields are larger. The input providing such subunits could come directly from the posterior thalamus (perhaps from W-cells in the C-laminae of the LGN) or indirectly from area 18.

Given the basic similarity of receptive fields of cells in PMLS to those of neurons in areas 17 and 18, it is somewhat surprising that there is no

equivalent of the simple class of cells found in the other two areas. Neurons in PMLS have non-linear spatial summation as soon as they begin to respond to visual stimuli and do not appear to go through a stage at which their receptive fields consist of only a single spatially-summating unit.

PMLS matures roughly in parallel with areas 17 and 18, but, if anything, slightly ahead. For the majority of neurons, some degree of stimulus selectivity is present as soon as they become visually responsive. This strongly suggests that this area is less dependent for its maturation on the effects of visual experience early in life, but further work will be needed to settle this point. Certainly the rapid maturation of PMLS seems to suit it well for the mediation of the kinds of simple visuomotor behaviour that first appear during the second and third weeks of life.

Acknowledgements

The work described here was funded by a Programme Grant (G7900491) from the Medical Research Council and by grants from the Wellcome Trust and the Science and Engineering Research Council. David Price held a Beit Memorial Fellowship and Thomas Zumbroich received support from the German National Scholarship Foundation (Bonn, F.R.G.), the Dr. Eberhard Kornbeck Foundation (Stuttgart, F.R.G.), the Dr. Carl Duisberg Foundation (Leverkusen, F.R.G.) and Wolfson College, Oxford. We thank John Eldridge, Duncan Fleming, John Mittell and Pat Cordery for their excellent technical help.

References

Albus, K. and Wolf, W. (1984) Early post-natal development of neuronal function in the kitten's visual cortex: a laminar analysis. *J. Physiol.*, 348: 153–185.
Barlow, H.B., Blakemore, C. and Pettigrew, J.D. (1967) The neural mechanism of binocular depth discrimination. *J. Physiol.*, 193: 327–342.
Bisti, S. and Sireteanu, R. (1986) Sensitivity to spatial frequen-

cy and contrast of cells in the cat superior colliculus. *Vision Res.*, 16: 247 – 251.

Blakemore, C. and Price, D.J. (1987a) The organization and post-natal development of area 18 of the cat's visual cortex. *J. Physiol.*, 384: 263 – 292.

Blakemore, C. and Price, D.J. (1987b) Effects of dark-rearing on the development of area 18 of the cat's visual cortex. *J. Physiol.*, 384: 293 – 309.

Blakemore, C. and Van Sluyters, R.C. (1975) Innate and environmental factors in the development of the kitten's visual cortex. *J. Physiol.*, 248: 663 – 716.

Blakemore, C. and Zumbroich, T.J. (1985) Spatial frequency selectivity in the lateral suprasylvian areas (PMLS/PLLS) of the cat visual cortex. *J. Physiol.*, 369: 40P.

Blakemore, C. and Zumbroich, T.J. (1987) Stimulus selectivity and functional organization in the lateral suprasylvian visual cortex of the cat. *J. Physiol.*, 389: 569 – 603.

Bonds, A.B. (1979) Development of orientation tuning in the visual cortex of kittens. In: R.D. Freeman (ed.), *Developmental Neurobiology of Vision*, pp. 31 – 41, Plenum Press, New York.

Camarda, R. and Rizzolatti, G. (1976) Visual receptive fields in the lateral suprasylvian area (Clare-Bishop area) of the cat. *Brain Res.*, 101: 427 – 443.

Cleland, B.G., Harding, T.H. and Tulunay-Keesey, U. (1979) Visual resolution and receptive field size: examination of two kinds of cat retinal ganglion cell. *Science*, 205: 1015 – 1017.

Di Stefano, M., Morrone, M.C. and Burr, D.C. (1985) Visual acuity of neurones in the cat lateral suprasylvian cortex. *Brain Res.*, 331: 382 – 385.

Eggers, H.M. and Blakemore, C. (1978) Physiological basis of anisometropic amblyopia. *Science,* 201: 264 – 267.

Flynn, J.T., Flynn, T.E., Hamasaki, D.I., Navarro, O., Sutija, V.G. and Tucker, G.S. (1977) Development of the eye and retina of kittens. In: S.J. Cool and E.L. Smith, III (Eds.), *Frontiers in Visual Science,* pp. 594 – 603. Springer, New York.

Guedes, R., Watanabe, S. and Creutzfeldt, O.D. (1983) Functional role of association fibres for a visual assocation area: the posterior suprasylvian sulcus of the cat. *Exp. Brain Res.,* 49: 13 – 27.

Hammond, P. and Andrews, D.P. (1978) Orientation tuning of cells in areas 17 and 18 of the cat's visual cortex. *Exp. Brain Res.,* 31: 341 – 351.

Hubel, D.H. and Wiesel, T.N. (1962) Receptive fields, binocular interaction and functional architecture in the cat's visual cortex. *J. Physiol.,* 160: 106 – 154.

Hubel, D.H. and Wiesel, T.N. (1963) Receptive fields of cells in striate cortex of very young, visually inexperienced kittens. *J. Neurophysiol.,* 26: 994 – 1002.

Hubel, D.H. and Wiesel, T.N. (1965) Receptive fields and functional architecture in two non-striate visual areas (18 and 19) of the cat. *J. Neurophysiol.,* 28: 229 – 289.

Hubel, D.H. and Wiesel, T.N. (1969) Visual area of the lateral suprasylvian gyrus (Clare-Bishop area) of the cat. *J. Physiol.,* 202: 251 – 260.

Ikeda, H. and Wright, M.J. (1976) Properties of LGN cells in kittens reared with convergent squint: a neurophysiological demonstration of amblyopia. *Exp. Brain Res.,* 25: 63 – 77.

McCall, M.A., Tong, L. and Spear, P.D. (1988) Development of neuronal responses in cat posteromedial lateral suprasylvian visual cortex. *Brain Res.,* in the press.

Morrone, M.C., Di Stefano, M. and Burr, D.C. (1986) Spatial and temporal properties of neurons of the lateral suprasylvian cortex of the cat. *J. Neurophysiol.,* 56: 969 – 986.

Movshon, J.A., Thompson, I.D. and Tolhurst, D.J. (1978a) Spatial summation in the receptive fields of simple cells in the cat's striate cortex. *J. Physiol.,* 283: 53 – 77.

Movshon, J.A., Thompson, I.D. and Tolhurst, D.J. (1978b) Receptive field organization of complex cells in the cat's striate cortex. *J. Physiol.,* 283: 79 – 99.

Movshon, J.A., Thompson, I.D. and Tolhurst, D.J. (1978c) Spatial and temporal contrast sensitivities in areas 17 and 18 of the cat's visual cortex. *J. Physiol.,* 283: 101 – 120.

Norton, T.T. (1974) Receptive field properties of superior colliculus cells and development of visual behavior in kittens. *J. Neurophysiol.,* 37, 674 – 690.

Norton, T.T. (1981) Development of the visual system and visually guided behavior. In: *Development of Perception,* vol. 2, pp. 113 – 156. Academic Press, New York.

Price, D.J., Zumbroich, T.J. and Blakemore, C. (1988) Development of stimulus selectivity and functional organization in the suprasylvian visual cortex of the cat. *Proc. Roy. Soc. Lond. Ser. B.,* in the press.

Raczkowski, D. and Rosenquist, A.C. (1980) Connection of the parvocellular C laminae of the dorsal lateral geniculate nucleus with the visual cortex in the cat. *Brain Res.,* 199: 447 – 451.

Raczkowski, D. and Rosenquist, A.C. (1983) Connections of the multiple visual cortical areas with the lateral posterior-pulvinar complex and adjacent thalamic nuclei in the cat. *J. Neurosci.,* 3: 1912 – 1942.

Shapley, R. and Hochstein, S. (1975) Visual spatial summation in two classes of geniculate cells. *Nature,* 256: 411 – 413.

Sherk, H. (1986) Location and connections of visual cortical areas in the cat's suprasylvian sulcus. *J. Comp. Neurol.,* 247: 1 – 31.

Smith, D.C. and Spear, P.D. (1979) Effects of superior colliculus removal on receptive-field properties of neurons in lateral suprasylvian visual area of the cat. *J. Neurophysiol.,* 42: 57 – 75.

Spear, P.D. and Baumann, T.P. (1975) Receptive-field characteristics of single neurons in lateral suprasylvian visual area of the cat. *J. Neurophysiol.,* 38: 1403 – 1420.

Spear, P.D. and Baumann, T.P. (1979) Effects of visual cortex removal on receptive-field properties of neurons in lateral

230

suprasylvian visual area of the cat. *J. Neurophysiol.,* 42: 31 – 56.

Sur, M. and Sherman, S.M. (1982) Linear and non-linear W-cells in C-laminae of the cat's lateral geniculate nucleus. *J. Neurophysiol.,* 47: 869 – 884.

Symonds, L.L. and Rosenquist, A.C. (1984) Corticocortical connections among visual areas in the cat. *J. Comp. Neurol.,* 229: 1 – 38.

Tolhurst, D.J. and Movshon, J.A. (1975) Spatial and temporal contrast sensitivity of striate cortical neurones. *Nature,* 257: 674 – 675.

Tong, L., Kalil, R.E. and Spear, P.D. (1982) Thalamic projections to visual areas of the middle suprasylvian sulcus in the cat. *J. Comp. Neurol.,* 212: 103 – 117.

Toyama, K. and Kozasa, T. (1982) Responses of Clare-Bishop neurones to three dimensional movement of a light stimulus. *Vision Res.,* 22: 571 – 574.

Toyama, K., Komatsu, Y., Kasai, H., Fujii, K. and Umetani, K. (1985) Responsiveness of Clare-Bishop neurons to visual cues associated with motion of a visual stimulus in three-dimensional space. *Vision Res.,* 25: 407 – 414.

von Grünau, M.W., Zumbroich, T.J. and Poulin, C. (1987) Visual receptive field properties in the posterior suprasylvian cortex of the cat: a comparison between the areas PMLS and PLLS. *Vision Res.,* 27: 343 – 356.

Wright, M.J. (1969) Visual receptive fields of cells in a cortical area remote from the striate cortex in the cat. *Nature,* 223: 973 – 975.

Zumbroich, T.J. and Blakemore, C. (1987) Spatial and temporal selectivity in the suprasylvian cortex of the cat. *J. Neurosci.,* 7: 482 – 500.

Zumbroich, T.J., Price, D.J. and Blakemore, C. (1988) Development of spatial and temporal selectivity in the suprasylvian visual cortex of the cat. *J. Neurosci.,* in press.

Zumbroich, T.J., von Grünau, M., Poulin, C. and Blakemore, C. (1986) Differences of visual field respresentation in the medial and lateral banks of the suprasylvian cortex (PMLS/PLLS) of the cat. *Exp. Brain Res.,* 64: 77 – 93.

T.P. Hicks and G. Benedek (Eds.)
Progress in Brain Research, Vol. 75
© 1988 Elsevier Science Publishers B.V. (Biomedical Division)

CHAPTER 21

Lens accommodation-related and pupil-related units in the lateral suprasylvian area in cats

Takehiko Bando, Haruo Toda and Takeo Awaji

Department of Physiology, Faculty of Medicine, Niigata University, Niigata 951 and Department of Physiology, Yamanashi Medical School, Tamaho, Nakakoma, Yamanashi 409-38, Japan

Introduction

It has been suggested that the lateral suprasylvian area (LSA) (Heath and Jones 1971; Palmer et al. 1978) of cats plays an important role in the central neuronal circuitry underlying lens accommodation, and this proposal has been based on two major results (Bando et al. 1981, 1984b). Firstly, many LSA units are known to discharge in synchrony with spontaneously-occurring lens accommodation (measured as fluctuations of the refractive power of the eye) and these were recorded in parts of the medial and lateral banks of the middle suprasylvian sulcus (MSS); an area corresponding to the postero-medial and postero-lateral subareas of LSA (PMLS and PLLS; Palmer et al. 1978). Secondly, the refractive power of the eye can be increased by intracerebral stimulation of parts of PMLS and PLLS. In addition, it has been reported that some unit activities in LSA are correlated with such visual stimuli as movements of visual targets, approaching or leaving the nose of the animal (Toyama et al. 1982, 1986). It is well known that these visual stimuli trigger lens accommodation (Davson 1972).

Pupillary constriction also can be induced by stimulating superficial parts of the medial bank of MSS, a region overlapping partly the lens accommodation-related area (Bando 1985). The close spatial arrangement between lens accommodation-related and pupillo-constrictor areas in LSA has been confirmed by the systematic microstimulation of the medial bank of MSS, while monitoring concurrently in the same preparation both the changes of refractive power of one eye, and the changes of pupillary area of the other eye (Bando 1986).

In view of the strong link between lens accommodation and pupillary constriction in the near reflex of the eye (Davson 1972), the overlapping arrangement of the lens-related and pupillo-constrictor areas in LSA suggests that this area may play an important role in coordinating these two intraocular muscular movements in processes underlying the near reflex of the eye.

In the present study, unit activities which were modulated in synchrony with spontaneously-occurring lens accommodation and/or pupillary constriction were sought in the medial bank of MSS, an area corresponding to PMLS in anesthetized cats. Nineteen of 146 units in PMLS discharged in synchrony with lens accommodation, pupillary constriction or pupillary dilation. These units were grouped by their synchronous activity both with intraocular muscular movements, and with the effects of electrical stimulation through the recor-

---

Correspondence to: Dr. Takehiko Bando, Department of Physiology, Faculty of Medicine, Niigata University, Niigata 951, Japan.

232

ding micro-electrode. The good correlation between these variables supports the notion that LSA contributes to the central nervous control of these intraocular muscular movements.

Methods

Materials

Eleven cats, weighing 2–3 kg, were anesthetized with α-chloralose (Wako, 40 mg/kg) and urethane (Sigma, 500 mg/kg). Additional doses were given if the pupillary area became larger than a medium oval size (10–50 mm²) (Bando 1985). After the surgical procedure, the animals were immobilized with gallamine triethiodide (Sigma) to permit the accurate measurement of lens accommodation and

the pupillary area. The right eye was dilated by a 10% solution of L-phenylephrine hydrochloride (Tokyo Kasei) to permit the accurate measurement of the refractive power of the eye.

The refractive power of the right eye was monitored by an infrared optometer (Campbell and Robson 1959; Hosoba et al. 1978; Bando et al. 1984a) in the dark, as a measure of lens accommodation. The pupillary area of the left eye was monitored by an infrared pupillometer (Ijichi et al. 1978; Bando 1985).

For unit recording and microstimulation in LSA, a tungsten-in-glass microelectrode was used. A train of 30 bipolar pulses (0.2 msec negative-going pulses followed by 0.1 msec positive-going pulses; intensity, 0.2–0.05 mA) was used for microstimulation. Unit activities, the refractive

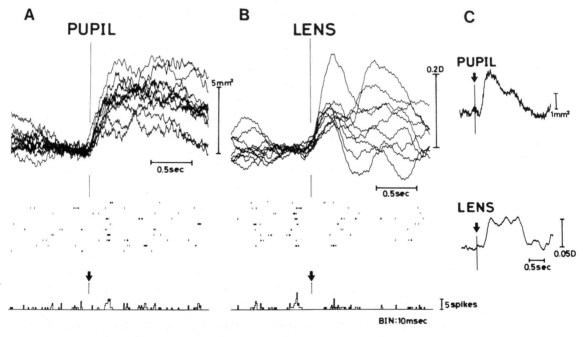

Fig. 1. A and B: the temporal relation of a LSA lens-related unit to spontaneously-occurring fluctations of pupillary area and lens accommodation, respectively. Top traces of A and B, traces of changes of pupillary area (A; upward deflection, decrease of the area) or refractive power of the eye (B; upward deflection, increase of the refractive power) superimposed in reference to the onset times of spontaneous responses (vertical lines, and downward arrows). Middle and bottom traces, raster displays and histograms of the onset times of spike potentials. C: pupillary (top) and lens (bottom) responses evoked by microstimulation at the recording site of the unit. Arrows in C show the timings of microstimulation. Calibration of pupillary area of 5 mm² for A, and that of 1 mm² for C are shown in A and C, respectively. Calibration of refractive power of 0.2 diopters (D) for B, and that of 0.05 D for C are shown in B and C, respectively.

power of the eye and pupillary area data were stored on magnetic tape for further off-line analysis (Bando et al. 1984a).

Results

Units related to lens accommodation and/or pupillary responses

Units were sought in the medial bank of the middle suprasylvian sulcus (MSS) whose activities were modulated in synchrony with spontaneously occurring fluctuations of the refractive power of the eye and/or with spontaneous changes of pupillary area. Nineteen of 146 units discharged in synchrony with spontaneous increases of the refractive power of the eye (lens accommodation) and/or

with changes of pupillary area, where the activity preceded the onset of these intraocular muscular movements by 250–650 msec.

These units were classified into four groups. Units in the first group discharged in synchrony with lens accommodation (Figs. 1B and 3B), but their activities were much less synchronized with changes of pupillary area (Figs. 1A and 3A). They were tentatively named 'lens-related' units (11 units). The second type of unit discharged in synchrony with pupillary constriction (Fig. 2A), but much less so with lens accommodation (Fig. 2B), and were assumed to be the class of 'pupillo-constrictor' units (4 units). Units in the third group discharged in synchrony with pupillary dilation, but not with pupillary constriction, nor with lens accommodation (pupillo-dilator units, 2 units). Units in the fourth group discharged in synchrony

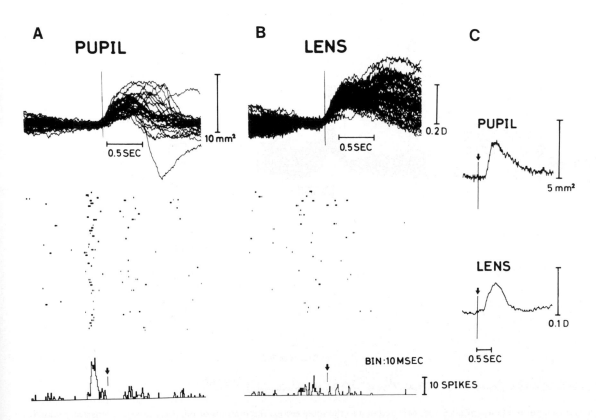

Fig. 2. A and B: temporal relation of a LSA pupillo-constrictor unit to the spontaneous changes of pupillary area and lens accommodation, respectively. Similar to Fig. 1. C: pupillary and lens responses evoked by microstimulation at the recording site of the unit.

234

both with lens accommodation and pupillary constriction (2 units).

Effect of microstimulation

Units again were classified in three groups based on the effect of microstimulation achieved through the recording microelectrode. At the recording sites of 9 units, both lens accommodation and pupillary constriction were evoked by microstimulation (Group I, Figs. 1C and 2C). At the recording sites of another 8 units, lens accommodation responses but not pupillary responses were evoked by microstimulation (Group II, Fig. 3C). At the recording sites of 2 other units, pupillary dilation was evoked by microstimulation (Group III).

Four of 9 Group I units discharged in synchrony with spontaneous fluctuations of lens accommodation (Fig. 1), but not with either pupillary constric-

tion or dilation. Activities of another 4 Group I units were synchronized with pupillary constriction, but much less so than with lens accommodation (Fig. 2). One Group I unit activity was synchronized both with lens accommodation and with pupillary constriction.

Seven of 8 Group II units discharged in synchrony with lens accommodation but not with pupillary responses (Fig. 3); and one with both lens accommodation and pupillary constriction. Activities of 2 Group III units were synchronized with pupillary dilation, and neither with pupillary constriction nor with lens accommodation. These results are summarized in Table 1.

Location of lens- and/or pupil-related units

Recording sites of lens-related and pupil-related units were located in histologically-reconstructed

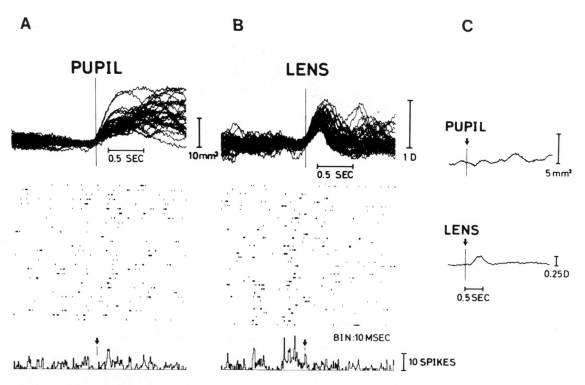

Fig. 3. A and B: temporal relation of a LSA lens-related unit to the spontaneous fluctuations of pupillary area and lens accommodation, respectively. Similar as in Fig. 1. C, pupillary and lens responses evoked by microstimulation at the recording site of the unit. Note that the scale for evoked lens response is different from that in Figs. 1 and 2.

tracks in frontal sections (Fig. 4). They were found in the deeper layers of the cortex. Pupillary constrictor units were located in the superficial parts of the medial bank of MSS, and lens-related units were distributed both superficially and in deep parts of the medial bank of MSS. Pupillo-dilation units were found in deep parts of the medial bank of MSS. The location of lens-related and pupillo-constrictor units were in agreement with the distribution of lens accommodation responses and that of pupillo-constriction responses evoked by systematic microstimulation in LSA (Bando 1985, 1986).

Discussion

In the present paper, units in LSA were shown which discharged in synchrony with spontaneously-occurring lens accommodation, pupillary constriction, and/or pupillary-dilation without the presentation of any visual stimulation. At the recording sites of these units, intraocular muscular movements were evoked, with which these units

were synchronized. For example, increased refractive power of the eye was evoked by electrical stimulation at the recording sites of lens-related units. Pupillary constriction was evoked by stimulating the recording sites of pupillo-constrictor

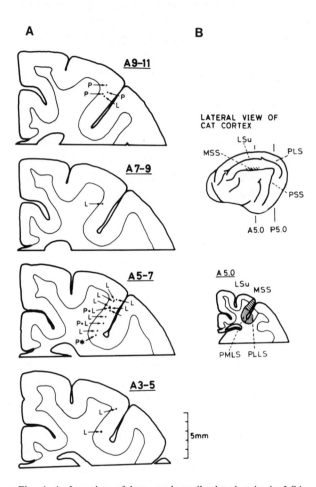

Fig. 4. A: Location of lens- and pupil-related units in LSA. Locations of units are shown as filled circles in four frontal sections. Stereotactic coordinates are given as the labels A9–11, A7–9, A5–7 and A3–5 above each section. P, pupillo-constrictor units; L, lens-related units; P + L, those units which discharged in synchrony with both pupillo-constriction and lens accommodation; P*, pupillo-dilator unit. Calibration of 5 mm applies to all sections. B: Top: lateral view of the cerebral cortex of the cat. LSu, lateral sulcus; MSS, middle suprasylvian sulcus; PLS, posterolateral sulcus; PSS, posterior suprasylvian sulcus. A5.0 and P5.0 indicate the stereotaxic coordinates. Bottom: a frontal section of cat occipital cortex at the stereotaxic coordinate A5.0. PMLS, postero-medial lateral suprasylvian area; PLLS, postero-lateral suprasylvian area.

TABLE 1

Unit activities and effects of microstimulation at the recording sites

	Effects of microstimulation			
	pc[a] + lens	Lens	pd + lens	Total
Lens-related units	4	7	0	11
Pupillo-con-strictor units	4	0	0	4
Pupillo-dilator units	0	0	2	2
Lens + pupillo-constriction units	1	1	0	2
Total	9	8	2	19

[a] pc, pupillary constriction; pd, pupillary dilation; lens, increased refractive power of the eye

units, and pupillary dilation was evoked at the recording sites of pupillo-dilator units. The locations of pupillo-constrictor units were in the superficial parts of the medial bank of MSS, and those of lens-related units, in both superficial and deep parts in agreement with results obtained by systematic microstimulation in a previous study (Bando 1985, 1986). The close parallelism of unit activities and effects of microstimulation favors the notion that LSA plays an important role in controlling intraocular muscular movements such as accompany lens accommodation and pupillary constriction.

Lens accommodation, pupillary constriction or pupillary dilation were synchronized only occasionally with each other in this study, which was conducted under anesthesia and without any visual stimulation. The activities of most of these units also discharged in prominent synchrony with only one of these three intraocular muscular movements. The desynchronized occurrence of these spontaneous movements argues against the possibility that they, and unit activities accompanying them, are reflective of generalized seizure activity, elicited during chloralose anesthesia.

Those units whose activities are related to the near response of the eye would be expected to be synchronized both with lens accommodation and with pupillary constriction, when both of these intraocular muscular movements are synchronized by presenting the visual targets approaching or departing from the nose of the animal. Similar experiments such as those described here, but with visual stimulation, now are under way.

Acknowledgement

This work was supported by a Grant-in-Aid for Scientific Research from the Japanese Ministry of Education, Sciences and Culture, and a grant from The Ichiro Kanehara Foundation. We thank Dr. J. Maeda for computer programs, and Mr. I. Kinno for technical assistance.

References

Bando, T. (1985) Pupillary constriction evoked from the postero-medial lateral suprasylvian (PMLS) area in cats. *Neurosci. Res.,* 2: 472 – 485.

Bando, T. (1986) Localization of lens accommodation-related and pupillary constriction-related regions in the lateral suprasylvian area in cats. *Abstracts 10th Jap. Neurosci. Meeting.*

Bando, T., Tsukuda, K., Yamamoto, N., Maeda, J. and Tsukahara, N. (1981) Cortical neurones in and around the Clare-Bishop area related with lens accommodation in the cat. *Brain Res.,* 225: 195 – 199.

Bando, T., Tsukuda, K., Yamamoto, N., Maeda, J. and Tsukahara, N. (1984a) Physiological identification of midbrain neurons related to lens accommodation in cats. *J. Neurophysiol.,* 52: 870 – 878.

Bando, T., Yamamoto, K. and Tsukahara, N. (1984b) Cortical neurons related to lens accommodation in posterior lateral suprasylvian area in cats. *J. Neurophysiol.,* 52: 879 – 891.

Campbell, F.W. and Robson, J.G. (1959) High-speed infrared optometer. *J. Opt. Soc. Amer.,* 49: 268 – 272.

Davson, H. (1972) *Physiology of the Eye,* Churchill Livingstone, Edinburgh, 643 pp.

Heath, C.J. and Jones, E.G. (1971) The anatomical organization of the suprasylvian gyrus of the cat. *Ergeb. Anat. Entwicklungsgesch.,* 45: 1 – 64.

Hosoba, N., Bando, T. and Tsukahara, N. (1978) The cerebellar control of lens accommodation of the eye in the cat. *Brain Res.,* 153: 495 – 505.

Ijichi, Y., Kiyohara, T., Hosoba, M. and Tsukahara, N. (1978) The cerebellar control of the pupillary light reflex in the cat. *Brain Res.,* 128: 69 – 79.

Palmer, L.A., Rosenquist, A.C. and Tusa, R.J. (1978) The retinotopic organization of lateral suprasylvian visual areas in the cat. *J. Comp. Neurol.,* 177: 237 – 256.

Toyama, K. and Kozasa, T. (1982) Responses of Clare-Bishop neurons to three dimensional movement of a light stimulus. *Vision Res.,* 22: 571 – 574.

Toyama, K., Komatsu, Y. and Kozasa, T. (1986) The responsiveness of Clare-Bishop neurons to motion cues for motion stereopsis. *Neurosci. Res.,* 4: 83 – 109.

T.P. Hicks and G. Benedek (Eds.)
Progress in Brain Research, Vol. 75
© 1988 Elsevier Science Publishers B.V. (Biomedical Division)

CHAPTER 22

Retinotopic order and functional organization in a region of suprasylvian visual cortex, the Clare-Bishop area

Helen Sherk

Department of Biological Structure, University of Washington, Seattle, WA, U.S.A.

Introduction

Traditionally, an area of visual cortex has been equated with a single representation of the visual hemifield (Talbot and Marshall 1941). The extensive visual cortex on the banks of the cat's suprasylvian sulcus was subdivided on this basis into a mosaic of at least eight distinct areas by Tusa et al. (1981), using conventional physiological mapping methods. On the other hand, it has also been assumed that a cortical area can be characterized by its set of extrinsic connections: all parts of an area should be connected to the same set of thalamic and cortical regions (e.g. Jones and Powell 1969; Graybiel and Berson 1981). In an earlier study of the suprasylvian cortex, I found that a connectional approach yielded a different set of cortical areas than those defined by physiological mapping (Sherk 1986a). One of these, referred to here as the Clare-Bishop area (Hubel and Wiesel 1969), was of particular interest because of its strong input from area 17 (Clare and Bishop, 1954). Its location, defined anatomically by its striate input, is shown in part in Fig. 1 (at the

posterior end of the suprasylvian sulcus, it also extends onto the ectosylvian gyrus, missing in this figure).

It is unclear how the Clare-Bishop area can be fitted into the scheme of retinotopically-defined areas of Tusa et al. (1981). One might expect that several of their small areas fall within the Clare-Bishop area. However, the latter area cuts across many physiologically-defined boundaries. For example, part of area 21a (Tusa and Palmer 1980) lies within it, and part outside. The same is true for some other areas, most notably the posterior medial lateral suprasylvian area (PMLS) of Palmer et al. (1978). This outcome is troubling because it is difficult to understand how one part of a visual area can receive a strong input from area 17, while the remainder receives none.

Because the Clare-Bishop area incorporated pieces of several retinotopically-defined areas, I was puzzled as to the organization of its map. I therefore carried out preliminary physiological mapping experiments, which revealed some discrepancies with the reports of Tusa et al. (1981). For example, a previously unrecognized representation of the upper vertical meridian was found on the posterior bank of the suprasylvian sulcus; likewise, an unreported representation of part of the lower vertical meridian was found running down the medial bank of the sulcus near its

Correspondence to: Helen Sherk, Dept. of Biological Structure, SM-20, University of Washington, Seattle, WA 98195, U.S.A.

238

posterior end. However, these data were too incomplete to determine the detailed organization of the map.

Perhaps the most striking feature of these experiments was the apparent retinotopic disorganization in the region, as noted by many previous experimenters (Hubel and Wiesel 1969; Spear and Baumann 1975; Turlejski and Michalski 1975; Tusa et al. 1981; Djavadian and Harutiunian-Kozak 1983; Zumbroich et al. 1986). Some electrode penetrations yielded relatively systematic progressions of receptive fields. Others, however, yielded erratic progressions that produced little net movement through the visual field, even across a distance of 3 – 4 mm of cortex. Two examples are shown in Fig. 2. If the Clare-Bishop area contains a single, continuous representation of the visual hemifield, as found in areas 17, 18 or 19, these erratic receptive field progressions indicate that there is considerable scatter in the fields at any given cortical site. Indeed, such data have led to a consensus that the map is rather disorderly (Hubel and Wiesel 1969; Spear and Baumann 1975; Turlejski and Michalski 1975; Tusa et al. 1981; Djavadian and Harutiunian-Kozak 1983; Zumbroich et al. 1986). However, the two assumptions stated above –

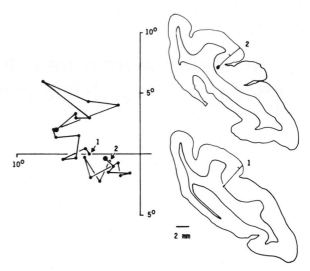

Fig. 2. Progressions of receptive fields along two penetrations in the cat's Clare-Bishop area. At left, the center of each field is marked with a dot. The first is indicated with a numbered arrow, and the terminal lesion, with a larger dot. At right are coronal sections containing the two electrode tracks. The first recording site on each track is marked with a dash. Midline is to the left.

that the map contains no repetitions, and that it is continuous – may be wrong. The map could be redundant, with multiple representations of a small part of the visual field embedded within it. Furthermore, 'fractures' might exist, so that some non-adjacent regions of visual field are represented side-by-side.

While physiological mapping methods have been extremely successful in revealing the retinotopic organization of areas 17, 18 and 19, they may fail in the Clare-Bishop area if the map is indeed complex. The resolution of mapping – that is, the spacing between sampling sites in the cortex – is often coarse in suprasylvian visual cortex. The chief reason is that the receptive fields of many cells cannot be defined accurately, so that often cortical recording sites are several hundred microns apart. Compressed, duplicate representations of a small part of visual field might go unrecognized. Likewise, a 'fracture' in the map would be difficult to detect.

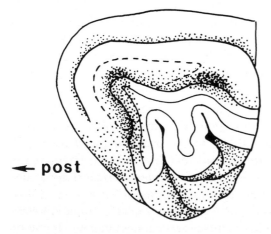

← **post**

Fig. 1. Lateral view of the posterior portion of the right hemisphere in a cat. The suprasylvian gyri have been removed to expose the medial and posterior banks of the suprasylvian sulcus. The Clare-Bishop area's approximate location is indicated by the dashed line.

I have turned to two other methods in order to investigate the organization of the map in the Clare-Bishop area. In the first, anterograde tracers were injected at sites in area 17 at which receptive fields had been plotted. The assumption, which is widely held regarding all visual pathways, was that only retinotopically-corresponding locations are interconnected. Any patches of label found in the suprasylvian cortex should represent the same visual field location as that injected in area 17 (see also Albus and Meyer 1981; Montero 1981).

Recently, I have used a novel physiological method in the Clare-Bishop areas of cats and also ferrets. (The ferret possesses a region of suprasylvian visual cortex that, at least superficially, resembles the Clare-Bishop area of the cat in its connectional and physiological characteristics (unpublished observations).) Some time ago I found that, in area 17, one can record directly from geniculate terminals after first silencing cellular responses by local injections of kainic acid. Kainic acid kills neurons but has no apparent effect on axons of passage or axon terminals (Coyle et al. 1978). This phenomenon was exploited by McConnell and LeVay (1984) to investigate the organization of geniculate afferents to the mink's area 17. I have now found that afferent terminals arising, apparently, from visual cortical areas can also be recorded in the Clare-Bishop area with this method.

Direct recording from afferent terminals has also allowed me to examine functional organization within the Clare-Bishop area, about which little is known. There is some disagreement as to whether neurons are orientation-selective, as initially described by Hubel and Wiesel (1969), or strictly direction-selective (Spear and Baumann 1975). As to their organization, the only suggestion is that of Hubel and Wiesel (1969), that cells are grouped according to preferred orientation. The final section below discusses the evidence regarding such an organization.

Tracer mapping of striate input to the Clare-Bishop area

Both data from my traditional physiological mapping experiments, and from tracer injections, indicated that the map has a simple overall layout. The upper field was located in the postero-lateral region, on the banks of the posterior suprasylvian sulcus. Anterior to the 'corner' where this sulcus meets the suprasylvian sulcus proper, the lower field was represented. The area centralis was found exclusively at the junction between the upper and lower fields, with no indication of additional representations located more anteriorly or laterally, as suggested previously by physiological recording (Palmer et al. 1978; Tusa and Palmer 1980; Updyke 1986).

In detail, however, the map appeared unexpectedly complex. A single tracer injection invariably yielded several patches of label within the Clare-Bishop area, as pointed out by Montero (1981) and as also seen in the monkey's area MT (e.g., Van Essen et al. 1981). Typical patches are illustrated in Fig. 3. The patchiness could not be explained by technical problems such as uptake by fibers of passage. What was particularly puzzling was the outcome when two different tracers were injected at different sites in area 17. If both sites had retinotopic locations in one quadrant, usually (in 11 of 16 cases) the two kinds of patches in the Clare-Bishop area were intermingled (Fig. 3D). If the injection sites were far apart retinotopically, however, there was no intermingling.

There are two ways these data might be interpreted. Either there is a single, non-redundant map that is quite messy, so that the target regions of two different sites in area 17 overlap. Alternatively, some segment of the visual field is represented more than once in the Clare-Bishop area's map.

There are objections to both interpretations. The second, retinotopic explanation seems unlikely to explain the full extent of patchiness. One tracer injection can yield numerous closely-spaced patches, and it is difficult to imagine that each one belongs to a distinct representation. However, patches that are widely separated might belong to duplicate representations, while closely-spaced patchiness might be caused by a different mechanism. Some previous work has supported this conclusion (Sherk 1986b).

The difficulties with the first interpretation are more serious. It predicts that unlabeled gaps be-

tween patches will represent the same region of visual field as the patches. But in two instances in which I have recorded from cells later found to lie within large unlabeled gaps, I have found that receptive fields did not correspond to those at the injection site in area 17. By contrast, when receptive fields were recorded within patches of label, there was a relatively good match between receptive fields in the Clare-Bishop area and those at the injection site in area 17.

Another difficulty stems from the large region of cortex over which patches arising from one striate injection may be scattered. According to the first interpretation, this entire region represents the retinotopic location involved by one injection in area 17. But when a second injection was made, the second set of patches often was intermingled with the first set, as noted above (see Fig. 3D). The first interpretation implies that the representations of these two different visual field loci overlap extensively in the Clare-Bishop area, producing a disorderly map. In the example of Fig. 3, input representing the point on the horizontal meridian (hatched) would be coextensive with input representing the site about 10° away on the vertical meridian (black). Such a degree of retinotopic chaos is incompatible with the outcome of tracer experiments, and, as described in the following section, with evidence from direct recording from afferent terminals.

Tracer experiments showed that, while patches of label from two different injections might be intermingled, the patches did not overlap with each other; hence, the labeled afferents must have remained segregated. This outcome was found in 9 experiments in which both injections' retinotopic locations were in the same quadrant, and the injection sites were not directly adjacent to each other. The lack of overlap was particularly striking in cases in which the two sets of patches were highly intermingled, as in Fig. 3. When the two injection sites were contiguous (3 experiments), there was some overlap between the two kinds of patches, but it was still modest. Although an absence of overlap might occur by chance in one or two ex-

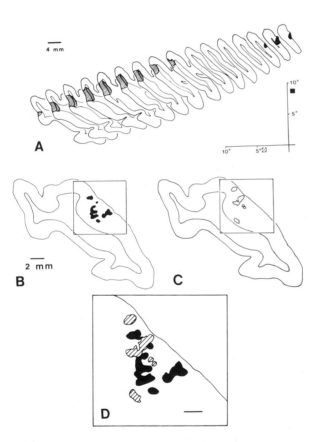

Fig. 3. Injections of two anterograde tracers in area 17, and the resulting patches of label in the Clare-Bishop area. A: The two injection sites are shown in a series of coronal sections, with the midline to the left. The corresponding retinotopic locations are indicated to the right. B: A coronal section through the Clare-Bishop area showing patches of one tracer. C: The adjacent section showing patches of the second tracer. D: The boxed region from these two coronal sections showing both kinds of patches. They are intermingled but non-overlapping. Calibration bar is 1 mm.

periments, it was seen so consistently that I think it unlikely to be accidental. A retinotopic segregation between the projections from the two injection sites seems the most plausible explanation, since the only consistent difference between the two injection sites in area 17 was their retinotopic location.

In these experiments, it was impossible to be certain of the exact region of visual field represented by the patches in the Clare-Bishop area, since I did not know to what extent of area 17's map had transported label. By recording directly from afferent terminals within Clare-Bishop, I hoped to assess their retinotopic locations more precisely, as discussed below.

Direct recording from cortical afferents to the Clare-Bishop area: retinotopic order

Obvious differences were apparent to the investigator when the cells in a region of cortex had been silenced by kainic acid. The noise level was low, and injury discharges were never seen. Spikes were of small amplitude and brief duration. In the Clare-Bishop area, there was a clear-cut laminar

zone within which visual responses could be recorded. This zone corresponded to that within which terminals from areas 17 and 18 end, comprising layers 3, 4 and possibly deep 2. At a given recording site, the signal appeared to be dominated by a small cluster of afferent terminals. Often one spike was well isolated, and, based on its distinctive waveform, receptive field, and response properties, seemed to correspond to the output of either a single neuron, or a few neurons with indistinguishable properties. The great majority of afferents appeared to originate in areas 17, 18, or possibly 19. They were either direction- or orientation-selective, with sharply defined receptive fields, and were usually binocular. The most striking characteristic of these afferents in both the ferret and cat was the vigor and reliability of their responses. Notably absent were ones with responses like those described in the cat's lateral posterior nucleus (Chalupa and Fish 1978; Mason 1978, 1981), which provides the dominant thalamic projection to the Clare-Bishop area (Graybiel 1970).

This approach is well-suited to the study of retinotopic organization because the cortex can be

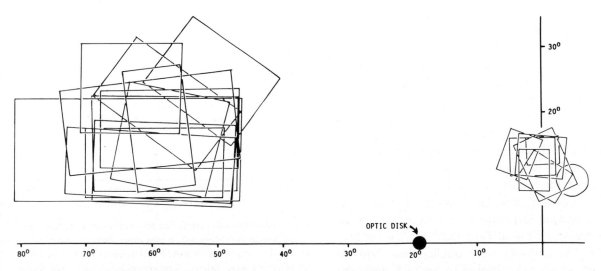

Fig. 4. Receptive fields in the ferret's suprasylvian visual cortex. These were recorded from afferent terminals, along two short penetrations that were approximately normal to the cortical surface. Cells had been silenced by kainic acid. These fields appeared to belong to afferents arising from other regions of visual cortex, except for the circular field, which had geniculate-like response characteristics.

sampled at a high degree of spatial resolution. Typically, response properties were tested at intervals of 10 μm, and receptive fields plotted whenever a shift in their position was detected. Discussed below are two measures of retinotopic order: the scatter of receptive fields recorded along a penetration normal to the cortical surface (Hubel and Wiesel 1974; Albus 1975) and receptive field size.

In the ferret, the scatter of fields in a surface-normal penetration was generally less than the fields' diameters, where diameter was taken to be the square root of a field's area. Two examples are shown in Fig. 4. In both cases, every field overlaps at least slightly with every other field in the penetration (excluding the single geniculate field); there are no major jumps in field position.

In the cat, the scatter in 77 receptive fields plotted along three penetrations was examined. The recording sites were close together, on average only 20 μm apart. The shifts between successively plotted fields were measured, and the average shift was taken as an estimate of scatter for that penetration. As in the ferret, field scatter was less than the diameter of the fields themselves: measured as a percentage of field diameter, it was 52% for one penetration, 43% for the second, and 33% for the third. This small scatter was impressive because the receptive fields themselves were modest in size.

On the whole, afferent fields in the cat were much smaller than those of cells in the Clare-Bishop area at the equivalent eccentricity. Afferent field diameters averaged 3.5°, versus 9 − 10° found by Zumbroich et al. (1986) when recording from cell bodies. Their sizes were compatible with the notion that they arose from areas 17, 18, and 19, which provide the driving visual cortical input to the Clare-Bishop area. On average, afferent fields were somewhat larger than those in area 17 in the same region of visual field (3.5° vs. 2.6° (Albus 1975)). The majority were smaller than fields in area 18, which are reported to be 2 − 3 times the size of those in area 17 (Tretter et al. 1975; Dreher et al. 1980). No comparison can be made with area 19, for which field sizes have not been reported.

These data thus suggest that the inputs from areas 17 − 19 to the Clare-Bishop are retinotopically well-ordered. What kind of map they form — that is, how they are organized tangentially — is not yet clear. However, these results appear more consistent with an orderly though complex map containing multiple representations of a small part of the visual field, and possibly discontinuities, than with a non-redundant but disorderly map.

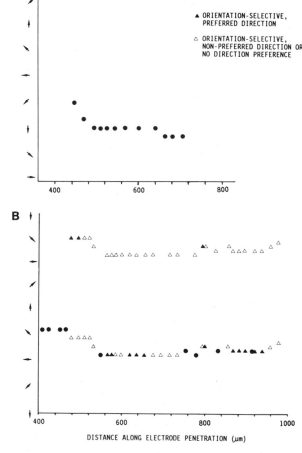

Fig. 5. Direction and orientation preferences of afferents to the Clare-Bishop area along two penetrations that were nearly normal to the cortical surface. A: Penetration in a ferret in which all afferents were strictly direction-selective, i.e., each had a null direction opposite to the preferred direction. B: In a cat, a penetration that encountered predominantly orientation-selective afferents. Note, however, that where there was a directional preference, it was almost always for the same direction.

Direct recording from cortical afferents to the Clare-Bishop area: functional organization

There was a striking organization of afferents according to both preferred orientation and direction of movement. In penetrations that were approximately normal to the cortical surface, it was common to find that all afferents had similar preferred directions, as illustrated in Fig. 5A. However, some columns instead appeared to be dominated by one optimal orientation, so that at many sites either direction of movement elicited brisk responses. Data from the penetration displaying the least degree of directional preference yet encountered are shown in Fig. 5B. Even in this penetration, however, direction preference seemed to be an important factor. At most sites where there was any bias for one direction over the other, the same direction was preferred throughout the penetration. I would conclude that, although there are regions where afferents are clearly orientation-selective, the dominant organizational parameter is preferred direction.

As one might expect, there was a tangential as well as columnar organization of preferred direction. Every penetration that cut across columns demonstrated an orderly progression of preferred direction and orientation. One of the most nearly tangential examples, from a ferret, is shown in Fig. 6. These data illustrate two other points. First, breaks in the progression of preferred direction or orientation did occur. At the arrow in Fig. 6, there was an abrupt jump from a preference for leftward horizontal movement, to upward right oblique movement. Second, regions dominated by orientation-selective afferents could be found adjacent to regions containing strictly direction-selective afferents.

It may well be that afferents to the Clare-Bishop area are organized according to additional response parameters. Afferents showed variation in other properties such as receptive field size, velocity preference, subfield organization, and ocular dominance. The most obvious feature of their organization, however, was the grouping according to preferred direction and orientation.

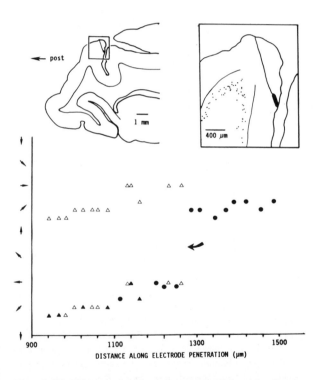

Fig. 6. Direction and orientation preferences of afferents recorded along a relatively tangential penetration in the ferret's suprasylvian visual cortex. At top is a parasagittal section containing the electrode track, which terminates in a lesion (black). In the enlarged view (upper right), small dots mark the large pyramidal cells of layer 5, while layer 4 is indicated by a line. The line is broken where cells were absent due to the kainic acid injection. The progression of preferred directions, below, shows an abrupt jump in preferred direction (arrow). Symbols as for Fig. 5.

Acknowledgements

This work was supported by grant EY04847 and by the Alfred P. Sloan Foundation. I greatly appreciate the comments of Dennis Dacey on the manuscript.

References

Albus, K. (1975) A quantitative study of the projection area of the central and the paracentral visual field in area 17 of the cat. I. The precision of the topography. *Brain Res.*, 24: 159 – 179.

Albus, K. and Meyer, G. (1981) Anatomical mapping of representations of the visual field in afferent projections to the visual cortex of the cat. *Neurosci. Abst.,* 7: 761.

Chalupa, L.M. and Fish, S.E. (1978) Response characteristics of visual and extravisual neurons in the pulvinar and lateral posterior nuclei of the cat. *Exp. Neurol.,* 61: 96 – 120.

Clare, M.H. and Bishop, G.H. (1954) Responses from an association area secondarily activated from optic cortex. *J. Neurophysiol.,* 17: 271 – 277.

Coyle, J.T., Molliver, M.E. and Kuhar, M.J. (1978) In situ injection of kainic acid: a new method for selectively lesioning neuronal cell bodies while sparing axons of passage. *J. Comp. Neurol.,* 180: 301 – 324.

Djavadian, R.L. and Harutiunian-Kozak, B.A. (1983) Retinotopic organization of the lateral suprasylvian area in the cat. *Acta Neurobiol. Exp.,* 43: 251 – 262.

Dreher, B., Leventhal, A.G. and Hale, P.T. (1980) Geniculate input to cat visual cortex: a comparison of area 19 with areas 17 and 18. *J. Neurophysiol.,* 44: 804 – 826.

Gattas, R. and Gross, C.G. (1981) Visual topography of striate projection zone (MT) in posterior superior temporal sulcus of the macaque. *J. Neurophysiol.,* 46: 621 – 638.

Graybiel, A.M. (1970) Some thalamocortical projections of the pulvinar-posterior system of the thalamus of the cat. *Brain Res.,* 22: 131 – 136.

Graybiel, A.M. and Berson, D.M. (1981) On the relation between transthalamic and transcortical pathways in the visual system. In: F.O. Schmitt, F.G. Worden and F. Dennis (Eds.), *The Organization of the Cerebral Cortex,* MIT Press, Cambridge, MA, pp. 286 – 319.

Hubel, D.H. and Wiesel, T.N. (1969) Visual area of the lateral suprasylvian gyrus (Clare-Bishop area) of the cat. *J. Physiol. (Lond.),* 202: 251 – 260.

Hubel, D.H. and Wiesel, T.N. (1974) Uniformity of monkey striate cortex: a parallel relationship between field size, scatter, and magnification factor. *J. Comp. Neurol.,* 158: 267 – 293.

Jones, E.G. and Powell, T.P.S. (1969) Connexions of the somatic sensory cortex of the Rhesus monkey. I. Ipsilateral cortical connexions. *Brain,* 92: 477 – 502.

Mason, R. (1978) Functional properties of the cat's pulvinar complex. *Exp. Brain Res.,* 31: 51 – 66.

Mason, R. (1981) Differential responsiveness of cells in the visual zones of the cat's LP-pulvinar complex to visual stimuli. *Exp. Brain Res.,* 43: 25 – 33.

McConnell, S.K. and LeVay, S. (1984) Segregation of on- and off-center afferents in mink visual cortex. *Proc. Natl. Acad. Sci. USA,* 81: 1590 – 1593.

Montero, V.M. (1981) Topography of the cortico-cortical connections from the striate cortex in the cat. *Brain Behav. Evol.,* 18: 194 – 218.

Palmer, L.A., Rosenquist A.C. and Tusa, R.J. (1978) The retinotopic organization of lateral suprasylvian visual areas in the cat. *J. Comp. Neurol.,* 177: 237 – 256.

Sherk, H. (1986a) Location and connections of visual cortical areas in the cat's suprasylvian sulcus. *J. Comp. Neurol.,* 247: 1 – 31.

Sherk, H. (1986b) Coincidence of patchy inputs from the lateral geniculate complex and from area 17 to the cat's Clare-Bishop area. *J. Comp. Neurol.,* 253: 105 – 120.

Spear, P.D. and Baumann, T.P. (1975) Receptive-field characteristics of single neurons in lateral suprasylvian visual area of the cat. *J. Neurophysiol.,* 38: 1403 – 1420.

Talbot, S.A. and Marshall, W.H. (1941) Physiological studies on neural mechanisms of visual localization and discrimination. *Am. J. Ophthalmol.,* 24: 1255 – 1263.

Tretter, F., Cynader, M. and Singer, W. (1975) Cat parastriate cortex: a primary or secondary visual area? *J. Neurophysiol.,* 38: 1099 – 1112.

Turlejski, K. and Michalski, A. (1975) Clare-Bishop area in the cat: location and retinotopic projection. *Acta Neurobiol. Exp.,* 35: 179 – 188.

Tusa, R.J. and Palmer, L.A. (1980) Retinotopic organization of areas 20 and 21 in the cat. *J. Comp. Neurol.,* 193: 147 – 164.

Tusa, R.J., Palmer, L.A. and Rosenquist, A.C. (1981) Multiple cortical visual areas. Visual field topography in the cat. In: C.N. Woolsey (Ed.) *Cortical Sensory Organization. Vol. 2, Multiple Visual Area,* Humana Press, Clifton, NJ, pp 1 – 31.

Updyke, B.V. (1986) Retinotopic organization within the cat's posterior suprasylvian sulcus and gyrus. *J. Comp. Neurol.,* 246: 265 – 280.

Van Essen, D.C., Maunsell, J.H.R. and Bixby, J.L. (1981) The middle temporal visual area in the macaque: myeloarchitecture, connections, functional properties and topographic organization. *J. Comp. Neurol.,* 199: 293 – 326.

Zumbroich, T.J., von Grünau, M., Poulin, C. and Blakemore, C. (1986) Differences of visual field representation in the medial and lateral banks of the suprasylvian cortex (PMLS/PLLS) of the cat. *Exp. Brain. Res.,* 64: 77 – 93.

T.P. Hicks and G. Benedek (Eds.)
Progress in Brain Research, Vol. 75
© 1988 Elsevier Science Publishers B.V. (Biomedical Division)

CHAPTER 23

Anterior ectosylvian visual area (AEV) of the cat: physiological properties

G. Benedek[2], L. Mucke[1], M. Norita[3], B. Albowitz[1] and O.D. Creutzfeldt[1]

[1] *Max-Planck-Institute for Biophysical Chemistry, Department of Neurobiology, Göttingen, F.R.G.,* [2] *Department of Physiology, University Medical School, Szeged, Hungary, and* [3] *Fujita-Gakuen University, Toyoake, Aichi, Japan*

The story of the AEV dates back to 1981, when Mucke and Creutzfeldt were searching for visual neurons in the feline claustrum. Several of the vertical penetrations aimed at the claustrum yielded cells with vigorous visual activity, and morphological examinations later showed that the cells often were located in the cortex along the anterior ectosylvian sulcus. This observation prompted a systematic study, the result of which was a description of the AEV (Mucke et al. 1982). The area was found and described practically simultaneously by Olson and Graybiel, whose published description, however, appeared one year later (Olson and Graybiel 1983).

According to the original descriptions, the cells in this area exhibit extraordinary visual properties. They are particularly sensitive to small stimuli moving at a fairly high speed in a particular direction in a rather large receptive field. Movement opposite to the preferred direction causes an inhibition of neuronal activity. As far as the receptive fields are concerned, the two groups reported conflicting results. Graybiel and Olson described a definite retinotopic register of the receptive fields. Our findings (Mucke et al. 1982) showed fairly uniform receptive fields that generally covered the area centralis, and hence no retinotopic tendency could be described. The physiological studies suggest that this visual area belongs to the extrageniculo-striate system; even removal of area 17 did not affect the functional properties of the cells.

The morphological connections of this area have been the topic of several studies (Mucke et al. 1982; Guldin and Markowitsch 1984; Higo and Kawamura 1984; Miceli et al. 1985; Olson and Graybiel 1985, 1987; Norita et al. 1986; Ptito et al. 1987). It has been found that the AEV receives visual inputs through two main routes: from the lateral suprasylvian visual area (LS) and from the extrageniculate visual thalamus, which consists of both the LPm (medial division of the lateral posterior nucleus) and the LM-Sg (nucleus lateralis medialis-nucleus suprageniculatus) complex. The AEV also receives afferents from the contralateral hemisphere. The main efferent pathways from the AEV are directed towards the LS and the extrageniculo-striate visual thalamus, and a rather dense efferent pathway also connects the AEV to the superior colliculus (SC). In addition to these, there are efferent connections towards the frontal eye fields and towards the amygdala, a structure heavily involved in limbic functions (Fig. 1).

Despite widespread research, several questions remain open, particularly concerning the functional importance of AEV. No direct evidence is yet available concerning this question. The high velocity and directional sensitivity suggest a role in motion perception. The following study was

---

Correspondence to: G. Benedek, Dept. Physiology, Dóm tér 10, H-6720 Szeged, Hungary.

designed to elucidate some physiological properties of the AEV neurons, and hence to facilitate the solution of questions concerning the physiological significance.

Methods

The study was performed on 22 cats. They were initially anaesthetized with ketamine hydrochloride (30 mg/kg i.m.). After cannulation of the trachea and the vena femoralis, the animals were placed in a stereotaxic headholder. The skull and dura were opened in order to allow a vertical approach to the AEV. The animals were then immobilized with

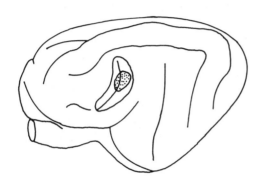

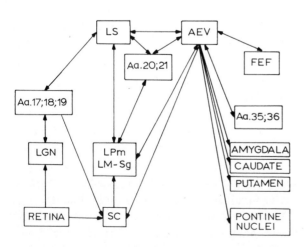

Fig. 1. Schematic presentation of the location of the AEV (top) and that of the AEV connections (after Norita et al. (1986) bottom). Interconnections between the areas are neglected. For abbreviations, see text.

gallamine triethiodide (Flaxedil, 20 mg/kg i.v), and anaesthesia was maintained with an infusion of pentobarbital (1.0 – 1.75 mg/kg/h) and Flaxedil (8 mg/kg/h) solution. Anaesthesia was repeatedly and carefully controlled by judging the effect of painful paw pinching on the arterial blood pressure. The end-tidal CO_2 level and the rectal temperature were monitored continuously and kept constant at 3.8 – 4.0% and 37 – 38°C, respectively. Phenylephrine and atropine eyedrops were administered repeatedly. The corneas were covered with contact lenses corrected to focus the vision on a tangent screen situated 35 cm in front of the approximate nodal point of the cat's eyes.

Light stimuli of 150 cd/m^2 were used against a homogeneous background of 5 – 10 cd/m^2. The light stimuli were presented through a computer-controlled projecting system. Stationary stimuli consisted of light squares 1.5 – 80° in width and were turned on and off for 1-sec periods.

Glass micropipettes filled with 2% pontamine sky blue served for the extracellular recording of neuronal activity. Electrical stimulation of the LS and the SC was carried out by means of bipolar concentric electrodes. Rectangular stimulus pulses (0.05 msec and 50 – 250 μA) were used for electrical stimulation.

At the end of the experiments the animals were deeply anaesthetized with pentobarbital and transcardially perfused with paraformaldehyde solution. The positions of the pontamine sky blue spots were correlated with microdrive readings made during the recordings and were used to reconstruct the positions of the cells.

Results

The AEV occupies at least the posterior two-thirds of the deep infolding of the anterior ectosylvian sulcus (Fig. 1). A definite rostral border was consistently observed around the 'elbow' of the sulcus, in agreement with the finding of Olson and Graybiel (1987). Occasionally, however, we found visual cells along the whole length of the sulcus. A total of 208 single units were recorded. Twenty-

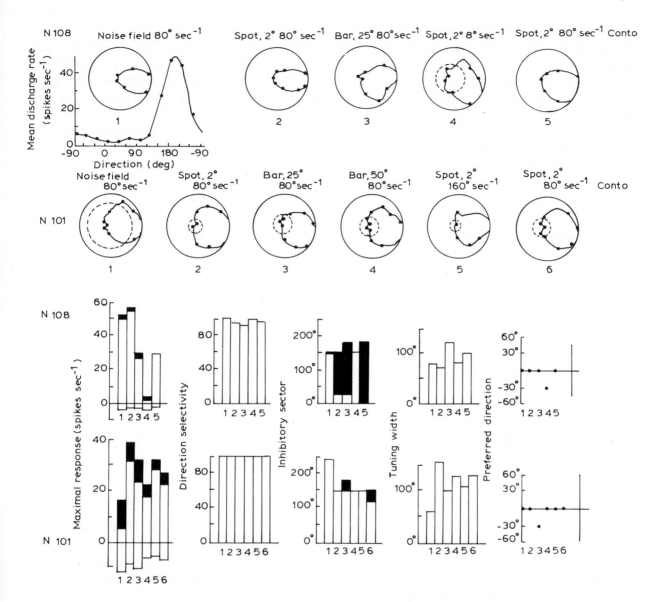

Fig. 2. Direction tuning characteristics as a function of stimulus parameters, exemplified in two AEV neurons. Upper half of the figure: direction tuning curves obtained with the stimulus indicated on top of each curve. In the diagram, upper left, the tuning curve is shown in both polar and cartesian coordinates. The dashed line corresponds to the average level of the SA. Each point in the polar diagrams represents the normalized response to motion in the corresponding direction, with the centre and perimeter of the circle representing minimal and maximal responses, respectively. The columns in the diagrams in the lower half of the figure were obtained from the direction tuning curves above. The number below each bar indicates the corresponding tuning curve above. *Maximal responses* are illustrated as the difference between maximal and minimal discharge rates (total upward bar height), and as the maximal discharge rate minus the SA (empty upward bar height), while the SA is represented in downward bars. The shaded areas indicate the degree of inhibition of the SA with movements in the least effective direction. The DS, inhibitory sector and tuning width are defined in the text. *Preferred directions:* differences in degrees from the preferred direction obtained with spot motion at 80°/sec. Vertical bars indicate the tuning width of the respective neuron, as obtained with spot stimulation.

four percent of the cells were recorded in the upper bank, and 76% of them in the lower bank of the sulcus.

A variety of visual stimuli were employed: squares (0.6 – 40° in width), round spots (2 – 4° in diameter), bars (7 – 60° in length and 1 – 8° in width), contrast edges, dark and light angles, crosses or stars, and also large fields of visual noise. These stimuli were moved across the visual field of the eye contralaterally to the recording site. A stimulus was considered to be effective if the neuronal response elicited was more than twice the resting, spontaneous discharge. With this criterion, each of the stimuli listed above was effective in at least some AEV neurons. Spots and squares were effective in all of the 208 neurons, bars over 25° in length were effective in only 29 of 42 neurons, and large fields of visual noise were effective in 61 of 93 neurons tested.

Stationary light stimulation, i.e., light squares 1.5 – 80° in width, flashed on and off over various parts of the receptive fields, was studied too. Of the 66 neurons tested, 32 reponded to stationary presentation of the light while 34 were insensitive to this type of stimulation.

Response latencies were generally rather short, ranging between 46 and 60 msec for both moving and stationary stimulation.

Direction tuning of the responses

Direction tuning curves were obtained for 53 neurons. Twelve different directions 30° apart were tested, and the mean discharge rate was calculated from 5 sweeps in each direction. The stimulus speed was usually 80°/sec, but could be varied from 8 to 160°/sec.

The tuning width was defined as the range of directions over which responses were at least half of the maximal response. The average was 96° and the values ranged between 38 and 170°.

The directional selectivity (DS) was quantified by the following index: DS $= 100 - (B/A \times 100)$ where A is the response above the spontaneous activity (SA) level in the preferred direction, and B is the response in the opposite direction.

Of 51 neurons tested, 37 displayed DS values above 90, and only 3 neurons had DS values below 50. Inhibition of the SA in the least preferred direction was a characteristic feature of 38 (75%) neurons.

The inhibitory sector, that set of directions producing inhibition of neuronal activity to values of less than the SA, ranged between 30 and 270°.

In 38 neurons, we investigated to what extent the direction tuning could be altered by changes in the stimulus parameters (Fig. 2). For 63 neurons, the DS was determined as a function of speed by comparing the responses in the preferred and opposite directions.

The maximal response, i.e., the maximal firing rate of the neurons in response to stimulus presentation, changed greatly upon different types of stimulation. Most neurons decreased their discharge rate when spot stimulation was replaced by noise fields or bars. Responses were enhanced upon increase of the speeds of the moving stimuli.

The DS values were not significantly affected upon change of the type of light stimulus used. The tuning width was also fairly independent of the stimulus used, although spot stimulation regularly yielded narrower direction tuning than noise stimulation. Noise fields systematically increased the inhibitory sectors.

Changes in the preferred direction were considered significant only if they were greater than the tuning width. In the 67 measurements listed in Table 1, 63 yielded no change at all in preferred direction.

In summary, whereas the maximal response and the extent of the inhibitory sector were dependent on the stimulus configuration, the DS and preferred direction were not greatly influenced by differing stimulus parameters.

Velocity sensitivity of cell responses

The velocity tuning, DS and direction tuning were studied as functions of the stimulus velocity. Spot stimulation was used as a stimulus in these experiments.

Velocity tuning to spot movements was evaluated in a total of 67 neurons. The effect of doubling the speed of the stimulus between 20 and 2560°/sec was listed. Mean discharge rates were calculated as counts per response duration, taking into account only the length of time that the response to the stimulus covered. All neurons tested responded vigorously to very high velocities. Stimulus speeds of 320 and 640°/sec elicited maximal response in 38 neurons (Fig. 3), whereas none of the cells tested at 20 and 40°/sec preferred such low speeds (Fig. 4). Although not all neurons had their maximal responses at the highest velocity tested, they all responded to visual events as short as 31 msec (2560°/sec).

In 23 neurons, the velocity tuning was determined with static broad band (2 – 20°) random binary noise fields. These stimuli extended beyond the receptive field borders at the end-positions, too. Noise motion tended to elicit maximal responses at lower speeds than spot motion (Fig. 3). Thus, of 23 neurons tested with noise, 16 preferred stimulus speeds between 80 and 320°/sec.

The DS was studied in 64 neurons. The high DS remained substantially unchanged over a wide range of velocities. DS was obvious even at a stimulus speed of 2560°/sec (Fig. 5). At very high speeds, however, there was a tendency for the DS values to diminish. In 45 neurons, the DS maximum occurred at the same velocity at which the discharge frequency was maximal; in 15 neurons, the DS was maximal at lower speed, and in only 3

TABLE 1

Effects of changes in stimulus configuration on different response characteristics of AEV neurons

Parameter compared	S → N (n = 22)	S → B (n = 24)	B → N (n = 17)	S → B → N (n = 17)	80 → 160°/sec (n = 11)
Maximal response	0 = 9 d = 9 i = 4	n = 11 d = 11 i = 2	0 = 9 d = 5 i = 3	0 = 3	0 = 5 d = 0 i = 6
Direction selectivity	0 = 18 d = 1 i = 3	0 = 17 d = 3 i = 4	0 = 15 d = 0 i = 2	0 = 12	0 = 11 d = 0 i = 0
Inhibitory sector	0 = 6 d = 5 i = 11	0 = 9 d = 6 i = 9	0 = 6 d = 4 i = 7	0 = 2	0 = 6 d = 0 i = 5
Tuning width	0 = 15 d = 4 i = 3	0 = 17 d = 7 i = 0	0 = 8 d = 3 i = 6	0 = 7	0 = 9 d = 1 i = 1
Preferred direction	0 = 20 c = 2	0 = 22 c = 2	0 = 14 c = 3	0 = 14	0 = 11 c = 0

Abbreviations: n = total number of neurons tested; S = spot or square; N = noise field; B = bar; d = decrease; i = increase; 0 = no change; c = change in either direction (as defined in text). The numbers represent neurons that were affected by the changes of the stimulus parameters indicated at the top of each column. Spots, squares, noise fields and bars were moved in the same direction and with the same amplitude for any given neuron. The stimulus velocity was 80°/sec, except in the last column where differences between 80°/sec and 160°/sec are presented.

neurons was the maximal value of DS at speeds higher than those of the respective discharge rates.

No definite changes could be found in the direction tuning curves upon change of the stimulus velocity (Table 1).

Receptive fields and the effect of small amplitude stimulation

Many AEV neurons responded clearly to spot motion when the usual 80° amplitude was substantially reduced. This allowed the drawing of receptive

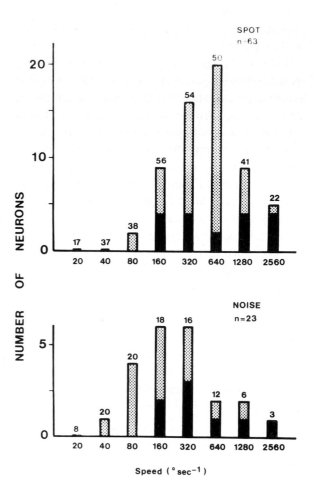

Fig. 4. Number of neurons with maximal response at different speeds indicated. Neurons were tested with spot ($n = 63$) and noise ($n = 23$) at 80° sweep amplitudes. The number above each column indicates the total number of neurons tested. The maximal response was determined by comparing the mean discharge rates calculated from the counts per response duration. Black columns indicate neurons that were not investigated at higher speeds.

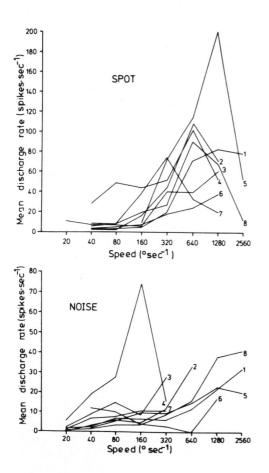

Fig. 3. Speed response curves for spot and noise stimuli for 8 different neurons tested with both stimuli (1–8). Mean discharge rates were calculated from counts per response duration from PSTHs obtained from 20 succesive sweeps at each of the different speeds tested.

field borders on the one hand, and the determination of the response characteristics to small amplitude versus large amplitude stimulation on the other.

Receptive field borders were determined repeatedly. As we reported earlier, the receptive fields were large: 20–40° in diameter. They consistently included area centralis and extended into the ipsilateral hemifield.

Small amplitude stimulation resulted in clear responses of the neurons, albeit with different intensities. A centre of the receptive field could be determined where small amplitude stimulation yielded the most intensive response, while stimulation at the peripheral parts of the receptive field elicited smaller responses. Habituation of the neuronal responses was a characteristic feature observed on repetitive stimulation. No change in the preferred direction was seen at small amplitude stimulation in different parts of the receptive field (Fig. 6).

The effect of stationary presentation of a light stimulus on AEV neurons

Light squares 1.5 to 80° in width were flashed on and off over various parts of the receptive fields. Of 66 neurons tested, 32 responded to at least one of the squares applied. Both on and off stimula-

tion were affected in most of the neurons. Maximal responses typically were obtained in the receptive field centre in concert with the effect of small amplitude stimulation (Fig. 6). The mean discharge rates elicited by on and off stimulation were 54 and 76 Hz, respectively.

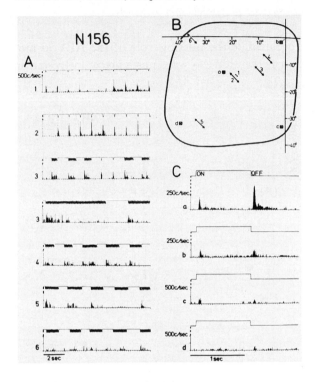

Fig. 6. Responses to small amplitude stimulation (A) and on-off stimulation (C) in different parts of the receptive field (B) of neuron 156 (contralateral eye stimulation). The centre of the coordinate system in B corresponds to the left area centralis, and the abscissa and ordinate represent the horizontal and vertical meridia, respectively. The moving stimuli in A and B were light spots 1.6° in diameter and swept at a speed of 500°/sec (A2 – 6) through parts of the receptive field. For stationary stimuli, a light square measuring 1.5 × 1.5° was turned on and off at 1-sec intervals. Arrows 1 – 6 in B indicate the position, amplitude and direction of the stimulus sweeps yielding the corresponding PSTHs in A. Squares a – d in B represent the position of the stationary stimulus and refer to the respective PSTHs in C. The analog signal above each histogram represents the stimulus movements (A) and the opening and closing of the shutter for on-off stimulation (C), respectively. PSTHs in A show neuronal responses to single stimulus sweeps. Note, however, that trains of forward/backward stimulus movements were also applied. The PSTHs in C give summed responses obtained from 20 successive stimulus presentations.

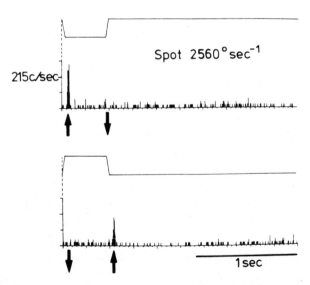

Fig. 5. Responses of an AEV neuron to spot motion at 2560°/sec. PSTHs were obtained from 20 successive stimulus sweeps. The upper traces represent the analog signal of the stimulus motion. c/sec = counts per second. The falling and rising parts of the trapezoid function indicate movement in the preferred and in the opposite directions, respectively. During the plateau phase and after the completion of the sweep, the stimulus was static and outside the receptive field in either end-position.

252

On increase of the size of the square-stimulus presented, the response duration decreased and the response intensity increased in 20 of the 26 neurons studied. An example is given in Fig. 7.

Responses to simultaneous presentation of moving spots and textured backgrounds

To elucidate the possible role of the AEV in motion perception we were particularly interested in

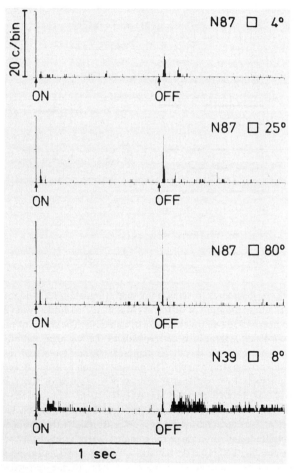

Fig. 7. Responses to on-off stimulation in 2 AEV neurons, N 87 (traces 1 – 3) and N 39 (trace 4). Each PSTH is composed of 20 successive stimulus presentations (1 sec on, 1 sec off). Traces 1 – 3 illustrate the effects of increasing the size of the light square from 4 to 80°, while trace 4 illustrates the inhibition and postinhibitory increase in discharge rate following the first response.

the interaction between small objects (round light spots 1.5 – 3° in diameter) and structured backgrounds (visual noise).

Of 36 neurons tested for the effect of a stationary noise background on the response to a moving spot, 13 showed a decrease of 17 – 58%, 11 showed an increase of 22 – 58%, and 12 neurons showed a change that was less than 10% of their spot response when the noise background was replaced by a homogeneous field of the same mean luminance.

Of 31 neurons in which the effect of a spot crossing a stationary noise-field was compared with spot-noise in-phase motion, 20 decreased their response by 14 – 90%, while 8 increased their response by 18 – 85%. In 3 neurons, the change was less than 12% when the noise background was moved in-phase with the spot.

Of 7 neurons tested with anti-phase motion, 5 decreased their response by 14 – 56%, and 2 neurons increased their response by 18 and 34%, respectively, compared to the spot motion at the same absolute velocity across a stationary background.

The algebraic sum of the spot response and the noise response in the corresponding directions was insufficient to predict the in-phase and anti-phase effect in all cases (Fig. 8).

In conclusion, the transformation of the simultaneously occurring motion of a small spot and a visual texture, two distinct visual stimuli, into an input signal by the AEV cells is characteristically non-linear, and differs among individual cells while it uniformly tends to preserve the high DS.

Electrical stimulation in SC and LS

The effect of electrical stimulation of the LS and/or SC was tested on 33 neurons. Orthodromic excitation of the AEV cells after LS stimulation was found after a latency of 2 – 4 msec. Orthodromic discharges were elicited by SC stimulation after slightly longer latencies than in the case of LS stimulation. Occasionally, the orthodromic response latencies to both SC and LS stimulation were roughly the same (neuron N 90, Fig. 9). Some responses followed SC stimulation after short, very constant latencies (Fig. 9), and frequently they were able to follow trains of at least 4 stimuli at 200 Hz. Such responses were probably elicited antidromically via the dense and direct projection from the AEV onto the SC demonstrated anatomically (Tortelly et al. 1980; Norita et al.

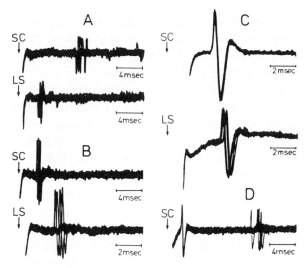

Fig. 9. Response of 4 AEV neurons (A–D) to electrical stimulation of the superior colliculus (SC) and the lateral suprasylvian visual area (LS). Each trace consists of 5 superimposed sweeps. Arrows indicate the time of electrical stimulation.

1986). A definite orthodromic response sometimes followed this antidromic one after a longer latency (Fig. 9).

Discussion

Our results confirmed the physiological properties described in the original reports (Mucke et al. 1982; Olson and Graybiel 1983). The main finding of this study seems to be the rather broad range of shapes, sizes and velocities of the stimuli that elicit excitation in AEV cells. Of these, the sensitivity of the AEV cells to visual noise is of considerable importance. Noise-sensitive cells have also been found in A 17/18 (Hammond and McKay 1977), in the superficial layers of the SC (Mason 1979) and in the striate-recipient part of the LP-pulvinar complex (Mason 1978). The LS is reportedly insensitive to noise; only a textured background was capable of changing the response of the neurons to structured stimuli (Von Grünau and Frost 1983).

Another peculiar feature of the AEV cells is their very high DS. The proportion of direction-selective cells is higher in the AEV than in any

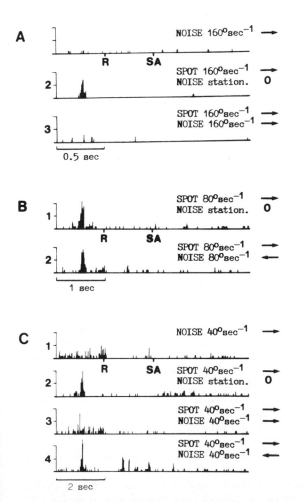

Fig. 8. Effects of spot and noise motion on the response of an AEV neuron (N 43). Each PSTH was obtained from 20 successive sweeps. R indicates the point of direction reversal, and SA the termination of the stimulus sweep. The SA was recorded with the stimuli in end-positions and visible. Spots were 3° in diameter and of 150 cd/m² luminance. Noise fields covered the receptive field of the neuron when stationary and also when moving, and had 5–10 cd/m² mean luminance. The spot remained within the noise field at all times.

other feline visual area (Godfraind et al. 1972; Camarda and Rizzollatti 1976; Mason 1978, 1981; Schoppmann and Hoffman 1979; Spear and Baumann 1979; Hicks et al. 1984).

Another striking finding of our study is that, although the response intensity is a function of the shape, size and velocity of the stimuli, other response characteristics of the AEV cells seem rather independent of these parameters. Thus, the preferred direction, direction tuning width and DS appear to be constant, irrespective of the kind of stimulation. This finding supports the notion expressed in our first paper (Mucke et al. 1982) that the AEV might take part in motion detection. This seems to be a general sensitivity towards moving objects in a rather large receptive field. Our findings also show that the quality of the background may influence the response of the cells. This suggests a rather elaborate mechanism, which may take part both in the orientation reaction of animals towards moving objects and in the adjustment of eye and body movements according to the environmental stimuli. The role of the AEV in orienting movement is supported by its sensitivity to small flashing spots, or to the on or off effect of stationary light stimuli.

This notion is further supported by the high velocity sensitivity of AEV cells, which is accompanied by a high DS. The velocity sensitivity is higher than in any other visual area. It has preferred velocities in a much higher range than the velocity domain where cats are capable of velocity discrimination (Vanderbussche et al. 1986). The high DS permits a distinction between objects moving along the same path but in opposite directions.

The anatomical connections described earlier (Norita et al. 1986) and which are supported by electrical stimulation data, provide further support for the notion of AEV acting as a system for detecting motion. The area appears to collect visual information from the LS area and the visual extrageniculate thalamus, both areas known for their sensitivity towards stimuli moving at high speed and having high DS, and provides a heavy output

to the LS and SC. This raises the possibility of a highly developed processing system in which both upstream and downstream information may flow. The output of the AEV towards the frontal eye fields and the limbic system provides further evidence for the participation of AEV in eye movements and in limbic functions.

Acknowledgement

G. Benedek was a recipient of an Alexander von Humboldt Followship.

References

Camarda, R. and Rizzolati, G. (1976) Visual receptive fields in the lateral suprasylvian area (Clare-Bishop area) of the cat. *Brain Res.*, 101: 427–443.

Godfraind, J.M., Meulders, M. and Veraart, C. (1972) Visual properties of neurons in pulvinar, nucleus lateralis posterior and nucleus suprageniculatus thalami in the cat. I. Qualitative investigation. *Brain Res.*, 44: 503–526.

Guldin, W.O. and Markowitsch, H.J. (1984) Cortical and thalamic afferent connections of the insular and adjacent cortex of the cat. *J. Comp. Neurol.*, 229: 393–418.

Hammond, P. and MacKay, D.M. (1981) Modulatory influences of moving textured backgrounds on responsiveness of simple cells in feline striate cortex. *J. Physiol.*, 319: 431–442.

Hicks, T.P., Watanabe, S., Miyake, A. and Shoumura, K. (1984) Organization and properties of visually responsive neurons in the suprageniculate nucleus of the cat. *Exp. Brain Res.*, 55: 359–367.

Higo, S. and Kawamura, S. (1984) Topographical linkage of tecto-thalamo-anterior ectosylvian sulcal cortex in the cat: an ^{125}I-WGA autoradiographic study. *Brain Res. Bull.*, 12: 647–655.

Mason, R. (1978) Functional organization in the cat's pulvinar complex. *Exp. Brain Res.*, 31: 51–66.

Mason, R. (1979) Responsiveness of cells in the cat's superior colliculus to textured visual stimuli. *Exp. Brain Res.*, 37: 231–240.

Mason, R. (1981) Differential responsiveness of cells in the visual zones of the cat's LP pulvinar complex to visual stimuli. *Exp. Brain Res.*, 43: 25–33.

Miceli, D., Reperant, J. and Ptito, M. (1985) Intracortical connections of the anterior ectosylvian and lateral suprasylvian visual areas in the cat. *Brain Res.*, 347: 291–298.

Mucke, L., Norita, M., Benedek, G. and Creutzfeldt, O.D. (1982) Physiologic and anatomic investigation of a visual cortical area situated in the ventral bank of the anterior ectosylvian sulcus of the cat. *Exp. Brain Res.*, 46: 1 – 11.

Norita, M., Mucke, L., Benedek, G. Albowitz, B., Katoh, Y. and Creutzfeldt, O.D. (1986) Connections of the anterior ectosylvian visual area (AEV). *Exp. Brain Res.*, 62: 225 – 240.

Olson, C.R. and Graybiel, A.M. (1983) An outlying visual area in the cerebral cortex of the cat. *Progr. Brain Res.*, 58: 239 – 245.

Olson, C.R. and Graybiel, A.M. (1987) Ectosylvian visual area of the cat: location, retinotopic organization and connections. *J. Comp. Neurol.*, 261: 277 – 294.

Ptito, M., Tassinari, G. and Antonini, A. (1987) Electrophysiological evidence for interhemispheric connections in the anterior ectosylvian sulcus in the cat. *Exp. Brain Res.*, 66: 90 – 98.

Schoppman, A. and Hoffmann, K.P. (1979) A comparison of visual response in two pretectal nuclei and in the superior colliculus of the cat. *Exp. Brain Res.*, 35: 495 – 510.

Spear, P.D. and Baumann, T.P. (1975) Receptive field characteristics of single neurons in lateral suprasylvian visual area of the cat. *J. Neurophysiol.*, 38: 1403 – 1420.

Tortelly, A., Reinoso-Suárez, F. and Llamas, A. (1980) Projections from non-visual cortical areas to the superior colliculus demonstrated by retrograde transport of HRP in the cat. *Brain Res.*, 188: 543 – 549.

Vanderbussche, E., Orban, G.A. and Maes, H. (1986) Velocity discrimination in the cat. *Vision Res.*, 26: 1835 – 1849.

Von Grünau, M. and Frost, B.J. (1983) Double-opponent- process mechanism underlying RF-structure of directionally specific cells of cat lateral suprasylvian visual area. *Exp. Brain Res.*, 49: 84 – 92.

T.P. Hicks and G. Benedek (Eds.)
Progress in Brain Research, Vol. 75
© 1988 Elsevier Science Publishers B.V. (Biomedical Division)

CHAPTER 24

AEV-insular axis: connectivity

David Emmans[1], Hans J. Markowitsch[1] and W.O. Guldin[2]

[1] *Department of Psychology, University of Konstanz, P.O. Box 7733, D-7750 Konstanz, F.R.G., and* [2] *Institute of Physiology, Free University, Arnimallee 22, D-1000 Berlin 33, Germany*

Introduction

Comparisons of morphological and functional properties of the insula (or insula Reilii) have been faced with problems of homology as well as of cytological boundaries. Using macroscopical criteria, the structure is well-demarcated in human, catarrhinic and cetacean brains, being covered by the frontal, temporal and parietal opercula within the sylvian fissure (Reil 1809; Marchand 1893; Clark 1896). Ontogenetically, general morphological areas are easily enough distinguished so as to show that different parts of the structure develop at various periods, the sylvian fissure, for example, already appearing in the second embryonic month (Clark 1896), while the opercula are not complete until post partem (Retzius 1902). A similar spread in development can be seen in myeloarchitecture: several areas (13, 20, and 25) begin to develop before birth, but are only complete afterwards, while area 32 does not begin myelination until after this time (Flechsig 1901). These two groups thus correspond to Flechsig's (1901) distinction between intermediary and terminal myeloarchitectural zones and give an a priori indication of a functional role in higher cognitive processing. Thus, in these animals the insula is a readily apparent, morphological unit.

However, although the area can be easily distinguished in such lobular, opercularized brains, there are obvious difficulties in finding homologous structures in other mammals (Marko-witsch and Pritzel 1978). Using the external landmark of the sylvian fissure is possible in gyrified species such as the dog and the cat (although this approach is only an approximation) but it is impossible in lissencephalic animals such as rodents. A different approach makes use of the claustrum (Meynert 1869; Holl 1899; Rose 1928; Brockhaus 1940) and identifies the insula as that part of the cortex overlying the claustrum, i.e. the 'claus-trocortex'. Admittedly, this definition is already problematical in species with clear-cut insular criteria: in humans, for example, the claustro-cortex is more extensive than the smaller insular triangle. Nonetheless, using the definition of insula as claustral cortex, Brodmann (1909) in fact considered the homologous structures in other mammals to be the most constant and obvious structural commonality throughout the whole mammalian line. Following this line of argumentation, the insula would appear as a principally distinguishable structure.

Cytoarchitectonically, however, there has been more cause for debate on cross-species homology (Sanides 1968; Stephan 1975). At the borders of the claustrum the cytoarchitectural extent of the insula becomes problematic (Brockhaus 1940). Nonetheless, Brodmann (1909) subdivided the 'insular main region' into areas 13 to 16, with an anterior granular and a posterior agranular half. However, as in other cytoarchitectural subdivisions, there is still a good deal of controversy as to the number of distinguishable fields belonging to the insula: Brockhaus (1940), for example, found 34, compared to Brodmann's 4. The isocortical parts, especially, have caused the greatest amount of definitional dispute (Brockhaus 1940).

While there is little controversy as to the extent of the primate insula, the above aspects of external morphology and cytoarchitecture become more problematic when considering work on particular species with less gyrification such as the cat.

For felines, an early definition was given by Holl (1899), including the basal part of the gyrus reuniens, the anterior part of the gyrus arcuatus II, the entire gyrus arcuatus I, and the 'trigonum sylvii'. But Winkler and Potter (1914) limited the insula to anterior levels, so that area 14 is within the anterior rhinal sulcus, and areas 14, 15 and 16 are dorsal to area 13. Furthermore, Brodmann did not publish any material on cats, but, because of the similarities between cats and Ursidae, his map of the kinkajou is usually considered as comparable, and shows the insular cortex extending over the sylvian fissure and the ventral part of the anterior sylvian gyrus.

Cytoarchitecturally, there is little information on the cat. Stephan (1975) pointed out that what is typically considered insular consists of allocortical, isocortical and even mesocortical tissue; and Mesulam and Mufson (1982a) re-titled such mixed tissue as paralimbic. While there is general agreement on the posterior insula bordering on area 35 (in the fundus of the rhinal sulcus) and area 36 (on and above its lateral bank), Woolsey (1961) included the anterior sylvian gyrus in the auditory cortex. Furthermore, the anterior border to area 8 in the prefrontal cortex is recognized as being very gradual. In general, there is agreement on an allocortical part in the rhinal and sylvian sulci and a (mainly) isocortical part covering the anterior sylvian gyrus.

A detailed map, in fact the only complete one developed explicitly on the cat cortex, was published by Gurewitsch and Chatschaturian (1928), who distinguished areas 13 (in the sylvian sulcus), 14 (the granular area covering the anteroventral part of the anterior sylvian gyrus), 15 and 16 (in the rhinal sulcus), and area 52 (the external surface of the sylvian gyrus). However, their map has been frequently contradicted on the basis of other studies (Winkler and Potter 1914; Muhs-Clement 1964; Sanides and Hoffmann 1969). Finally, Krettek and Price (1977), who in turn had only extrapolated or adapted Rose's map (1928) of the rabbit and lemur insula for cats, found a large granular field (covering the larger part of the anterior sylvian gyrus), a dorsal agranular field (ventral to the granular insula), a ventral agranular area (in the anterior rhinal sulcus), a posterior agranular area (partly in the rhinal sulcus and the sylvian sulcus), and finally a dorsal agranular area.

Due partly to the difficulty in reaching the surface of the insula at the base of the skull without substantially damaging the overlying opercula, and partly to our lack of knowledge on loss of function after insular lesions, little data are available on the afferents and efferents of the cat's insula (Avanzini et al. 1969; Benevento and Loe, 1975; Cranford et al. 1976). There was good material only on the connections of the posterior thalamus (Heath and Jones, 1971a; Jones and Powell 1971; Graybiel 1972, 1973; Hughes 1980; Updyke 1981). In this work, and in that of others on the rat (Guldin and Markowitsch 1983), the hamster (Reep and Winnans 1982), and on the monkey (Roberts and Akert 1963; Mufson et al. 1981; Mesulam and Mufson 1982a,b; Mufson and Mesulam 1982, 1984), the lateral suprageniculate complex and the medial geniculate nucleus were recognized as contributing afferents.

With the introduction of horseradish peroxidase (HRP), Mufson and Mesulam (1984) found a gradient in the thalamic connectivity of the primate insula: the more anterior parts were found to be connected with medial nuclei of the thalamus (such as the nuclei reuniens, parafascicularis, mediodorsalis, and centralis medialis) the more posterior parts were connected with the suprageniculate, the medial pulvinar and the ventroposterior inferior nucleus. This work basically confirmed the results of Benjamin and Burton (1968), Chow and Pribram (1956), Roberts and Akert (1963), Wirth

(1973), and Burton and Jones (1976).

But compared to other cortical areas, there was still little detailed information on the interconnections of the insula, or its cytoarchitectural parcellation. In recent years, however, the work of Mesulam and Mufson (1982a,b), Reinoso-Suárez (1985), Mucke et al. (1982), Olson and Graybiel (1981, 1983, 1987), and our own laboratory has added considerable detail to our knowledge of the feline and primate insula. In the following, some of our results will be reviewed.

Methods

For the afferents to the cat's insula we examined 12 cats, using unilateral HRP injections into the insula (Guldin and Markowitsch 1984).

In our work on the efferents from the feline insula, we examined 20 cats using unilateral injections of HRP into different regions of the cerebral cortex (Guldin and Markowitsch 1984; Guldin et al. 1986).

With respect to the primate, while investigating the afferents and efferents to the temporal pole and to the lateral premotor cortex, we found efferents from the insula, using in total 4 rhesus and 9 squirrel monkeys, and 11 marmosets, with small injections of HRP used throughout the greater part of the cerebral cortex (Markowitsch et al. 1985, 1987).

Results

Afferents to the cat's insula

With respect to the cat's insula, the strongest thalamo-insular projections were from the suprageniculate and parts of the posterolateral nucleus; projections to the anterior insula also included especially the intralaminar nuclei and the ventromedial posterior nucleus, and those to the posterior insula were from the medial and dorsal parts of the medial geniculate nucleus. The mediodorsal nucleus (MD) projected only to the anterior and most ventral insula. Projections to the anterior sylvian gyrus came from the prefrontal cortex, the inferotemporal region, and from the presylvian, suprasylvian and splenial sulci; the cortico-insular afferents arose mainly from sulcal areas next to the prefrontal, parietal and cingulate cortices, that is, from association cortex adjacents.

The thalamic sources formed a band from the ventromedial nucleus, to the intralaminar nuclei within (and including parts of) the MD, to the lateral dorsal nucleus. In the anterior-posterior direction, the band continued from the posterior MD, to the lateral posterior complex, through the suprageniculate and the posterior nuclei, the magnocellular division of the medial geniculate complex, ending in the dorsal division.

The cortical sources to areas around the anterior sylvian gyrus were distributed throughout the cerebral cortex, excluding only the posterior visual cortex. On the other hand, afferents to within the anterior sylvian gyrus were generally limited to cerebral sulci and to the prefrontal and cingular cortices.

Importantly, cells from the 'anterior ectosylvian visual area' (Olson and Graybiel 1981, 1983, 1987; Mucke et al. 1982) were found projecting to the more anterior parts of the anterior sylvian gyrus and to the orbital region. A large injection into the anterior ectosylvian gyrus (reaching the somatosensory field) revealed a diffuse distribution of cells in the ectosylvian and sylvian gyrus and the medial surface of the cruciate gyrus, with a considerable spread of the cells over the gyri. There were also cells marked in the whole lateral prefrontal fields, especially the proreal and coronal gyri, and in the frontal and cingulate gyri. Injections into the ventral bank of the ectosylvian sulcus revealed labeled cells in the central medial nucleus, the suprageniculate nucleus and in various subnuclei of the posterior complex. A somewhat more anterior injection also marked cells in the principal ventromedial nucleus, while the more posterior injection did so in the magnocellular part of the medial geniculate.

Efferents from the cat insula

For the efferents from the cat insula, after applying 20 small injections along the lateral and medial regions of the cortical hemisphere, all injections revealed labeling in the insula, with the exception of the six injections placed along the lateral gyrus, that is, within the visual cortex. Thus most parts of the cat's cerebral cortex (including prefrontal, parietal, temporal and cingulate regions) are well reached. We found absolutely no evidence for monosynaptic interconnections between the insula and occipital areas 17 or 18.

Insular labeling was typically less intense and originated in fewer areas than that from the adjacent claustrum. Similarly, the topographical organization of these insular efferents was also less stringent than that from the claustrum, thus indicating a functional (and probably also different ontogenetic) role for the two structures, and thereby somewhat making relative the importance of either structure in homologous definitions of the other. Interestingly, the efferent connections from the insula were quite similar to those originating in the prefrontal cortex. Our results basically confirmed and extended those of Cranford et al. (1976).

In detail, the efferents from the cat's insula included:

(1) a major projection to the medial frontal cortex (including the gyrus rectus, infralimbic area 25, and the anterior cingular and posterior cruciate gyrus). The connection was to bilateral parts of the insula after the injections in the infralimbic, cingular and cruciate sites;

(2) a major ipsilateral and minor contralateral connection with areas adjacent to the claustro-cortex;

(3) a moderate projection to the suprasylvian sulcus with a clear anterior-posterior gradient and only slight contralateral labeling. The projections thus reached areas 5, 7 and 22 (covering the Clare-Bishop area), and area 20;

(4) a moderate bilateral projection to the coronal sulcus and a minor, unilateral one to the middle of area 36;

(5) very sparse projections to the splenial gyrus (areas 18 and 30), to the border between areas 2 and 53, and to the dorsal end of the anterior sylvian sulcus in area 50, and the ventral part of area 4, all with but few contralateral, labeled cells;

(6) and, finally, no labeled cells whatever from any of the four injections along the lateral sulcus in areas 17 and 18, or from the two injections in area 21 or the occipital pole (area 20).

From these results a very tentative overview of the cat's insular-cortical efferents can be advanced:

The anterior dorsal area, belonging to the allocortex, projects to (1) the peri-auditory association belt region (Heath and Jones 1971a,b); (2) the suprasylvian sulcal area; (3) the prefrontal cortex; (4) the cingulate and claustral areas; and (5) the auditory and sensory-motor areas.

The ventral and posterior areas, likewise allocortical tissue, project to supragenual, infralimbic cortex. The allocortical dorsal rhinal and sylvian areas project to the supplementary motor area ($6a\beta$), as does the allocortical posterior rhinal area. Finally, the isocortical dorsal area, extending from the upper rhinal sulcus to the ectosylvian and orbital sulci, projects to the supplementary motor area as well.

Efferents from the monkey insula

For the efferents in monkeys we found (1) an insulo-temporal, and (2) an insulo-premotor cortical projection. With regard to the temporal targets, the earlier finding by Mesulam and Mufson (1982) of a major connection from the insula to the temporal pole in macaques was confirmed and extended by our finding of a major connection to the temporal pole in the rhesus monkeys, a major one in squirrel monkeys, and only a minor one in marmosets. Only in the rhesus monkey was a very minor contralateral connection observed. With regard to the premotor projection a major number of afferents from the insula to the lateral premotor cortex was found in four of six squirrel monkeys. The ipsilateral connection was major, moderate or minor, while the contralateral connection was minor. This is similar to the results published by Sanides (1968) using staining techniques for anterograde degeneration.

Discussion

There are differences as well as similarities between the different species we have examined so far for insular connectivity. Comparing the present findings with those we found on the rat (Guldin and Markowitsch, 1983) and those of Saper (1982), the cat would appear to take on an intermediate position between the rat and the monkey in the degree of insular connectivity: the rat possesses but minor insular connections with somatosensory, motor, and parietal areas, and stronger ones to infralimbic, cingulate and prefrontal cortices. In the monkey, the efferents to parietal and temporal association and sensory areas become more important. As mentioned above, the size of the isocortical region increases with increasing encephalization (see Brodmann (1909); Krieg (1946), for the

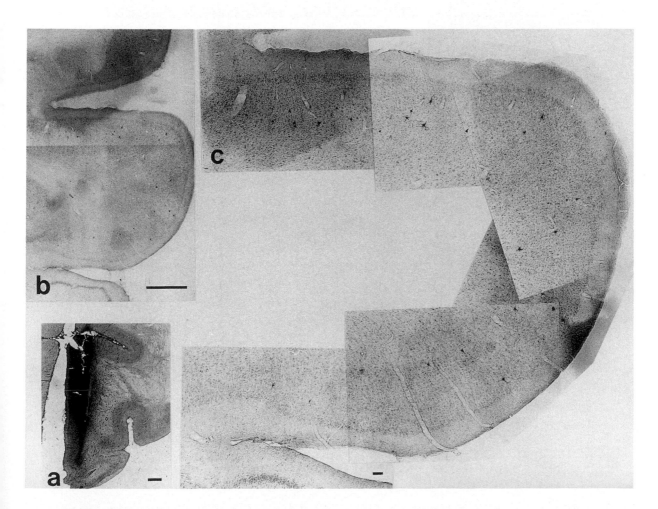

Fig. 1. Labeled cells in the cat's insular cortex after an injection of HRP into the medial prefrontal cortex. (a) Coronal section through the center of the injection locus; scale bar = 1 mm. (b) Coronal section through the area of the anterior ectosylvian cortex where the labeled cells magnified in c were found; scale bar = 1 mm. (c) Labeled cells from b under higher magnification; scale bar = 100 μm.

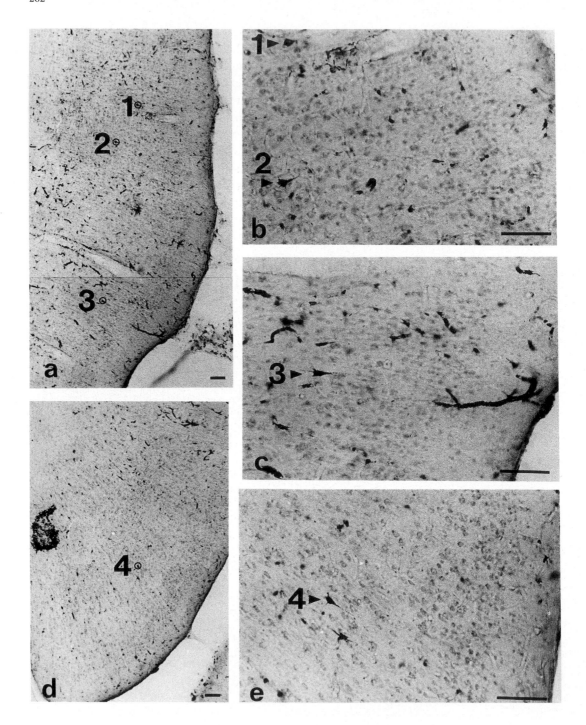

Fig. 2. Labeled cells in the insular cortex of the rhesus monkey after an injection of HRP into the temporopolar area. (a) Coronal section through the insula (upper area 13); scale bar = 100 μm (b) and (c). Cells shown in (a) under higher magnification; scale bar = 10 μm. (d) Coronal section in insular region; scale bar = 100 μm. (e) Cell shown in (d), under higher magnification; scale bar = 100 μm.

rat; Krettek and Price (1977), for the cat; Mesulam and Mufson (1982a), for the macaque; and Brockhaus (1940), for humans).

On the other hand, all three species share the tendency for anterior insular regions to be connected with orbital and infralimbic cortex while posterior regions project preferentially to cingular, parietal and sensory areas of the cerebral cortex. In all species there is a strong similarity in the connectivity patterns and the cytoarchitecture of both in-

sular and prefrontal cortices, although they differ in that the insula has direct afferents from thalamic sensory association nuclei.

The pattern of connectivity to and from the insula is certainly so highly variable that a similarly broad functional distribution would be expected, as is already indicated by the large number of sensory stimuli that can evoke electrophysiological responses in the insula: auditory, somatosensory, visual, olfactory and visceral (Loe and Benevento

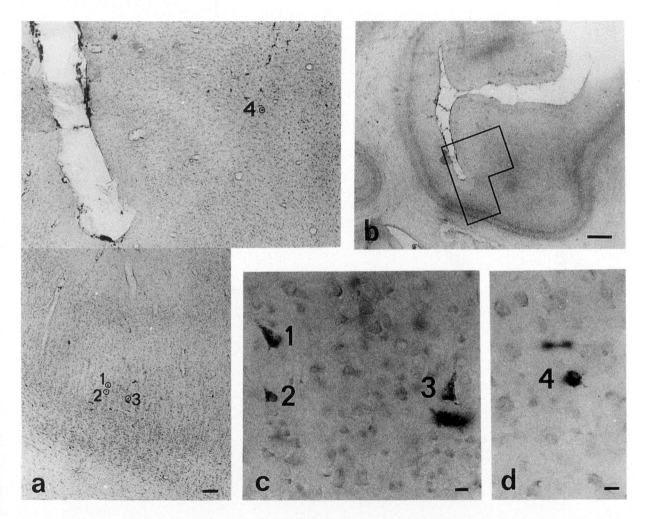

Fig. 3. Labeled cells of posterior insular cortex of rhesus monkey after an injection of HRP into the temporal pole. (a) Coronal section; scale bar = 100 μm. (b) Coronal section with inset marking the region magnified in (a); scale bar = 500 μm. The orientation of microphotograph (b) shows the ventral portion of the cortex at the left of the picture and the medial portion at the bottom. (c) Coronal section reproducing the cells shown in (a) under higher magnification; scale bar = 10 μm. (d) Coronal section, showing cell from (a) under higher magnification; scale bar = 10 μm.

1969; see also Kaada et al. 1949, for further responses).

Specific visual functions: if, as we assume (Markowitsch et al. 1985), the temporal pole is a limbic integrating cortex for complex, preprocessed visual (from area 20 and 21) and auditory (from area 22) information, then the major connection from the insula is a possible preliminary indication of prior modality-oriented processing in the insula. The large size of the insular-temporal projection

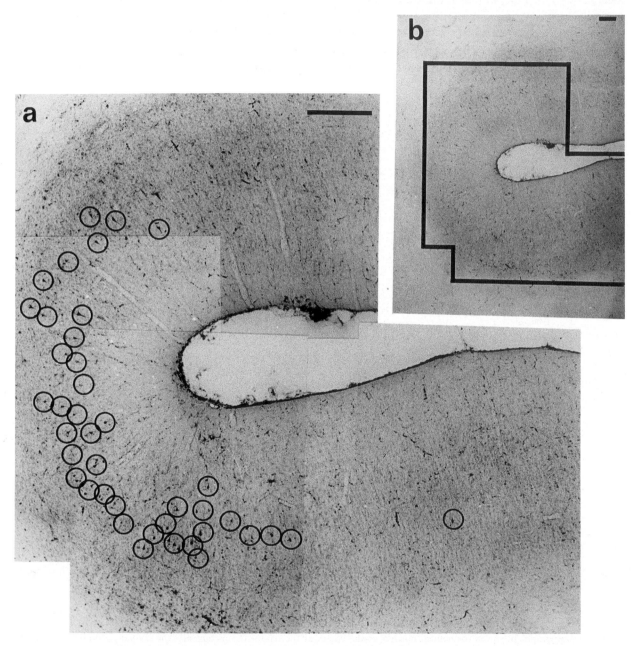

Fig. 4. Labeled neurons (encircled in a) in the insular cortex of a rhesus monkey following an injection of HRP in the ipsilateral temporopolar cortex; the area magnified in (a) is outlined in (b); scale bars = 500 μm.

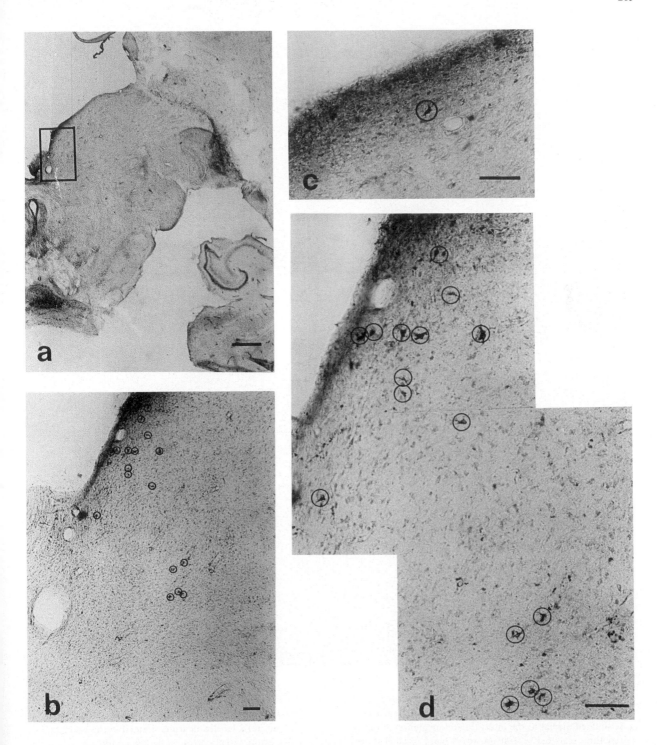

Fig. 5. Labeled cells in the nucleus pulvinaris of the thalamus after an injection of HRP into the temporopolar cortex. (a) Coronal section through the posterior thalamus; the insert marks the area magnified in (b); scale bar = 1 mm; (b) Labeled cells (encircled) in the pulvinar nucleus; scale = 100 μm; (c, d). The labeled cells from (b) under higher magnification; scale bars = 100 μm.

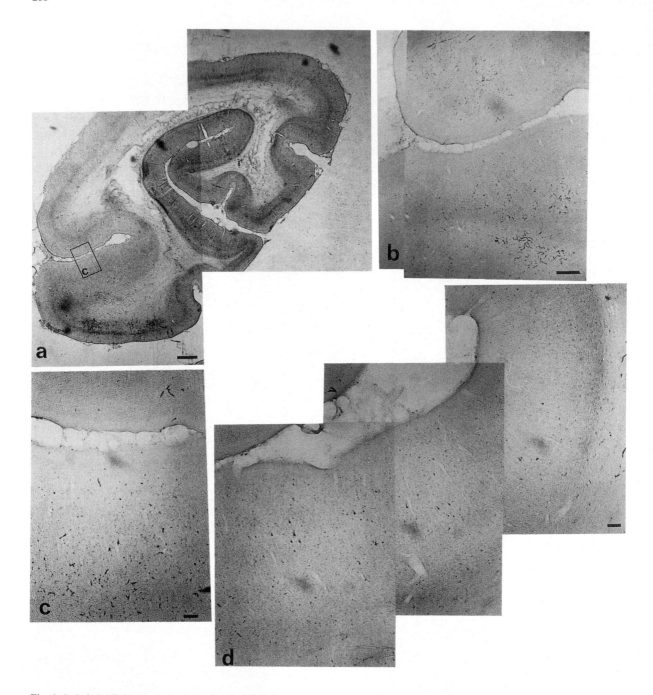

Fig. 6. Labeled cells in the squirrel monkey's occipital cortex following an injection of HRP into the lateral premotor cortex. (a) Coronal section through the occipital cortex; the insert marks the area magnified in (c); scale bar = 1 mm. (b) Magnification of the area situated medial to the insert (c) and magnified in (d); scale bar = 100 μm. (c) 2 labeled neurons situated in the lower half of the picture; scale bar = 100 μm. (d) A band of labeled neurons in layer III of the visual cortex; scale bar = 100 μm.

would indicate that these efferents from the insula are not the vestigial rest of a transitory neonatal projection. Nor would such a large connection fit a mere activating role of one 'pre-processing unit' on the subsequent stage (which might explain the surprising, very minor projection that we found between occipital area 17 and the temporal pole: see Markowitsch et al. 1987). On the contrary, an important role in the joint visual and auditory functions of the temporal pole could reasonably be expected to be mediated through the strong insular afferents. Similarly, the fact that premotor cells respond to visual signals (Wiesendanger et al. 1985; Kurata and Tanji 1986) can be partly explained by the significant occipital-premotor innervation that we found (Markowitsch et al. 1987), and would not necessitate the insular connection; but the involvement of the premotor area in multimodal integrative functions (Gemba et al. 1981; Weinrich and Wise 1982; Godschalk et al. 1985; Halsband and Passingham 1985; Kurata and Tanji 1985; Wiesendanger et al. 1985) makes a prior stage of sensory pooling likely which may be similar to that for the temporal pole: again a limbic intermediate stage for joint-input pooling. In fact we found several other limbic system-related structures with afferent input to the premotor area, an indication of the stage of pre-processing likely to be found in the insular input, including visual-related material. Thus, for both the temporal pole and the premotor cortex, there is a substantial direct input from geniculate visual sources as well as a substantial input from extrageniculate ones, namely the insula. Whether the insular function is, however, the same for the two target sites could well be tested for by simultaneous bilocal single cell recording.

Some degree of functional parallelism or even identity for the insula with respect to these two target sites is perhaps indicated by the fact that our results on the insulo-temporal projection confirm a classification made by Mesulam and Mufson (1982a): based on similarities in cytoarchitecture the lateral orbito-frontal cortex, the temporal polar cortex and the insula constitute a family of related paralimbic structures, while the retrosplenial, cingulate and parahippocampal regions constitute another.

Furthermore, the connections between the insula and the temporal pole and the lateral premotor region again corroborate the frequent finding that adjacent areas have similar connections as well as strong interconnections with each other (Jones and Powell 1970).

References

Avanzini, G., Manzia, D. and Pelliccioli, G. (1969) Ascending and descending connections of the insular cortex of the cat. *Arch. Ital. Biol.*, 107: 696–714.

Benevento, L.A. and Loe, P.R. (1975) An intracellular study of thalamocortical synapses in the orbitoinsular cortex. *Exp. Neurol.*, 46: 634–643.

Benjamin, R.M. and Burton, H. (1968) Projection of taste nerve afferents to anterior opercular-insular cortex in squirrel monkey *(Saimiri sciureus). Brain Res.*, 7: 221–231.

Brockhaus, H. (1940) Die Cyto- und Myeloarchitektur des Cortex claustralis und des Claustrum beim Menschen. *J. Psychol. Neurol. (Leipzig)*, 49: 249–348.

Brodmann, K. (1909) *Vergleichende Lokalisationslehre der Grosshirnrinde in ihren Prinzipien dargestellt auf Grund des Zellbaues*, Barth, Leipzig.

Burton, H. and Jones, E.B. (1976) The posterior thalamic region and its cortical projections in the new world and old world monkeys. *J. Comp. Neurol.*, 168: 249–302.

Clark, T.E. (1896) The comparative anatomy of the insula. *J. Comp. Neurol.*, 6: 59–100.

Cranford, J.L., Laderer, S.J., Campbell, C.B.G. and Neff, W.D. (1976) Efferent projections of the insular and temporal neocortex of the cat. *Brain Res.*, 117: 195–210.

Chow, K.L. and Pribram, K.H. (1956) Cortical projections of the thalamic ventrolateral nuclear group in monkeys. *J. Comp. Neurol.*, 104: 57–75.

Flechsig, P. (1901) Developmental (myelogenetic) localization of the cerebral cortex in the human subject. *Lancet*, i: 1027–1029.

Gemba, H., Hashimoto, S. and Sasaki, K. (1981) Cortical field potentials preceding visually initiated hand movements in the monkey. *Exp. Brain Res.*, 42: 435–441.

Godschalk, M., Lemon, R.N., Kuypers, H.G.J.M. and Van der Steen, J. (1985) The involvement of monkey premotor cortex neurones in preparation of visually cued arm movements. *Behav. Brain Res.*, 18: 143–157.

Graybiel, A.M. (1972) Some ascending connections of the pulvinar and nucleus lateralis posterior of the thalamus in the cat. *Brain Res.*, 44: 99–125.

Graybiel, A.M. (1973) The thalamo-cortical projection of the so-called posterior nuclear group: a study with anterograde degeneration methods in the cat. *Brain Res.*, 49: 229–244.

Guldin, W.O. and Markowitsch, H.J. (1983) Cortical and thalamic afferent connections of the insular and adjacent cortex of the rat. *J. Comp. Neurol.*, 215: 135–153.

Guldin, W.D. and Markowitsch, H.J. (1984) Cortical and thalamic afferent connections of the insular and adjacent cortex of the cat. *J. Comp. Neurol.*, 229: 393–418.

Guldin, W.O., Markowitsch, H.J., Lampe, R. and Irle, E. (1986) Cortical projections originating from the cat's insular area and remarks on claustrocortical connections. *J. Comp. Neurol.*, 243: 468–487.

Gurewitsch, M. and Chatschaturian, A. (1928) Zur Cytoarchitectonik der Grosshirnrinde der Feliden. *Z. Ges. Anat. I*, 87: 100–138.

Halsband, U. and Passingham, R. (1985) The role of premotor and parietal cortex in the direction of action. *Brain Res.*, 240: 269–277.

Hassler, R. and Muhs-Clement, K. (1964) Architektonischer Aufbau des somatosensorischen und parietalen Cortex der Katze. *J. Hirnforsch.*, 6: 377–420.

Heath, C. and Jones, E.G. (1971a) An experimental study of ascending projections from the posterior group of thalamic nuclei in the cat. *J. Comp. Neurol.*, 141: 397–426.

Heath, C. and Jones, E.G. (1971b) The anatomical organization of the suprasylvian gyrus of the cat. *Ergeb. Anat. Entwichlungsgesch.*, 45: 1–64.

Holl, M. (1899) Ueber die Insel des Carnivorengehirnes. *Arch. Anat. Physiol. Anat. Abt.*, 217–266.

Hughes, H.C. (1980) Efferent organization of the cat pulvinar complex with a note on bilateral claustrocortical and reticulo-cortical connections. *J. Comp. Neurol.*, 193: 937–963.

Jones, E.G. and Powell, T.P.S. (1971) An analysis of the posterior group of thalamic nuclei on the basis of its afferent connections. *J. Comp. Neurol.*, 143: 185–216.

Kaada, B.R., Pribram, K.H. and Epstein, J.A. (1949) Respiratory and vascular responses in monkeys from temporal pole, insula, orbital surface and cingulate gyrus. *J. Neurophysiol.*, 12: 347–355.

Krettek, J.E. and Price, J.L. (1977) Projections from the amygdaloid complex to the cerebral cortex and thalamus in the rat and cat. *J. Comp. Neurol.*, 172: 687–722.

Krieg, W.J.S. (1946) Connections to the cerebral cortex. I. The albino rat. A. Topography of the cortical areas. *J. Comp. Neurol.*, 84: 221–275.

Kurata, K. and Tanji, J. (1985) Contrasting neuronal activity in supplementary and precentral motor cortex of monkeys. II. Responses to movement triggering vs. nontriggering sensory signals. *J. Neurophysiol.*, 53: 142–152.

Kurata, K. and Tanji, J. (1986) Premotor cortex neurons in macaques: activity before distal and proximal forelimb movements. *J. Neurosci.*, 6: 403–411.

Loe, P.R. and Benevento, L.A. (1969) Auditory-visual interaction in single units in the orbito-insular cortex of the cat. *Electroenceph. Clin. Neurophysiol.*, 26: 395–398.

Marchand, F. (1893) *Die Morphologie des Stirnlappens und der Insel der Antropomorphen*, G. Fischer, Jena.

Markowitsch, H.J. and Pritzel, M. (1978) The insular region: part of the prefrontal cortex? *Neurosci. Biobehav. Rev.*, 2: 271–276.

Markowitsch, H.J., Emmans, D., Irle, E., Streicher, M. and Preilowski, B. (1985) Cortical and subcortical afferent connections of the primate's temporal pole: a study of rhesus monkeys, squirrel monkeys, and marmosets. *J. Comp. Neurol.*, 242: 425–458.

Markowitsch, H.J., Irle, E. and Emmans, D. (1987) Cortical and subcortical afferent connections of the squirrel monkey's (lateral) premotor cortex: evidence for visual cortical afferents. *Intern. J. Neurosci.*, in press.

Mesulam, M.-M. and Mufson, E.J. (1982a) Insula of the old world monkey. I. Architectonics in the insulo-orbito-temporal component of the paralimbic brain. *J. Comp. Neurol.*, 212: 1–22.

Mesulam, M.-M. and Mufson, E.J. (1982b) Insula of the old world monkey. III. Efferent cortical output. *J. Comp. Neurol.*, 212: 38–52.

Meynert, T.C. (1869) *Der Bau der Grosshirnrinde und seine örtlichen Verschiedenheiten nebst einem pathologisch-anatomischen Corollarium*, Heuser'sche Buchhandlung, Neuwied.

Mucke, L., Norita, M., Benedek, G. and Creutzfeldt, O. (1982) Physiologic and anatomic investigation of a visual cortical area situated in the ventral bank of the anterior ectosylvian sulcus of the cat. *Exp. Brain Res.*, 46: 1–11.

Mufson, E.J. and Mesulam, M.-M. (1982) Insula of the old world monkey. II. Afferent cortical input. *J. Comp. Neurol.*, 212: 23–37.

Mufson, E.J. and Mesulam, M.-M. (1984) Thalamic connections of the insula in the rhesus monkey and comments on the paralimbic connectivity of the medial pulvinar nucleus. *J. Comp. Neurol.*, 227: 109–120.

Mufson, E.J. Mesulam, M.-M. and Pandya, P.N. (1981) Insular interconnections with the amygdala in the rhesus monkey. *Neuroscience*, 6: 1231–1248.

Olson, C.R. and Graybiel, A.M. (1981) A visual area in the anterior ectosylvian sulcus of the cat. *Soc. Neurosci. Abstr.*, 7: 831.

Olson, C.R. and Graybiel, A.M. (1983) An outlying visual area in the cerebral cortex of the cat. In: J.-P. Changeaux, J. Glowinski, M. Imbert and F.E. Bloom (Eds.), *Molecular and Cellular Interactions Underlying Higher Brain Functions, Progress in Brain Research, Vol. 58*, Elsevier, Amsterdam, pp. 239–245.

Olson, C.R. and Graybiel, A.M. (1987) Ectosylvian visual area of the cat: location, retinotopic organization, and connections. *J. Comp. Neurol.*, 261: 277–294.

Reep, R.L. and Winnans, S.S. (1982) Afferent connections of

the dorsal and ventral agranular insular cortex in the hamster *Mesocricetus auratus. Neuroscience*, 7: 1256 – 1288.

Reil, J.C. (1809) Die sylvische Furche. *Arch. Physiol. (Halle)*, 9: 195 – 208.

Reinoso-Suárez, F. and Roda, J.M. (1985) Topographical organization of the cortical afferents to the cortex of the anterior ectosylvian sulcus in the cat. *Exp. Brain Res.*, 59: 313 – 324.

Retzius, G. (1902) Zur Morphologie der Insula Reili. *Biol. Unters.*, 10: 15 – 20.

Roberts, T.S. and Akert, K. (1963) Insular and opercular cortex and its thalamic projections in *Macaca mulatta. Schweiz. Arch. Neurol. Neurochir. Psychiatr.*, 92: 1 – 43.

Rose, M. (1928) Die Inselrinde des Menschen und der Tiere. *J. Psychol. Neurol. (Leipzig)*, 37: 467 – 624.

Sanides, F. (1968) The architecture of the cortical taste nerve areas in squirrel monkey *(Saimiri sciureus)* and their relationships to insular and prefrontal regions. *Brain Res.*, 8: 97 – 124.

Sanides, F. and Hoffmann, J. (1969) Cyto- and myeloarchitecture of the visual cortex of cat and surrounding integration cortices. *J. Hirnforsch.*, 11: 79 – 104.

Saper, C.B. (1982) Convergence of autonomic and limbic connections in the insular cortex of the rat. *J. Comp. Neurol.*, 210: 163 – 173.

Stephan, H. (1975) *Allocortex. Handbuch der Mikroskopischen Anatomie des Menschen, Vol. IV/9*, Springer, Berlin.

Updyke, B.V. (1983) A reevaluation of the functional organization and cytoarchitecture of the feline lateral posterior complex, with observations on adjoining cell groups. *J. Comp. Neurol.*, 219: 143 – 181.

Weinrich, M. and Wise, S.P. (1982) The premotor cortex of the monkey. *J. Neurosci.*, 2: 1329 – 1345.

Wiesendanger, M., Hummelsheim, H. and Bianchetti, M. (1985) Sensory input to the motor fields of the agranular frontal cortex: a comparison of the precentral, supplementary motor cortex. *Behav. Brain Res.*, 18: 89 – 94.

Winkler, C. and Potter, A. (1914) *An Anatomical Guide to Experimental Research on the Cat's Brain*, W. Versluys, Amsterdam.

Wirth, F.B. (1973) Insular-diencephalic connections in the macaque. *J. Comp. Neurol.*, 150: 361 – 392.

Woolsey, C.N. (1961) Organization of cortical auditory sytem. In: W.A. Rosenblith (Ed.), *Sensory Communication*, MIT Press, Cambridge, MA, pp. 235 – 257.

T.P. Hicks and G. Benedek (Eds.)
Progress in Brain Research, Vol. 75
© 1988 Elsevier Science Publishers B.V. (Biomedical Division)

CHAPTER 25

The visual insular cortex of the cat: organization, properties and modality specificity

G. Benedek* and T.P. Hicks

Department of Medical Physiology, Faculty of Medicine, The University of Calgary, 3330 Hospital Drive N.W., Calgary, Alberta, Canada T2N 4N1

Introduction

Insular cortex of the cat is the newest member of a growing family of extrageniculo-striate visual areas. Long considered by anatomists and physiologists to be the archetypic association cortex in monkey and man (Mesulam and Mufson 1985), the insula now appears to possess a subregion which is unimodally-responsive for vision, having a specific thalamic input, and therefore which no longer fits the general rubric of 'association' cortex. Recent anatomical findings that the visually responsive areas of the suprageniculate nucleus receive their strongest afferent connections from the insula (Hicks et al. 1986) prompted us to assess in detail the physiological, or functional, response properties of the cells of this area, as regards receptive field properties, modality sensitivity and other electrophysiological and neuropharmacological aspects of neuronal behaviour. Our findings support the view that the insula of the cat is an independent cortical region which contains unimodal, visually responsive cells. This area may play a functional role in goal-directed visual orienting behaviours or in visuo-affective integration.

---

* *Permanent address:* Dept. of Physiology, University Medical School, Dòm tèr 10, H-6720 Szeged, Hungary.
Correspondence to: T.P. Hicks, at the above address.

Extracellular recordings have been made from 415 neurones within the insular cortex of barbiturate-anaesthetized cats prepared as described previously (Benedek et al. 1986). The area sampled with our microelectrodes comprised that region lying anterior to the ventral bank of the rostrally-curving anterior ectosylvian sulcus, posterior to the front half of the ventral bank of the orbital sulcus, and ventrolateral to the previously-mentioned sulcal infoldings: that is, the cortex within the crown of the anterior sylvian gyrus (Fig. 1). The presence of regions containing visually insensitive cells surrounding this area aided in defining these borders; of particular note was the consistent observation that the anterior ectosylvian visual area (AEV) (Mucke et al. 1982; Olson and Graybiel 1983) was segregated spatially from this visual insular area. Visual stimuli consisted of bars of light of various lengths, moving at $60°$ sec^{-1} or $600°$ sec^{-1}, oriented in various directions, and of drifting grating stimuli presented at various spatial and temporal frequencies. Neurones were classified according to their preferred velocities, directional and orientation preferences, length sensitivities, modality specificities, responses to electrical stimulation of various visually-responsive brain regions and responses to light stimulation in the presence of microiontophoretically administered bicuculline methiode (BMI). Velocity has been expressed as a quotient to indicate the relative degree of preference for a fixed value, chosen here as $60°$

sec^{-1}. The peak firing rate elicited with a stimulus of 60° sec^{-1} was divided by that with 600° sec^{-1}, therefore the closer the quotient is to one, the less selective is the cell for the different velocities. Quotients much less than one indicate relative preferences for velocities > 60° sec^{-1}; those exceeding one represent preferences for relatively slower moving stimuli than 60° sec^{-1}.

Physiological response properties

Insular cells within the first 600 μm of cortex situated along the ventral banks of the anterior ectosylvian sulcus and orbital sulcus were exclusively unimodally responsive for vision, and exhibited a preference for stimuli moving at 600° sec^{-1} as opposed to 60° sec^{-1}, whereas those visually responsive cells in deeper laminae (within the next visually-responsive band of cells at 1100–1800 μm, or in the lower zone, at 2000–2500 μm) generally preferred lower velocity movements. In the entire population, irrespective of cortical location, velocity preference was about evenly divided between the two values tested. Most neurones (75%; 104 of 139 cells) studied proved to be either directionally selective or directionally sensitive, having peak firing rates in the preferred direction more than twice as great as in the non-preferred direction. Almost all cells displayed a preference for certain directions of movement within the 360° arc, suggesting the existence of a dynamic orientation sensitivity. A substantial portion of the cells

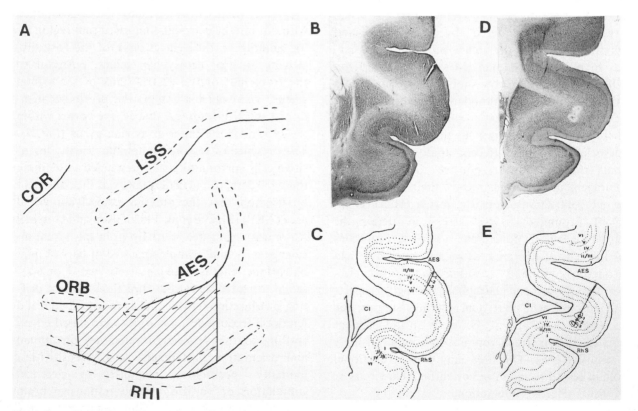

Fig. 1. Location of the region of insula within which the modality-specific cortical visual area can be found. Left: lateral view of the cortical surface. Vertical lines represent the rostral-most and caudal-most penetrations where visually-responsive neurons were found. Right: representative coronal sections and corresponding drawings of reconstructed electrode tracks. (Top: photographs; bottom: schematic drawings.) Each drawing of the electrode track shows locations of three visually responsive neurons encountered in the penetrations.

encountered exhibited end-inhibition: using bars of light of 1.5° width and lengths of 1.5°, 10° and 30°, the 135 cells sampled fell into the following categories of length preference: preferring 1.5° (spot-like stimulus) = 58 cells (43%), preferring 10° = 55 cells (41%), and preferring 30° = 22 cells (16%). A marked preference for the spot-like (1.5° × 1.5°) stimulus was shown by the cells which had strong direction selectivities and these

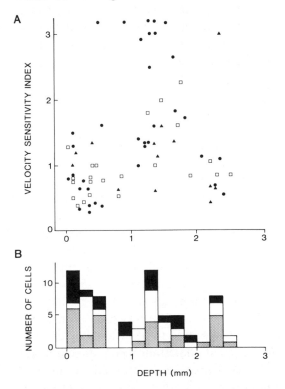

Fig. 2. The relationship between the physiological responses of insular neurones to light and their location along the penetration track. Upper part of the figure shows the relationship of velocity sensitivity (expressed as an index: peak firing frequency at 60° s⁻¹ stimulation/peak firing frequency at 600° s⁻¹ stimulation) to cortical depth where the neurone was found. See text for further explanation of velocity sensitivity index. Each symbol corresponds to one unit recorded. The following symbols represent the direction sensitivity of the cells: □ = 90−100; ▲ = 51−90; ● = 0−50; where 90−100 = directionally selective, 51−90 = directionally sensitive, and 0−50 = nondirectionally sensitive. (B) shows the distribution of length sensitivity along the electrode tracks (▨▨▨ = preference to 1.5° stimulus; ▭ = preference to 10° stimulus; ■■■ = preference to 30° stimulus). Abscissa denotes cortical depth within the penetrations.

cells virtually always preferred the higher velocity stimulus. Those cells lying in the middle layers of the cortex (located between 1100 μm and 1800 μm) strongly preferring 60° sec⁻¹ velocities (velocity quotient of > 2), were non-directionally sensitive. These interactions of response variables are shown for a representative sampling of neurones in Fig. 2.

Visuotopy

As an important issue in determining the organization of extrageniculo-striate visual systems, we were anxious to assess the question of retinotopy of visually responsive insular cortex. Confounding this effort was the realization that cells exhibiting very large receptive fields, often producing after-discharges to stimulation and having direction and orientation sensitivity as well as response lability even to optimal stimuli, cause great difficulties in accurately making receptive field maps. This point was particularly acute when it became obvious that virtually every neurone encountered contained the area centralis within its receptive field boundaries. Accordingly, we refrained deliberately from attempting to represent the area visuotopically and instead concentrated on examining the role of area centralis in the cells' responsiveness.

Area centralis was masked from view by a 3° × 3° black square and following testing, the mask was removed and replaced by an occlusion of the entire receptive field which previously had been visible, but now with the central 3° × 3° square visible. Clear visual responses were obtained in both situations although important differences were evident in the nature of the responses. As is apparent from Fig. 3, allowing viewing exclusively of the area centralis region caused only a minor reduction of response magnitude, and reversing the visual occlusion produced a qualitatively different response, one showing a split peak, or a bimodal response, having a variant latency when compared with the former two conditions. Direction preference was maintained in 82% of the cases during viewing only of the central region; in the reverse situation it was maintained in just 55% of the cases. Similarly, when considering the variable of orientation sensitivity, this property was maintained when the cell's receptive field was masked all but for the area centralis region, and orienta-

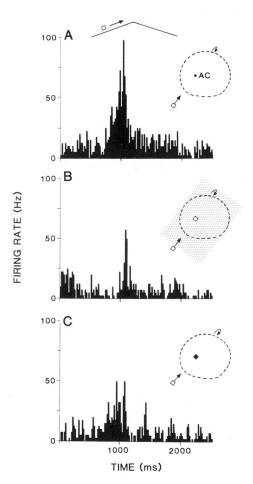

Fig. 3. Peristimulus time histograms of the responses of a cell to a light slit moving across: (A) an unobstructed receptive field; (B) the same receptive field almost completely blocked from view save for a 3° × 3° unoccluded region encompassing area centralis; (C) the same receptive field, but having only the small 3° × 3° region surrounding area centralis blocked from view. Inserts by each psth illustrate these different conditions schematically. Diagonally sloping line above the column of histograms represents the stimulus trajectory moving forward (upward slope) across the receptive field and backward (downward slope) along the same path but in the return direction, with the corresponding cell response appearing beneath. AC, area centralis. Each psth is the record of 20 stimulus repetitions.

tion sensitivity was lost in all but 12% of the cases when area centralis viewing only was blocked. Further emphasizing the important role of this feature of insular cells' receptive fields was the temporal constancy of responses afforded the cells by virtue of stimulation of area centralis. As was noted from the responses shown in Fig. 3, the stimulation of this region was a prerequisite not only for the vigorous excitatory response to be elicited, but also for it to occur at a fixed, time-locked latency after area centralis stimulation. This pertained however only to responses evoked by stimuli moving in the preferred direction for the cell.

Role of inhibition

As immunocytochemical experiments had shown that GABA-positive neurones were present in insula and distributed relatively evenly throughout all cortical laminae (Fig. 4A), and since many response properties examined such as end-inhibition, direction and velocity selectivity and response to gratings (see below), suggested the existence of an inhibitory influence, we employed a neuropharmacological approach using the micro-iontophoretic administration of BMI to block the effects of intrinsic GABA. Based on results from 77 cells, there appeared to be little if any effect of GABA mediated inhibition upon direction sensitivity or length preference and only a minor effect upon velocity selectivity. BMI did however exert potent effects on visual responsiveness. Thus a substantial number of cells showing no response to light prior to the ejection of BMI produced a vigorous discharge to the same stimulus during the presence of low levels of the antagonist. As shown by Fig. 4B, which illustrates a lack of selective effect upon length and velocity preference of an insular cell, the most pronounced effect of the antagonist was an overall enhancing of the vigour of visual responsiveness, causing an increase in response-to-background ratio. As well, significant elevations of spontaneous firing usually accompanied the ejection of BMI. This finding stands in marked contrast to the results of Sillito (1984) with bicuculline obtained in striate cortex, where the drug produces quite selective effects upon specific response properties (direction and orientation sensitivity, length preference, etc.).

Spatial frequency: responsiveness to periodic stimuli

The assessment of cell responses to moving and stationary periodic stimuli at various frequencies

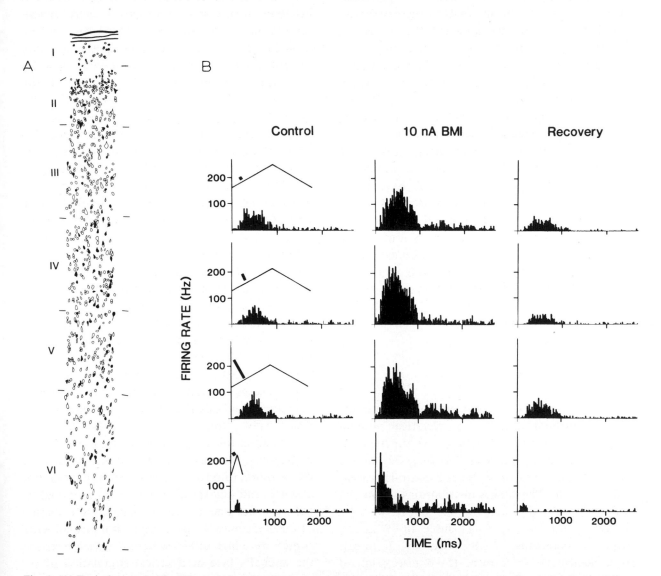

Fig. 4. (A) Typical example of a 232-μm wide strip of cortex traced through a drawing tube at 25×, showing the laminar positions of each cell body staining positively for immunoreactive GABA (filled-in cells) and the outlines of non-GABA-positive cells (cell profiles not filled-in). (B) Peristimulus time histograms of the responses of a neurone to a moving stimulus before (left column), during (central column) and after (right column), the microiontophoretic ejection of 10 nA of BMI. Each histogram represents the responses of the cell to 20 consecutive stimulus presentations. Top row: 60° sec^{-1} stimulus velocity; slit size, 1.5° × 1.5°. Second row: 60° sec^{-1} velocity; slit size, 10° × 1.5°. Third row: 60° sec^{-1} velocity; slit size, 30° × 1.5°. Bottom row: 600° sec^{-1} velocity; slit size, 1.5° × 1.5°. Diagonally sloping lines follow the convention described in the legend of Fig. 3.

can help to determine the resolving power and stimulus integrating capacity of visually responsive cells. We sampled the responses of 60 neurones to drifting square wave gratings at frequencies varying between 0.05 and 1.5 cycles per degree. When the spatial frequency was varied at a particular drift velocity, this meant that an increased temporal cycle length accompanied the decreasing spatial frequency for that grating pattern.

Most cells displayed a well modulated and phase-locked discharge and alteration of spontaneous firing in response to grating stimulation. Despite the large receptive field sizes of these cells, all spatial frequencies between 0.05 and 1.5 cycles produced response modulation irrespective of the number of stimulus contours present within the receptive fields, showing that the units have resolving powers well beyond the constraints which would be expected, based on receptive field dimension. Most vigorous responsiveness was to the lowest frequencies, with the diminishing preference following a smoothly-progressing monotonic function to increasing frequencies, until inhibitions were elicited by the gratings, evident as a responsiveness modulated below the rate of spontaneous activity.

Synaptic activation

Visually responsive insular neurones were activated orthodromically by electrical stimuli delivered to the optic nerve ($n = 33$), superior colliculus ($n = 28$), suprageniculate ($n = 32$), lateral suprasylvian cortex ($n = 28$) and contralateral insula ($n = 16$). The latency distributions and modal values (in parentheses) for the above were as follows: optic nerve, $5 - 11$ msec ($8 - 9$ msec); superior colliculus, $3 - 8$ msec ($6 - 7$ msec); suprageniculate, $2 - 7$ msec ($5 - 6$ msec); lateral suprasylvian area, $2 - 6$ msec ($3 - 4$ msec); and insula, $2 - 11$ msec ($4 - 5$ msec). With stimulation of the optic nerve there was a strong correlation between visual responsiveness and synaptic activation by electrical stimulation: 33 of 37 synaptically activated cells were visually responsive.

Modality specificity

Reports exist that insular cells display multimodal properties (Benevento and Loe 1975; Fallon and Benevento 1977) and anatomical studies are consistent with these reports as they show the presence of afferents arising from a variety of heterogenous sensory nuclei of the diencephalon and mesencephalon, and from regions themselves reported to be polymodally responsive (Rose and Woolsey 1943; Heath and Jones 1971; Cranford et al. 1976). It must be borne in mind, however, that the demonstration of an input by anatomical means, while a prerequisite for proving communication between two sites, does not of itself indicate the existence of a functional interaction between such sites; this requires a physiological demonstration. Whether the insula is a region multimodal with respect to single cells or is so only at a population level, where for example groups of cells or subregions retain sensory specificity but as a whole represent a variety of modalities, was addressed by a series of experiments on 111 neurones.

Stimuli were divided into two types: those using natural means to excite cells at levels considered to be within normal, physiologically-relevent intensities, and those using electrical stimulation of nerves or brain pathways or using natural means but at exceedingly intense levels. These are called here physiologically relevant or non-physiological, respectively. Physiologically relevant levels of stimuli were, for the visual modality, moving spots or bars of light presented to a tangent screen; for the auditory modality, bursts of white noise at about 40 dB; and for the somatosensory modality, light touches and gentle mechanical deformation of the skin, muscles and joints. Non-physiological stimuli were high intensity light flashes directed to the animal's face or electrical stimulation of the optic nerve; clicks and white noise at $80 - 100$ dB (0.1 msec) intensity; and electrical stimulation of the radial nerve by bipolar cuff electrodes.

Cells situated in dorsal insular regions, along the upper banks of the cortex lying along the ventrolateral lip of the anterior ectosylvian sulcus and orbital sulcus were responsive exclusively to visual stimuli when physiologically relevant levels of stimulation were employed. Responses in this region to somatosensory or auditory stimulation were observed only when non-physiologically relevant levels of stimulation were delivered. In these cases, apparent polymodality could be demonstrated with single neurones on some occasions. With cells situated in more ventral regions of the

insula, a very few instances were noted where bimodal responses could be elicited from single neurones using physiologically relevant levels of stimulation (3 of 111 cells) although again, when very intense forms of natural stimulation or when electrical activation was performed, considerable apparent polymodality could be observed (44 cells of 111 studies). As well as recording from single neurones during non-physiological levels, or forms, of stimulation, evoked field potential recordings were made from the same loci as the single cell records were taken. Field potential recordings revealed widely overlapping representations of all modalities in both dorsal and ventral insular regions, irrespective of the sensitivity displayed by the local neuronal response. A typical example is provided in Fig. 5, where evoked fields from all three modalities were recorded from the same point in cortex, using non-physiological stimulation. When the amplifier filters were adjusted for extracellular recording however, the unit responses obtained at this site were selective for specific modalities. Thus, two distinct groups of action potentials differing in amplitude were recorded; both were unresponsive to radial nerve stimulation but the large spike responded to optic nerve stimulation and a moving light bar, whereas the smaller spikes were elicited only by a loud click (80 dB) stimulus, i.e., a non-physiologically relevant level of auditory stimulation. This example typifies the main result of this section; that is, that many sites within the insula, on the basis of evoked field potentials and of non-physiologically relevant levels of 'sensory' stimulation at the single cell level, appear to receive convergent or polymodal inputs. Yet, when stimuli from different modalities are presented to the same cells within normal, physiologically relevant intensities, or forms, only unimodal responses are recorded. This calls into serious question the reports of others of a multimodal sensory representation of this cortical area, and requires a careful reconsideration of the use of the term, association cortex, to describe the insula (Avendaño and Llamas 1984; Mesulam and Mufson 1985; Pandya and Yeterian 1985).

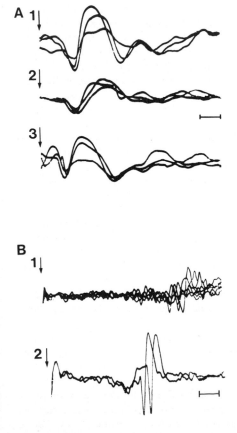

Fig. 5. (A) Field potentials (arrow indicates time of stimulation) of all three modalities tested at a single recording site (depth = 2200 μm). Each illustrated oscillographic record is of 3 successive sweeps. From top to bottom: (1) click, (2) radial nerve, (3) optic nerve. Calibration bar: 10 msec. (B) Two oscillographs of evoked responses from different cells, recorded at the same site. B₁: 3 sweeps, auditory stimulation by loud ~ 80 dB) click; B₂: 2 sweeps, visual stimulation by electrical activation of the optic nerve. Calibration bar: 2 msec.

Summary and conclusions

We describe here, for the first time, a detailed survey of the response properties, modality specificity and organization of a new visual area of the cat's extrastriate cortex. The area is in close functional and anatomical association with the AEV and has strong connectional inter-relationships with other members of the extrageniculo-striate cortex and limbic structures (Russchen 1982; Guldin et al. 1986). These findings together point towards a likely functional role of this area as an integrative centre between visual and emotive brain systems. Nevertheless, the modality specificity at the level of the single cell, together with the strong and specific diencephalic connections with unimodal regions argues against the view that this area is association cortex as defined classically. These observations and conclusions underscore the need to consider very carefully redefining not only this area, but also other functionally similar regions of 'non-primary' sensory cortex, in terms other than merely associational.

References

Avendaño, C. and Llamas, A. (1984) Thalamic and non-thalamic direct subcortical projections to association areas of the cat's cerebral cortex. In: F. Reinoso-Suárez and C. Ajmone-Marsan (Eds.), *Cortical Integration: Basic, Archicortical, and Cortical Association Levels of Neural Integration, IBRO Monograph Series, Vol. II*, Raven Press, New York, pp. 195 – 221.

Benedek, G., Jang, E.K. and Hicks, T.P. (1986) Physiological properties of visually responsive neurones in the insular cortex of the cat. *Neurosci. Lett.*, 64: 269 – 274.

Benevento, L.A. and Loe, P.R. (1975) An intracellular study of thalamocortical synapses in orbito-insular cortex. *Exp. Neurol.*, 46: 634 – 643.

Cranford, J.L., Ladner, S.J., Campbell, C.B.G. and Neff, W.D. (1976) Efferent projections of the insular and temporal neocortex of the cat. *Brain Res.*, 117: 195 – 210.

Guldin, W.O., Markowitsch, H.J., Lampe, R. and Irle, E. (1986) Cortical projections originating from the cat's insular area and remarks on claustrocortical connections. *J. Comp. Neurol.*, 243: 468 – 487.

Fallon, J.H. and Benevento, L.A. (1977) Auditory-visual interaction in cat orbito-insular cortex. *Neurosci. Lett.*, 6: 143 – 149.

Heath, C. and Jones, E.G. (1971) An experimental study of ascending connections from the posterior group of thalamic nuclei in the rat. *J. Comp. Neurol.*, 141: 397 – 426.

Hicks, T.P., Stark, C.A. and Fletcher, W. (1986) Origins of afferents to visual suprageniculate nucleus in the cat. *J. Comp. Neurol.*, 246: 544 – 554.

Mesulam, M.-M. and Mufson, E.J. (1985) The insula of Riel in man and monkey. Architectonics, connectivity, and function. In: A. Peters and E.G. Jones (Eds.), *Cerebral Cortex, Vol. 4, Association and Auditory Cortices*, Plenum Press, New York and London, pp. 179 – 226.

Mucke, L., Norita, M., Benedek, G. and Creutzfeldt, O. (1982) Physiologic and anatomic investigation of a visual cortical area situated in the ventral bank of the anterior ectosylvian sulcus of the cat. *Exp. Brain Res.*, 46: 1 – 11.

Olson, C.R. and Graybiel, A.M. (1983) An outlying visual area in the cerebral cortex of the cat. In: J.-P. Changeaux, J. Glowinski, M. Imbert and F.E. Bloom (Eds.), *Molecular and Cellular Interactions Underlying Higher Brain Functions, Progress in Brain Research, Vol. 58*, Elsevier, Amsterdam, pp. 239 – 245.

Pandya, D.N. and Yeterian, E.H. (1985) Architecture and connections of cortical association areas. In: A. Peters and E.G. Jones (Eds.), *Cerebral Cortex, Vol. 4, Association and Auditory Cortices*, Plenum Press, New York and London, pp. 3 – 61.

Rose, J.E. and Woolsey, C.N. (1943) A study of thalamo-cortical relations in the rabbit. *Johns Hopkins Hosp. Bull.*, 73: 65 – 128.

Russchen, F. (1982) Amygdalopetal projections in the cat. I. Cortical afferent connections. A study with retrograde and anterograde tracing techniques. *J. Comp. Neurol.*, 206: 159 – 169.

Sillito, A.M. (1984) Functional considerations of the operation of GABAergic inhibitory processes in the visual cortex. In: E.G. Jones and A. Peters (Eds.), *Cerebral Cortex, Vol. 2, Functional Properties of Cortical Cells*, Plenum Press, New York and London, pp. 91 – 118.

T.P. Hicks and G. Benedek (Eds.)
Progress in Brain Research, Vol. 75
© 1988 Elsevier Science Publishers B.V. (Biomedical Division)

CHAPTER 26

Some extra-striate corticothalamic connections in macaque monkeys

S. Squatrito[1], M.G. Maioli[1], C. Galletti[2] and P.P. Battaglini[1, *]

[1] *Istituto di Fisiologia Umana and* [2] *Cattedra di Fisiologia Generale, Università di Bologna, Piazza di Porta S. Donato 2, 40127 Bologna, Italy*

Introduction

One of the most challenging ideas in recent years on the organization of the central nervous system is that the brain centers are not linked in a series of successive functional units, each of which serially processes the incoming flow of information, but rather it is organized as a distributed system of modules, widely interconnected in parallel, in which cognitive and motor processes emerge from the interactions of large numbers of simple processing units (see Mountcastle 1982).

The extrageniculo-striate visual system seems to be a representative model of the above mentioned organizing principle. In fact, the discovery of an ever increasing number of cortical visual areas and subcortical visual centers, each with its internal modular organization, along with the identification of intricate interconnections between areas and centers, supports the idea of a distributed parallel system. Apart from the intrinsic organization of each of these modules, one aspect of this principle is the way in which several modules are interconnected in parallel networks. For instance, corticosubcortical connections are known to form re-entrant loops anatomically linking cortical fields involved in related integrative functions,

often paralleling the associative connections. In this respect, study of the bulky anatomical connectivity can provide the wiring substrate for these integrated operations.

In the macaque monkey the caudal half of the superior temporal sulcus (STS) is an important cortical station of the extrageniculo-striate visual system in which discrete visual areas have been identified. Among these, the middle temporal (MT) area is reputed to play a key role in visual motion analysis because of the property of its neurons to selectively respond to the direction and speed of moving visual stimuli (Zeki 1974; Maunsell and Van Essen 1983a). Areas surrounding MT are less defined as to their anatomical limits, connections, and functions. Nevertheless, there is some general agreement on their involvement in visual processes (Maunsell and Van Essen 1983b; Desimone and Ungerleider 1986). In this paper, we will describe some corticothalamic connections of the MT area and the neighbouring, MT-recipient, visual region situated in the fundus and upper bank of STS of the macaque monkey. These connections turned out to be part of a parallel network reciprocally linking sensory structures to cortical and subcortical formations, that from anatomical and electrophysiological investigations appear to be involved in the neural control of directionally oriented eye movements, as well as in the orientation of visual attention. The

---

* *Present address:* Istituo di Fisiologia, Università di Trieste, Via Fleming 34, 34127 Trieste, Italy.

wide connectivity among these structures might, in our opinion, support the model of a distributed parallel system processing these functions.

Methods

Experiments were carried out on 9 Java monkeys (*Macaca fascicularis*). The animals were deeply anaesthetized with Nembutal and a mixture of L-

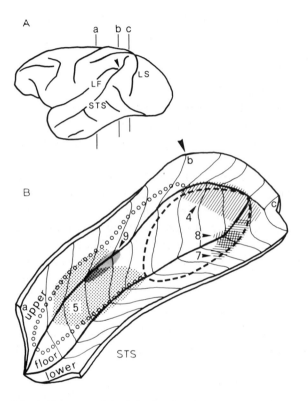

Fig. 1. Summary of the injection sites in STS. A: Lateral view of the left hemisphere of macaque monkey. B: Caudal half of the superior temporal sulcus (STS) reconstructed from layer IV outlines of coronal sections of an exemplary case. Three of these sections are marked by lines (a, b, c) to compare their location on the brain drawing in A. The large arrow head points to the region where the lateral fissure joins the STS. Stippled and hatched areas correspond to the injection zones of the 5 animals considered for the results. Dashed line marks the border of the densely myelinated area corresponding to MT. This limit was reconstructed for each animal and then adjusted to the MT border of the case shown in the illustration. Small circles delimit the gross area receiving projections from the MT-injected cases M-4, M-7 and M-8. LF, lateral fissure; LS, lunate sulcus; STS, superior temporal sulcus.

[5-³H]proline (14 Ci/mmol, 45 μCi/μl and L-[4,5-³H]leucine (188 Ci/mmol, 45 μCi/μl) was injected using a 10-μl Hamilton syringe fitted with a 26S gauge needle. Each animal usually received in the same area 1 – 3 injections of 0.8 – 1 μl. In order to locate the MT area, and then the neighbouring cortex in the STS, the results of two animals in which area 17 had been injected were used, and the regions of projection in STS of striate cortex were extrapolated to the other animals. The amino acids were released over a period of 20 min, the experimenter waiting an additional 15 min before withdrawing the needle. After 7 days the animals were re-anaesthetized and 7 stainless steel rods (3 antero-posterior and 4 vertical) were inserted in the brains at precise stereotaxic points, in order to calculate brain shrinkage and have landmarks in the assessment of the stereotaxic planes. Animals were then killed. After removal and further fixation (15 days) the brains were embedded in paraffin, sectioned serially at 8 – 10 μm in frontal planes and then treated according to the autoradiographic technique. The sections were exposed for 8 weeks and then developed and fixed. Toluidine blue or cresyl violet was used to counterstain the autoradiographically treated sections. In addition, several sections across the injection zones, and adjacent to those treated, were stained for fibers. All histological preparations were observed under bright- and dark-field microscopy, and selected sections were drawn by camera lucida.

Results

Location of injection zones

In delimiting the injection sites we considered the areas of cortex around the puncture tracks that, with bright-field microscopy, appeared uniformly black, and the surrounding zone in which grain density was unambiguously higher on the cell somata than on the neuropil. Location of the functional areas in STS was identified post-mortem by extrapolating the maps described by other authors, and by finding the specific myeloarchitectonic features and known connections with other structures. Of the 7 animals that received injections in STS, 5 revealed uptake regions mainly inside identifiable visual areas, 2 involved non-visual structures, or were obviously spread over more than one area, and these were discarded from the analysis.

Fig. 1 shows a summary of the locations and the extent of injection sites in the 5 animals considered in the results. Three animals had injection areas mainly inside the myeloarchitectonic limits of MT, with only minor invasion of the neighbouring cortex. In no case was the whole extent of the area covered. In the other two animals, the uptake area was totally outside of area MT. In one case (M-5), the area covered a patch of cortex anterior to MT, including the floor of STS and part of the upper wall of the sulcus. Spreading of the injection to the lower wall was negligible, and limited to the first two cortical layers. In the other case (M-9), the uptake region was much smaller and restricted to the junction of the floor with the upper bank of the sulcus. We refer to the whole region covered by these two injection sites as AMST (anteromedial superior temporal). We believe that this area is still part of the visual STS in that (i) we found that it was entirely within a region corresponding to a labeled field in the cases in which we injected the MT area (Fig. 1B, small circles). (ii) We did not find any relevant connection linking this area to sensory specific structures other than to visual ones.

Projections from the MT area

In all cases with injections in the MT area we found consistent grain accumulations in the pulvinar inferior (PLI) and the pulvinar lateralis (PLL). Fig. 2 shows an exemplary case of these findings. In this case (M-7), the injection site was entirely inside the limits of the densely myelinated area corresponding to MT (Figs. 1B and 2A). Labeled fibers approach the dorsal pole of the PLL, penetrate the nucleus and form several multiform patches of terminal grains, distributed over almost all the anteroposterior extent of the nuclear subdivision (Fig. 2C, stippled area). The terminal grain accumulation zone continues without interruption into the PLI, where it forms a patch that occupies the dorsal-most part of the subdivision, at the boundary between the PLI and the PLL. The other two animals injected in the MT showed qualitatively similar results. The only remarkable point is that in case M-4 almost the whole dorsoventral extent of PLI was uniformly labeled, especially in the cranial-most sections. In none of the 3 cases did we see label in the medial portion of the pulvinar.

In addition to these projections to the pulvinar, other thalamic targets of the MT were found, namely the intralaminar nuclei (ILN), the nucleus reticularis thalami (R) and the pregeniculate nucleus (PG). The intralaminar nuclei found labeled after injections in the MT were the paracentral (Pc), the central lateral (CL) and the centre median (CM). Pc was the most evidently and consistently labeled nucleus. Grains were found in it in all 3 cases with injections in the MT, and in all of them, the grain accumulation covered almost the entire anteroposterior extent of the nucleus. Nevertheless, the grain density was much sparser than that seen in the pulvinar. Terminal accumulations in CL and CM were less consistent and much less extended. They were found in only 2 of the 3 cases (M-4 and M-7), and the label was followed for only a few sections. Fig. 3a,b shows the appearance of the described labels in selected sections. The nucleus reticularis thalami was labeled in all the cases of MT injections. We found grains in the part of the nucleus crossed by the labeled fibers directed to the pulvinar (Fig. 2D). Since the terminal labeling in this nucleus is intermingled with labeled fibers, it is difficult to say whether the terminal fields are uniform, or are present in some particular pattern of distribution. Grain accumulations were also found in the pregeniculate nucleus. We have already described these projections in a previous paper (Maioli et al. 1984).

282

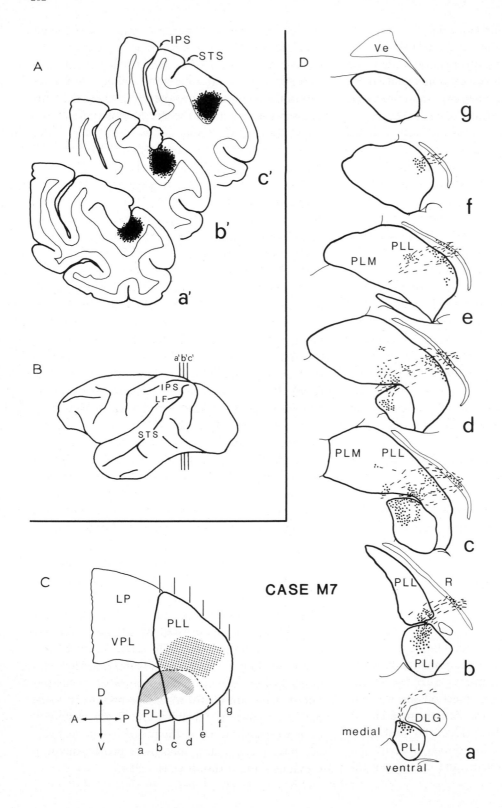

CASE M7

Projections of the AMST

All the MT targets described above were also reached by fibers coming from the AMST. In addition, we found 4 more thalamic targets of this region: the pulvinar medialis (PLM), the supra-geniculate nucleus (SG), the medial dorsal nucleus (MD) and the lateral dorsal nucleus (LD). Figures 3c,f and 4 show the results of the case with the largest injection in the AMST (case M-5). In PLL we found several patches of terminal labels, often irregular in shape, sometimes forming a band-like

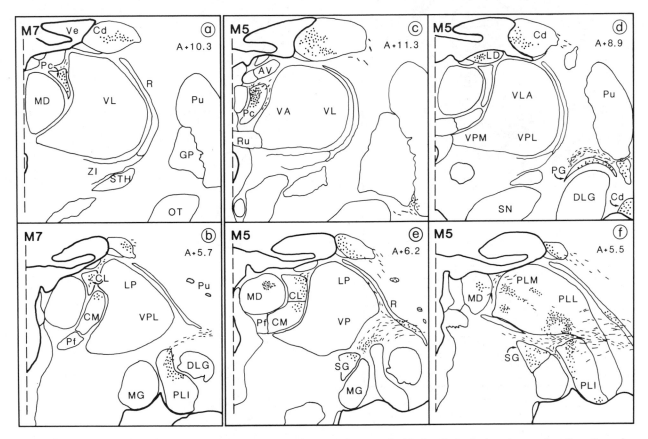

Fig. 3. Projections from MT and AMST to several thalamic nuclei. a – f: camera lucida drawings of selected coronal sections through the thalamus and adjacent basal ganglia. Computed stereotaxic levels are reported at the top right of each panel. For each section the midline is indicated by an interrupted vertical line. AV, anteroventral nucleus; Cd, caudate; CL, central lateral n.; CM, centre median n.; GP, globus pallidus; MD, medial dorsal n.; MG, medial geniculate n.; OT, optic tract; Pc, paracentral n.; Pf, parafascicular n.; PG, pregeniculate n.; Pu, putamen; Ru, n. reuniens; SG, suprageniculate n.; SN, substantia nigra; STH, sub-thalamic n.; VA, ventral anterior n.; VL, ventral lateral complex; VLA, ventral lateral anterior n.; VP, ventral posterior complex; VPL, ventral posterolateral n.; VPM, ventral posteromedial n.; ZI, zona incerta. Other abbreviations as in the previous legends.

Fig. 2. MT-pulvinar projections. A: Selected coronal sections through the injection site (black area). B: Lateral view of the left hemisphere, with lines (a′ – c′) marking the levels of the sections shown in A. C: Orthographic projection of the caudal part of the thalamus, showing the lateral aspect of the pulvinar subdivisions and the labeled regions in PLI (hatched area) and PLL (stippled area). The interrupted line traces the caudal border of the PLI hidden underneath PLL. D: camera lucida drawings of coronal sections of the pulvinar whose levels are reported in C (small letters). The dot density is roughly proportional to the silver grain density in the terminal fields. IPS, intraparietal sulcus; DLG, dorsal lateral geniculate; LP, n. lateralis posterior; PLI, inferior pulvinar; PLL, lateral pulvinar; PLM, medial pulvinar; R, n. reticularis thalami; Ve, ventriculus; A, anterior; D, dorsal; P, posterior; V, ventral.

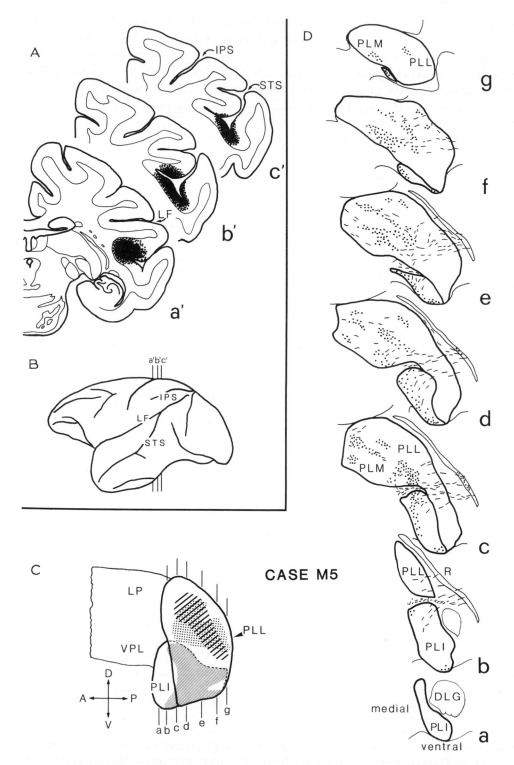

Fig. 4. AMST-pulvinar projections. Same as in Fig. 2. Note that in C the thick-hatched area represents the PLM projection zone seen as a shadow overlapping the PLL projection zone.

arrangement. This sort of labeling occupied a large part of the anteroposterior (A-P) extent of the nucleus (Fig. 4C, stippled area). PLI showed preferential labeling of the medial and ventral border of the nucleus (Fig. 4De). This labeling, more uniform than that seen in PLL, occupied almost the entire anteroposterior dimension of the nucleus, sparing only its cranial pole (Fig. 4C, thin hatched area). Label in PLM was found in both cases injected in the AMST. The labeled zone in this subdivision was continuous, in a lateromedial direction, with that seen in PLL, and showed the same arrangement. In case M-5 it occupied almost the entire extent of the nucleus.

The ILN and the nucleus reticularis thalami were labeled in the same way as described for the MT-injected cases (Fig. 3c – e). In the SG the grain accumulation occupied the whole anteroposterior extent of the nucleus, with a diffuse pattern (Fig. 3e – f). This nucleus was labeled in both cases with injections in the AMST. The nuclei LD and MD were found unambiguously labeled only in case M-5, the one with a large injection site. In this case, the terminal accumulation zone in MD consisted of a heavily-labeled spot of grains, with clear-cut limits, visible for at least 3 mm A-P (Fig. 3e – f), and situated entirely in the non-magnocellular portion of the nucleus. In LD we found a monopatched label extending for about 1.5 mm A-P, in the oral half of the nucleus (Fig. 3d). In case M-9, the one with a much smaller AMST injection site, only very sparsely labeled fibers and a slight, above-background grain density at observation with high magnification were found in the same MD and LD regions.

Discussion

Thalamic projections of MT

The MT area has a well-recognizable myeloarchitectonic characteristic (Van Essen et al. 1981) that makes detection of its limits on myelin-stained sections quite reliable. Although we failed to inject the whole extent of this area, injection sites in cases M-4, M-7 and M-8 covered a significant part of MT. The results obtained in these animals suggest that the MT area of the macaque sends important efferents to the inferior and lateral subdivisions of the pulvinar. These projections virtually cover the entire extent of these nuclear masses, though the pattern of distribution, especially in PLL, is rather patchy. Similar results have been described already (Maunsell and Van Essen 1983b; Standage and Benevento 1983) although there has been some disagreement as to the extent of the MT-recipient pulvinar area. Our results, showing that most of PLI and PLL are labeled, are closer to the findings of Maunsell than to those of Standage.

Projections of MT to the reticular nucleus of the thalamus have already been reported (Maunsell and Van Essen 1983b; Ungerleider et al. 1984). Our results are in quite good agreement with these descriptions.

MT efferents to the ILN, though rather sparse, are consistent in our cases, especially those to Pc. The lack of similar findings in other works on subcortical projections of the MT area might be due to the different extent of the injection zones between these and the other experiments. In our past experience with the autoradiographic tracing technique, it was found that the extent of the uptake region is one of the crucial factors for the detection of all the targets of a given field. When the projection systems are rather diffuse, as is probably the case with cortical connections with intralaminar nuclei, restricted injection sites might not be sufficient to detect the terminal fields.

Thalamic projections of the AMST

The region of cortex medially and anteriorly surrounding the MT area has been investigated both anatomically and functionally. Attempts have been made to define several subregions in this cortex, on the basis of criteria such as the extent of the projections from the MT area, the existence in this cortex of distinct retinotopic representations and the finding of sets of neurons specifically excited by a given stimulus quality. While Maunsell and

Van Essen (1983b) describe a single MT-recipient area, situated medially and anteriorly to MT in the upper bank and in the fundus of STS, Desimone and Ungerleider (1986) subdivide this region into multiple areas. In particular, they consider the cortex of the fundus of STS in front of MT as a separate area called FST, with its own myeloarchitecture and response specificity. Actually, the limits of these areas are not completely defined by the criteria mentioned. In fact, the retinotopic representation has been reported as being rough in this region. The characteristic myeloarchitecture of the fundus of STS is gradually lost anteriorly in the sulcus, whereas with respect to the projections from MT, which are distributed in several patches, there is disagreement between the authors on the need to subdivide this region into multiple areas on such a basis. Accordingly, while the rough localization of these areas can be assessed with some reliability following the guideline of the border of MT, their precise regional limits must be taken with some degree of approximation. One more cause for uncertainty is added in our cases, because extrapolated anatomical localization does not take into account the individual variability between animals. Bearing this in mind, we can attempt to compare the injection sites of cases M-5 and M-9 with the areas surrounding MT. None is coextensive with MST or FST: injection of M-9 might have been inside the limits of FST, since it is situated in the fundus of STS a few millimeters from the border of MT. The injections of M-5, being again anterior to the border of the MT but transversely covering almost the entire fundus of the sulcus and extending also to part of its upper bank, could occupy most of FST and part of MST. According to the definition of Maunsell and Van Essen (1983b), since our injections are in a region most probably MT-recipient, the closest approximation of our injected zone is with the anterior part of these authors' MST. Therefore by analogy we refer to this region as AMST (anteromedial superior temporal). This does not imply that the region we injected is a separate subarea of MST.

Thalamic projections from this region of the macaque cortex traced with autoradiography are not reported in the literature. Our results, although obtained only from two cases, seem rather consistent: the MT-recipient area surrounding the MT medially and anteriorly shares the same targets with MT, and, in addition, its efferents reach other nuclei like the PLM and SG. The projections of AMST to MD and LD are a point of uncertainty in our results because we found them only in case M-5. We impute the failure in finding manifest grain accumulations in these nuclei (also in case M-9) to insufficient uptake of marker by the cell somata due to the small extent of the injection site. Since at least MD has a set of interconnections with the superior colliculus (SC) and the prefrontal cortex (PFC) consistent with those of PLM and SG (see below), the origin of these projections from the whole MT-recipient region of cortex seems convincing. Nevertheless we cannot rule out the possibility that the source of these connections is restricted to an area not covered by the small injection in M-9.

The cortico-thalamo-cortical network and its functional interpretation

Inferior (PLI) and lateral (PLL) pulvinar are reciprocally connected with visual striate and prestriate areas (Benevento and Rezak 1976; Ogren and Hendrickson 1976; Trojanowsky and Jacobson 1976; Benevento and Davies 1977), and they receive a major input from the superficial layers of the superior colliculus (Benevento and Fallon 1975; Benevento and Rezak 1976; Harting et al. 1980). Moreover PLI receives fibers also from the pretectum (Carpenter and Pierson 1973) and a small contingent of axons from the retina (Campos-Ortega et al. 1970; Mizuno et al. 1982). The output of these subdivisions is directed mainly to cortical targets. In addition to the reciprocal connections with striate and prestriate cortex, referred to above, PLI and PLL send fibers to the parietal lobe (areas 5 and 7; Trojanowsky and Jacobson 1976), and to the temporal lobe (areas 20 and 21; Benevento and Rezak 1976; Mauguière and Baleydier 1978). These reciprocal connections with visual sensory structures are met by functional features of these areas. Bender (1982), recording neuronal responses to visual stimuli from PLI, demonstrated that most of the cells of this structure are sensitive either to stimulus orientation or to the direction of stimulus movement. Moreover, Petersen et al. (1985) found that, in addition to the properties described by Bender, pulvinar (PLI and PLL) neurons have eye movement modulation, and a particular dorsomedial subdivision of PLL also has attentional modulation. PLI and PLL then receive a parallel input from visual sensory structures which may account for the characteristic responsiveness of their neurons. This leads us to believe that these subdivisions are stations of a mainly sensorial cortico-thalamo-cortical parallel system, especially related to functions for detecting moving visual stimuli as well as the orientation of visual attention. The new issue is the contribution of fibers given to this system by AMST.

An outstanding result of this work is the finding that AMST, besides sending efferents to PLI and PLL, also projects to PLM, a pulvinar subdivision formerly excluded from the visual system. Several reports have shown that PLM is reciprocally connected with the dorsal prefrontal cortex (PFC), that includes the frontal eye field (FEF) (Trojanowsky and Jacobson 1974, 1976; Barbas and Mesulam 1981; Leichnetz 1981). Furthermore it receives some input from the deep layers of the SC (Benevento and Fallon 1975), the same layers that receive axons from FEF (Astruc 1971; Leichnetz 1981). Interestingly, in our cases, with injections in AMST, we found dense labels in the dorsal PFC, in a region much larger than that seen after injections in the MT (Maioli et al. 1983b). These projections affected, with distinct patches of terminals, not only both banks of arcuate sulcus and the gyrus in front of it but also the caudal part of the principal sulcus. Furthermore, in the same cases we saw labels also in the intermediate and deep layers of SC (unpublished observations). This suggests that, apart from other sources, PFC may receive visual signals, also from cortical visual fields such as the AMST, both directly and through the thalamic − SC influenced − relay of PLM. On the whole, deep SC, PLM, FEF and AMST are all reciprocally interconnected in an anatomical network.

Comments made for PLM seem to apply to other thalamic targets of frontal AMST, i.e., MD, SG, and intralaminar nuclei Pc, CL and CM, in that they all receive afferents from deep layers of SC and are reciprocally connected with the prefrontal cortex (PFC). The MD has one of its main targets in PFC, including the FEF (Tobias 1975; Trojanowsky and Jacobson 1976) and receives fibers from this cortex (Astruc 1971; Kunzle and Akert 1977). Additionally, it also receives afferents from the deep layers of the superior colliculus (Harting et al. 1980). Also SG contributes fibers to PFC (Trojanowsky and Jacobson 1976; Leichnetz 1982) and an input to SG from deep SC has been described (Benevento and Fallon 1975). The ILN are reciprocally connected with PFC (Astruc 1971; Kunzle and Akert 1977; Barbas and Mesulam 1981; Leichnetz 1981), and receive afferents from deep SC (Benevento and Fallon 1975; Harting et al. 1980). Accordingly, these non-pulvinar thalamic nuclei appear to be part of the network that has been described which interconnects SC, PLM, PFC and AMST.

The pattern of interconnections of PLM, ILN, SG and MD with PFC is similar to the scheme of the connections of these nuclei with the inferior parietal lobule (area 7). In fact, this area, in the macaque, besides being reciprocally connected with the dorsal PFC (Mesulam et al. 1977; Barbas and Mesulam 1981) is also reciprocally linked with PLM (De Vito and Simmons 1976; Divac et al. 1977; Mauguière and Baleydier 1978) and sends fibers to ILN, SG and MD (De Vito and Simmons 1976; Divac et al. 1977). It is worth mentioning that we found direct projections from AMST to a region of the inferior parietal lobule closely resembling that which, according to Lynch et al. (1985), sends fibers to the deep layers of the SC

(Squatrito et al. in preparation). In summary, the thalamic nuclei PLM, ILN, SG and MD, all receiving afferents from AMST and deep layers of SC, show a common set of connections with the dorsal part of PFC and with area 7. Figure 5 summarizes these observations, emphasizing the broad parallelism of the connections discussed.

We still know little about the specific functional role of each of these structures. Nevertheless, there are consistent pieces of information suggesting that some of them have functional features in common: the dorsal PFC and deep layers of the SC play a key role in the neural control of voluntary initiation of saccadic eye movements (Schiller et al.

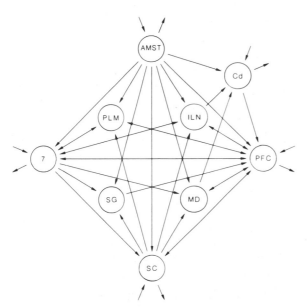

Fig. 5. Possible network of tele-diencephalic interconnections in macaque. The drawing summarizes the intricate interconnections linking some thalamic nuclei targets of AMST to other cortical and subcortical structures involved in initiation of saccades and direction of attention. Note the common connections of these thalamic nuclei with both PFC and area 7. Note also the common ascending and descending paths from SC and AMST respectively. Short arrows lacking the second target suggest the presence of several other channels of input and output to and from this network, according to the theoretical model of a parallel distributed system. PFC in this scheme refers to the dorsal part of the prefrontal cortex. Similarly, SC is restricted to the deep layers of the superior colliculus and ILN refers to the intralaminar nuclei Pc, CL and CM. 7, area 7. Other abbreviations as in previous legends.

1980), and PFC and area 7 are associated both with the occurrence of elicited saccades, and the direction of visual attention toward a target (Lynch et al. 1977; Mountcastle 1981; Bruce and Goldberg 1985). In addition, some neurons of ILN have been found to be directionally selective and to fire during and before saccadic eye movements (Schlag and Schlag-Rey 1984), We lack detailed information on the functions of PLM, MD and SG in monkeys but the described interconnections with the deep layers of the SC, the dorsal part of PFC and area 7 suggest some involvement of these nuclei in oculomotor and attentional mechanisms.

The mentioned visual connections of ILN call into play other non-thalamic complementary pathways to these circuits passing through the basal ganglia, a major ILN-recipient structure. Involvement of this telencephalic formation in visual processes has been suggested by the connectionally-based finding that the tail and body of the caudate nucleus of the macaque evidently receive input from the MT area (Maioli et al. 1983a; Ungerleider et al. 1984). In addition, we have found that AMST projects over a wider area of the basal ganglia than does MT, affecting not only the tail and body, but also part of the head of the caudate (unpublished observations). Recently, it was demonstrated that firing of neurons of the caudate nucleus precedes saccadic eye movements directed to a target (Hikosaka and Sakamoto 1986), thus confirming the anatomical suggestion of there being some participation of basal ganglia in visual functions. Thus, cortical visual messages relevant for oculomotor and attentional functions come from MT and AMST to reach PFC, besides other pathways, and also route through caudate or ILN-caudate intermediation. Incidentally, also the MD contributes fibers to the head of caudate nucleus (Tobias 1975), adding one more element to the circuits connecting these related structures. The position of AMST in this complex circuit seems particularly relevant. In fact, since it is connected with the MT area as well as with PLI and PLL, and it distributes efferents to several structures engaged in the neural circuits controlling eye movements and the direction of attention, it must act as some cortical link between sensory visual and oculomotor attentive functions.

Projections from MT and AMST to PG would appear to be extraneous to these circuits. Although PG is related to saccadic eye movements (Buttner and Fuchs 1973), and inputs from SC (Benevento and Fallon 1975; Harting et al. 1980) and STS visual areas (Maunsell and Van Essen 1983b; Maioli et al. 1984) might reflect this involvement, it lacks connections, however, with cortical area 7 or PFC, as well as with other subcortical structures related to attentive behavior.

A final remarkable result is the finding of projections from AMST to LD. This nucleus is a 'gate' for the limbic system and has been shown to be a way of introducing visual signals arising from both prestriate cortex (Benevento and Davis 1977) and the retina (Itaya et al. 1986) to limbic structures. It is significant that projections from AMST to LD are paralleled by associative fibers arising from the same area to the cingulate gyrus (Squatrito et al., in preparation). These pathways therefore may be part of the interface linking limbic functions to attentional processes.

Comparison with cats

The main reciprocal projection link with cortex of the LP-pulvinar complex in cats is the lateral suprasylvian visual area (LSVA). Attempts to delineate in detail the connections between individual subregions of the LP-pulvinar complex and the several subareas of LSVA have shown that there is a wide overlap of the cortical projections to the thalamus, but significant quantitative differences do exist. From a very general point of view the posteromedial (PMLS) and the anteromedial (AMLS) lateral suprasylvian areas are preferentially connected with the pulvinar and the more laterally-situated portions of the nucleus lateralis posterior (LP), while the posterolateral (PLLS) and anterolateral (ALLS) areas are preferentially connected with the more medially-situated parts of LP (Updyke 1981). This general

subdivision has a correspondence in the collicular connections of this cortical region, in that the lateral bank of the middle suprasylvian sulcus is preferentially connected with the deep layers of the SC, whereas the medial bank privileges the connections with the superficial layers (Segal and Beckstead 1984). These considerations would lead us to think of the medial-most part of the LP complex as the analogue of the medial pulvinar of the monkeys. Consequently, the lateral bank of the medial suprasylvian sulcus of the cat might be the analogue of the MST area of the macaque. One difference between the two systems is that there are no described connections between the medial portions of LP and FEF in the cat, and projections from the LSVA to frontal cortex are limited to the ventral bank of cruciate sulcus (Battaglini et al. 1980), considered a supplementary FEF (see Hartwich-Young and Weber 1986). On the other hand, the extreme medial portion of LP, which is connected with the deepest layers of SC, has its main cortical target in the anterior ectosylvian visual area (AEV), abundantly connected with the main part of FEF in the presylvian sulcus (Norita et al. 1986). Thus, if we restrict the analogy of monkey PLM to the part of LP connected with the deep SC, we should associate AEV with AMST. This view would be supported also by the fact that AMST is, by definition, the main forward corticocortical target of MT, just as AEV is the main forward target of LSVA (Squatrito et al. 1981; Mucke et al. 1982). These speculations are not conclusive and the whole matter appears to need more evidence to be solved.

As to the other, non-LP, thalamic nuclei involved in the described circuits, there is a wide range of reports that demonstrate in the cat, circuits and functions similar to those outlined in this paper for the monkey. Intralaminar nuclei of the cat have been proved to receive fibers from the intermediate and deep layers of the SC (Graham 1977; Kaufman and Rosenquist 1985b), and to project to the FEF (see Kaufman and Rosenquist 1985a, for refs). Involvement of these nuclei with eye movements and attentive behavior has also been consistently

described (Schlag-Rey and Schlag 1977). Cats'
MD, whose involvement in visual functions is suggested by its afferents from areas 18, 19 and 20
(Markowitsch et al. 1982), receives, in its lateral
portion, fibers from deep SC and sends projections
to FEF (Velayos and Reinoso-Suárez 1982). SG
shows also a set of similar connections since it
receives some input from intermediate and deep
SC (Graham 1977; Hicks et al. 1986) and projects
to AEV (Norita et al. 1986). It is significant that
visual responsive neurons in cat SG, being especially sensitive to high stimulus velocities, have been
interpreted as functionally related to saccadic eye
movements and attentional behavior (Hicks et al.
1984). It seems from these considerations that also
in the cat, as in the monkey, a set of cortical and
thalamic structures functionally related to similar
tasks, are interconnected.

Conclusions

The pieces of evidence highlighted in this paper
suggest that the extrageniculo-striate corticothalamic system involving the superior temporal
cortex is an intimate part of a complex network of
functional units. This system might supply signals
carrying information on the location and direction
of visual stimuli to the circuits controlling voluntary eye movements and, most likely, some form
of visual attention. Figure 5 summarizes the circuits that may form part of the anatomical basis of
these functions in the macaque. It is evident how
these functionally-related structures are connected
in parallel, suggesting that the functions must be
processed in this way.

It should be pointed out that the picture is not
intended to be exhaustive of all the possible interconnections between the units that cooperate in
these functions, neither does it imply that all these
structures participate equally and unspecifically in
all aspects of the functions they process. Preferential circuits in this framework might be activated in
relation to specific aspects of the broad field of
visual functions discussed in this paper. In this
respect a weak point of this scheme is that some of

the units in the circuits are too wide to be considered as units. Structures such as PFC, MD,
AMST and so on, will probably be subdivided into
a number of functional modules on the basis of
physiological and anatomical criteria. Moreover,
although a lot of these parallel connections have
broad overlapping regions on the target areas, we
do not know to what extent they impinge upon the
same neurons, nor what is the internal connectivity
of each module. The picture in Fig. 5 has to be
taken as a working scheme, to be further completed and detailed. Rather than to suggest specific
operations, it tends to stimulate more research in
the direction of the parallel distributed processing
models of the visual system.

References

Astruc, J. (1971) Corticofugal connections of area 8 (frontal
eye field) in *Macaca mulatta*. *Brain Res.*, 33: 241 – 256.
Barbas, H. and Mesulam, M.M. (1981) Organization of af-
ferent input to subdivisions of area 8 in the rhesus monkey.
J. Comp. Neurol., 200: 407 – 431.
Battaglini, P.P., Squatrito, S., Galletti, C., Maioli, M.G. and
Riva Sanseverino, E. (1980) Autoradiographic evidence of
visual cortical projections to the frontal cortex in the cat.
Arch. Ital. Biol., 118: 189 – 195.
Bender, D.B. (1982) Receptive-field properties of neurons in the
macaque inferior pulvinar. *J. Neurophysiol.*, 48: 1 – 17.
Benevento, L.A. and Davis, B. (1977) Topographical projections of the prestriate cortex to the pulvinar nuclei in the
macaque monkey: an autoradiographic study. *Exp. Brain
Res.*, 30: 405 – 424.
Benevento, L.A. and Fallon, J. (1975) The ascending projections of the superior colliculus in the rhesus monkey (*Macaca
mulatta*). *J. Comp. Neurol.*, 160: 339 – 362.
Benevento, L.A. and Rezak, M. (1976) The cortical projections
of the inferior pulvinar and adjacent lateral pulvinar in the
rhesus monkey (*Macaca mulatta*): an autoradiographic
study. *Brain Res.*, 108: 1 – 24.
Bruce, C.J. and Goldberg, M.E. (1985) Primate frontal eye
fields. Single neurons discharging before saccades. *J.
Neurophysiol.*, 53: 603 – 635.
Buttner, U. and Fuchs, A.F. (1973) Influence of saccadic eye
movements on unit activity in simian lateral geniculate and
pregeniculate nuclei. *J. Neurophysiol.*, 36: 127 – 141.
Campos-Ortega, J.A., Haỹhow, W.R. and Cluver, de V. (1970)
A note on the problem of retinal projections to the inferior
pulvinar nucleus of primates. *Brain Res.*, 22: 126 – 130.
Carpenter, M.B. and Pierson, R.J. (1973) Pretectal region and

pupillary light reflex. An analysis in the monkey. *J. Comp. Neurol.*, 149: 271–300.

Desimone, R. and Ungerleider, L.G. (1986) Multiple visual areas in the caudal superior temporal sulcus of the macaque. *J. Comp. Neurol.*, 248: 164–189.

De Vito, J.L. and Simmons, D.M. (1976) Some connection of the posterior thalamus in monkey. *Exp. Neurol.*, 51: 347–362.

Divac, I., LaVail, J.H., Rakic, P. and Winston, K.R. (1977) Heterogeneous afferents to the inferior parietal lobule of the rhesus monkey revealed by retrograde transport method. *Brain Res.*, 123: 197–207.

Graham, J. (1977) An autoradiographic study of the efferent connections of the superior colliculus in the cat. *J. Comp. Neurol.*, 173: 629–654.

Harting, J.K., Huerta, M.F., Frankfurter, A.J., Strominger, N.L. and Royce, G.J. (1980) Ascending pathways from the monkey superior colliculus: an autoradiographic analysis. *J. Comp. Neurol.*, 192: 853–882.

Hartwich-Young, R. and Weber, J.T. (1986) The projection of frontal cortical oculomotor areas to the superior colliculus in the domestic cat. *J. Comp. Neurol.*, 253: 342–357.

Hicks, T.P., Watanabe, S., Miyake, A. and Shoumura, K. (1984) Organization and properties of visually responsive neurones in the suprageniculate nucleus of the cat. *Exp. Brain Res.*, 55: 359–367.

Hicks, T.P., Stark, C.A. and Fletcher, W.A. (1986) Origins of afferents to visual suprageniculate nucleus of the cat. *J. Comp. Neurol.*, 246: 544–554.

Hikosaka, O. and Sakamoto, M. (1986) Cell activity in monkey caudate nucleus preceding saccadic eye movements. *Exp. Brain Res.*, 63: 659–662.

Itaya, S.K., Van Hoesen, G.W. and Benevento, L.A. (1986) Direct retinal pathways to the limbic thalamus of the monkey. *Exp. Brain Res.*, 61: 607–613.

Kaufman, E.F.S. and Rosenquist, A.C. (1985a) Efferent projections of the thalamic intralaminar nuclei in the cat. *Brain Res.*, 335: 257-279.

Kaufman, E.F.S. and Rosenquist, A.C. (1985b) Afferent connections of the thalamic intralaminar nuclei in the cat. *Brain Res.*, 335: 281–296.

Kunzle, H. and Akert, K. (1977) Efferent connections of cortical area 8 (frontal eye field) in *Macaca fascicularis*. A reinvestigation using the autoradiographic technique. *J. Comp. Neurol.*, 173: 147–164.

Leichnetz, G.R. (1981) The prefrontal cortico-oculomotor trajectories in the monkey. *J. Neurol. Sci.*, 49: 387–396.

Leichnetz, G.R. (1982) Connections between the frontal eye field and pretectum in the monkey: an anterograde/retrograde study using HRP gel and TMB neurochemistry. *J. Comp. Neurol.*, 207: 394–402.

Lynch, J.C., Mountcastle, V.B., Talbot, W.H. and Yin, T.C.T. (1977) Parietal lobe mechanisms for directed visual attention. *J. Neurophysiol.*, 40: 362–389.

Lynch, J.C., Graybiel, A.M. and Lobeck, L.J. (1985) The differential projection of two cytoarchitectonic subregions of the inferior parietal lobule of macaque upon the deep layers of the superior colliculus. *J. Comp. Neurol.*, 235: 241–254.

Maioli, M.G., Squatrito, S., Battaglini, P.P., Rossi, R. and Galletti, C. (1983a) Projections from the visual cortical region of the superior temporal sulcus to the striatum and claustrum in the macaque monkey. *Arch. Ital. Biol.*, 121: 259–266.

Maioli, M.G., Squatrito, S., Galletti, C., Battaglini, P.P. and Riva Sanseverino, E. (1983b) Cortico-cortical connections from the visual region of the superior temporal sulcus to frontal eye field in the macaque. *Brain Res.*, 265: 294–299.

Maioli, M.G., Galletti, C., Squatrito, S., Battaglini, P.P. and Riva Sanseverino, E. (1984) Projections from the cortex of the superior temporal sulcus to the dorsal lateral geniculate and pregeniculate nuclei in the macaque monkey. *Arch. Ital. Biol.*, 122: 301–309.

Markowitsch, H.J., Irle, E. and Streicher, M. (1982) The thalamic mediodorsal nucleus receives input from thalamic and cortical regions related to vision. *Neurosci. Lett.*, 32: 131–136.

Mauguière, F. and Baleydier, C. (1978) Topographical organization of medial pulvinar neurons sending fibres to Brodmann's areas 7, 21 and 22 in the monkey. *Exp. Brain Res.*, 31: 605–607.

Maunsell, J.H.R. and Van Essen, D.C. (1983a) Functional properties of neurons in middle temporal visual area of the macaque monkey. I. Selectivity for stimulus direction, speed and orientation. *J. Neurophysiol.*, 49: 1127–1147.

Maunsell, J.H.R. and Van Essen, D.C. (1983b) The connections of the middle temporal visual area (MT) and their relationship to a cortical hierarchy in the macaque monkey. *J. Neurosci.*, 3: 2563–2586.

Mesulam, M.M., Van Hoesen, G.W., Pandya, D.N. and Geshwind, N. (1977) Limbic and sensory connections of the inferior parietal lobule (area PG) in the rhesus monkey: a study with a new method for horseradish histochemistry. *Brain Res.*, 136: 393–414.

Mizuno, N., Itoh, K., Uchida, K., Uemura-Sumi, M. and Matsushima, R. (1982) A retino-pulvinar projection in the macaque monkey as visualized by the use of anterograde transport of horseradish peroxidase. *Neurosci. Lett.*, 30: 199–203.

Mountcastle, V.B. (1981) Functional properties of the light-sensitive neurons of the posterior parietal cortex and their regulation by state controls: influence on excitability of interested fixation and the angle of gaze. In: O. Pompeiano and C. Ajmone Marsan (Eds.), *Brain Mechanisms of Perceptual Awareness and Purposeful Behavior*, Raven Press, New York, pp. 67–106.

Mountcastle, V.B. (1982) An organizing principle for cerebral function: the unit module and the distributed system. In: G.E. Edelman and V.B. Mountcastle (Eds.), *The Mindful Brain*, MIT Press, Cambridge, MA, pp. 7–50.

Mucke, L., Norita, M., Benedek, G. and Creutzfeldt, O. (1982) Physiologic and anatomic investigation of a visual cortical area situated in the ventral bank of the anterior ectosylvian sulcus of the cat. *Exp. Brain Res.*, 46: 1 – 11.

Norita, M. and Katoh, Y. (1986) Cortical and tectal afferent terminals in the suprageniculate nucleus of the cat. *Neurosci. Lett.*, 65: 104 – 108.

Norita, M., Mucke, L., Benedek, G., Albowitz, B., Katoh, Y. and Creutzfeldt, O.D. (1986) Connections of the anterior ectosylvian visual area (AEV). *Exp. Brain Res.*, 62: 225 – 240.

Ogren, M.P. and Hendrickson, A.E. (1976) Pathways between striate cortex and subcortical regions in *Macaca mulatta* and *Saimiri sciureus*: evidence for a reciprocal pulvinar connection. *Exp. Neurol.*, 53: 780 – 800.

Petersen, S.E., Robinson, D.L. and Keys, W. (1985) Pulvinar nuclei of behaving rhesus monkey: visual responses and their modulation. *J. Neurophysiol.*, 54: 867 – 886.

Schiller, P.H., True, S.D. and Conway, J.L. (1980) Deficits in eye movements following frontal eye-field and superior colliculus ablations. *J. Neurophysiol.*, 44: 1175 – 1189.

Schlag, J. and Schlag-Rey, M. (1984) Visuomotor functions of central thalamus in monkey. II. Unit activity related to visual events, targeting and fixation. *J. Neurophysiol.*, 51: 1175 – 1195.

Schlag-Rey, M. and Schlag, J. (1977) Visual and presaccadic neuronal activity in thalamic internal medullary lamina of cat: a study of targeting, *J. Neurophysiol.*, 40: 156 – 173.

Segal, R.L. and Beckstead, R.M. (1984) The lateral suprasylvian corticotectal projection in cats. *J. Comp. Neurol.*, 225: 259 – 275.

Squatrito, S., Galletti, C., Maioli, M.G. and Battaglini, P.P. (1981) Cortical visual input to the orbito-insular cortex in the cat. *Brain Res.*, 221: 71 – 79.

Standage, G.P. and Benevento, L.A. (1983) The organization of connections between the pulvinar and visual area MT in the macaque monkey. *Brain Res.*, 262: 288 – 294.

Tobias, T.J. (1975) Afferents to prefrontal cortex from the thalamic mediodorsal nucleus in the rhesus monkey. *Brain Res.*, 83: 191 – 212.

Trojanowsky, J.Q. and Jacobson, S. (1974) Medial pulvinar afferents to frontal eye fields in rhesus monkey demonstrated by horseradish peroxidase. *Brain Res.*, 80: 395 – 411.

Trojanowsky, J.Q. and Jacobson, S. (1976) Areal and laminar distribution of some pulvinar cortical efferents in rhesus monkey. *J. Comp. Neurol.*, 169: 371 – 392.

Ungerleider, L.G., Desimone, R., Galkin, T.W. and Mishkin, M. (1984) Subcortical projections of area MT in the macaque. *J. Comp. Neurol.*, 223: 368 – 386.

Updyke, B.V. (1981) Projections from visual areas of the middle suprasylvian sulcus onto the lateral posterior complex and adjacent thalamic nuclei in cat. *J. Comp. Neurol.*, 201: 477 – 506.

Van Essen, D.C., Maunsell, J.H.R. and Bixby, J.L. (1981) The middle temporal visual area in the macaque: Myeloarchitecture, connections, functional properties and topographic organization. *J. Comp. Neurol.*, 199: 293 – 326.

Velayos, J.L. and Reinoso-Suárez, F. (1982) Topographic organization of the brainstem afferents to the mediodorsal thalamic nucleus. *J. Comp. Neurol.*, 206: 17 – 27.

Zeki, S.M. (1974) Functional organization of a visual area in the posterior bank of the superior temporal sulcus of the rhesus monkey. *J. Physiol. (Lond.)*, 236: 549 – 573.

T.P. Hicks and G. Benedek (Eds.)
Progress in Brain Research, Vol. 75
© 1988 Elsevier Science Publishers B.V. (Biomedical Division)

CHAPTER 27

Two cortical visual systems in Old World and New World primates

Rosalyn E. Weller

Department of Psychology, 201 Campbell Hall, University of Alabama at Birmingham, Birmingham, AL 35294, U.S.A.

Introduction

Two quite different syndromes are seen in humans with damage to posterior parietal cortex and inferior temporal cortex (for review, see Mountcastle et al. 1975; Levine 1982; Maunsell and Van Essen 1987). Patients with posterior parietal lobe injury have visual impairments in tracking, localizing, and even noticing stimuli. Injury to inferior temporal cortex, in contrast, results in visual agnosia, a deficit in recognizing visual stimuli. Deficits similar to these are also found in macaque monkeys with ablations of posterior parietal or inferior temporal cortex (for review, see Mishkin 1966; Gross et al. 1972; Ungerleider and Mishkin 1982). The visual impairments seen in humans and macaque monkeys have led to the suggestion that posterior parietal cortex is specialized in primates for spatial perception, or locating *where* an object is, and inferior temporal cortex is specialized for object perception, or identifying *what* an object is (Mishkin 1972; Pohl 1973; but see Maunsell and Van Essen 1987).

Receptive field properties of neurons in posterior parietal and inferior temporal cortex of macaque monkeys support their hypothesized functions (e.g., Gross et al. 1972; Hyvärinen and Poranen 1974; Desimone and Gross 1979). Neurons in posterior parietal cortex have large receptive fields that emphasize peripheral vision and are most responsive to moving stimuli. They

are relatively insensitive to variations in stimulus shape and form. In contrast, neurons in inferior temporal cortex have large receptive fields that invariably include the fovea and are selectively responsive to visual stimuli of particular shapes or forms.

Visual cortex is divided into multiple subdivisions, or areas, in the brains of advanced mammals such as primates. Each visual area has a distinctive and complex pattern of cortical connections. A valuable insight was the observation made by Ungerleider and Mishkin (1982) that connections between areas of visual cortex in macaque monkeys form two major diverging pathways. Both pathways originate at the level of cortex from striate cortex. One pathway relays through a number of areas rostral to striate cortex and terminates in cortex of the posterior parietal lobe. The other pathway relays through a number of (largely) different areas and terminates in inferior temporal cortex. Both posterior parietal and inferior temporal cortex depend for their normal functioning on the visual input they receive from striate cortex, which is, with minor exception, the sole target of the retinogeniculate system in primates (e.g., Hendrickson et al. 1978). This dependence has been most conclusively demonstrated in macaque monkeys. Preventing the relay of visual information from striate cortex to either inferior temporal or posterior parietal cortex produces a deficit as severe as that found after damage to inferior temporal or posterior parietal cortex itself (Mishkin 1966; Mishkin and Ungerleider 1982).

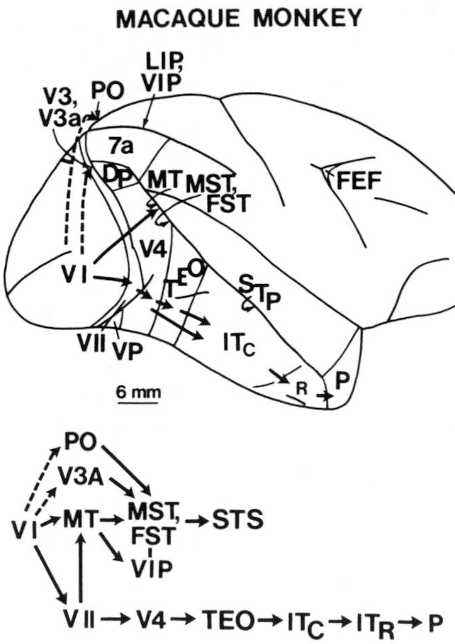

MACAQUE MONKEY

Fig. 1. Subdivisions of visual cortex of macaque monkeys and some of their connections. Locations and borders of areas are taken from Desimone and Gross (1979), Van Essen (1979, 1985), Spiegler and Mishkin (1981), and Maunsell and Newsome (1987). Small arrows indicate the locations of areas not visible on the lateral view of cortex. Large arrows indicate projections that terminate in a 'feedforward' laminar pattern (see text). Dashed lines represent sparser connections. Connections shown on the lateral view of the brain at top are also shown more fully below in 'two cortical visual systems' format. The connections between MST and FST, and VIP, are represented by a line rather than an arrow because they have an 'intermediate' laminar pattern. The connections shown for V4 are for parts of V4 representing central, not peripheral, vision. For simplicity, some connections are not shown; these are projections from foveal V I to V4, from V I to V3, V3 to both MT and V4, and MST and FST to LIP. Although IT cortex has traditionally been considered a single area in macaques (distinct, however, from area TEO), it appears to contain at least caudal (C) and rostral (R) subdivisions. DP, dorsal prelunate area; FEF, frontal eye field; FST, an area found in the fundus of the superior temporal sulcus; IT$_C$ and $_R$, caudal and rostral subdivisions of inferior temporal cortex (IT; both together correspond to area TE of von Bonin and Bailey 1947); LIP, lateral intraparietal area; MST, medial superior temporal area; P, polar cortex; PO, parieto-occipital area; STP, superior temporal polysensory area; STS, superior temporal sulcus, which includes but is not limited to area STP; VIP, ventral intraparietal area; VP, ventroposterior area. See text for details.

When Ungerleider and Mishkin (1982) formulated the 'two cortical visual systems' concept, many details were lacking about the courses of the two pathways. Subsequent anatomical experiments done in macaque monkeys over the past five years have revealed connections that support and extend their scheme (for review, see Van Essen 1985; Ungerleider and Desimone 1986; Maunsell and Newsome 1987). Some of the new anatomical information, however, also indicates that the two systems are not completely separate.

Multiple areas of visual cortex are also found in other primates, and some of these areas are undoubtedly homologous to areas found in macaques. The presence of some of the same visual areas in different primates raises the possibility that these areas may also have similar connections. An obvious question is, how general is the parallel processing scheme described for macaque monkeys? Do these pathways exist in all primates, or only in certain groups? The answer to this question is not only of interest for comparative issues, but can also be used to infer the evolutionary origin of the pathways in the primate lineages.

In order to address the question asked above, we need to examine visual cortical connections in a range of primates. This chapter describes results of anatomical studies done in Old World macaque monkeys; in three different species of New World monkeys, owl monkeys, squirrel monkeys, and marmosets; and in an Old World prosimian primate, galago. Similarities in the connections of visual cortex in these distantly related primates suggest that two cortical visual systems exist in all primates. The existence of a similar pattern of connections in prosimians also suggests that these cortical systems arose early in the evolution of primates.

The organization of visual cortex in macaque monkeys

The subdivisions of visual cortex of macaque monkeys and some of their connections are shown in Fig. 1. Almost twenty visual areas have been described in the cortex of macaque monkeys (for review, see Van Essen 1979, 1985; Weller and Kaas 1981; Maunsell and Newsome 1987). Areas V I, V II (V2), V3, VP, V3A, V4, MT, and PO have been electrophysiologically mapped. Other areas, such as MST, VIP, and STP, are defined on the basis of distinctive receptive field characteristics or patterns of connections. If all the known connections between visual areas were shown in Fig. 1, the result would be an extremely complex and difficult to interpret wiring diagram that might suggest that all areas are connected to almost all others. However, a simplifying principle was used to illustrate connections in Fig. 1 and subsequent figures. With one or two exceptions explained in the text, the only connections shown (large arrows) are those known to terminate in layer IV of cortex. This laminar pattern is assumed to indicate that one area is providing 'feedforward', or the primary activating input, to another area (Tigges et al. 1977, 1981; Wong-Riley 1978; Rockland and Pandya 1979; Weller and Kaas 1981; Maunsell and Van Essen 1983). In contrast, projections that terminate in layers superficial and deep to layer IV, but not in IV, are assumed to provide 'feedback' or 'modulatory' input to an area. These latter connections are not shown in the figures. The laminar locations of cells sending cortical projections have also been used to characterize pathways as feedforward or feedback, with cells located predominantly in superficial layers thought to provide feedforward connections and cells located predominantly in infragranular layers or in both supra- and infragranular layers thought to provide feedback connections (Wong-Riley 1978; Rockland and Pandya 1979; Tigges et al. 1981).

Because the two cortical pathways have been previously described in detail for macaque monkeys (Ungerleider and Mishkin 1982; Ungerleider and Desimone 1986; Maunsell and Newsome 1987), they will be described here only briefly, with emphasis placed on recently discovered connections. Both pathways originate at the level of cortex from striate cortex. (The two pathways may, in fact, originate before the level of cortex, in the X and Y ganglion cells of the retina; Maunsell and Newsome 1987; Weller and Kaas

1987). All parts of striate cortex project to V2 and MT (Kuypers et al. 1965; Cragg and Ainsworth 1969; Zeki 1969; Jones and Powell 1970; Rockland and Pandya 1979; Ungerleider and Mishkin 1979; Weller and Kaas 1983; Van Essen et al. 1986). It is actually different populations of cells in V I that relay to V2 and MT (for review, see Maunsell and Newsome 1987). Striate cortex representing the lower visual hemifield also projects to V3, foveal striate cortex also projects to V4, and peripheral V I projects to V3A and PO (Zeki 1978, 1980; Colby et al. 1983; Van Essen et al. 1986). All of these projections terminate with a feedforward laminar pattern.

The major targets of V2 are V3, V4, and MT (Zeki 1971; Ungerleider et al. 1983; Felleman and Van Essen 1983). Thus, V2, like V I, projects to areas belonging to both the parietal and temporal pathways (see below). The projections to V4 and MT, at least, originate from separate subsets of cells in V2 (DeYoe and Van Essen 1985; Shipp and Zeki 1985). V3 also appears to be involved in both the parietal and temporal pathways, because it projects in a feedforward pattern to both MT and V4 (Felleman and Van Essen 1983; Ungerleider and Desimone 1986).

V4 is the only target of V2 known to project to inferior temporal cortex. It does so, in a feedforward manner, both directly and indirectly through a relay in TEO (Seltzer and Pandya 1978; Desimone et al. 1980; Felleman and Van Essen 1983; Felleman et al. 1986). The additional relay in TEO is included only when projections originate from parts of V4 representing the central visual field (Ungerleider et al. 1986). V4 also projects to cortex in ventral inferior temporal cortex (architectonic area TF) and provides a feedback projection to V2 (Felleman and Van Essen 1983; Ungerleider et al. 1986). Parts of V4 representing the peripheral visual field have somewhat different connections than those just described. Peripheral V4 provides a stronger projection to TF and also projects to areas related to the posterior parietal pathway (areas V3A, DP, VIP, and PO; see below; Ungerleider et al. 1986).

Although 'IT', the area coextensive with architectonic area TE of von Bonin and Bailey (1947), has traditionally been considered a single area in macaque monkeys, an increasing amount of evidence suggests that it contains at least caudal and rostral subdivisions (e.g., Bolster and Crowne 1979; Desimone and Gross 1979; Felleman et al. 1986; see Weller and Kaas 1987, for review). Anatomical evidence in support of these subdivisions is that V4 projects to caudal but not rostral IT, caudal IT projects to rostral IT, and rostral IT projects to polar cortex (Seltzer and Pandya 1978; Felleman and Van Essen 1983).

When Ungerleider and Mishkin (1982) presented their dual processing model, little was known about how visual information reached posterior parietal cortex. We now know that this pathway involves MT and its targets, as well as some of the areas that receive minor projections from striate cortex. The major feedforward projections of MT are to two areas that border it in the superior temporal sulcus, MST and FST, and to an area in the intraparietal sulcus of posterior parietal cortex, VIP (Maunsell and Van Essen 1983b; Ungerleider and Desimone 1986). Other targets of MT projections are V I, V2, V3, VP, V4, V3A, perhaps PO, and, weakly, the frontal eye field. Projections to V I, V2, V3, and VP are of the feedback type, while those to V4, V3A, and PO have a columnar laminar pattern, characterized by Maunsell and Van Essen (1983b) as 'intermediate' to feedforward and feedback.

The connections of MST and FST have been recently described (Boussaoud et al. 1987). MST and FST receive input from MT, V3A, TF, and, for MST only, PO and the cingulate gyrus. MST and FST have strong feedforward projections to areas further rostral in the superior temporal sulcus, which appear to include STP. MST and FST also possess major connections with VIP and LIP, as well as with surrounding areas of posterior parietal cortex. The laminar patterns of connections between MST-FST and VIP-LIP are of the 'intermediate' type (Boussaoud et al. 1987). MST and FST also have connections with the frontal eye field, and weak and inconsistently observed connections with V4, TEO, the caudal sylvian fissure, and area 7a.

The physiological significance of the anatomical pathways relaying to posterior parietal and inferior temporal cortex can be seen in the similarities between the receptive field properties of neurons in posterior parietal cortex and in MT, MST, and STP, and between those of neurons in inferior temporal cortex and V4 (Bruce et al. 1981; Newsome and Wurtz 1982; Maunsell and Van Essen 1983a; Saito et al. 1986; Desimone and Schein 1987).

In summary, the pathway from striate cortex to inferior temporal cortex involves V2, V3, central V4, and TEO. The relay from striate cortex to posterior parietal cortex also involves V2 and V3, as well as peripheral V4, MT, and targets of MT. MT projects to bordering areas in the superior temporal sulcus, MST and FST, and to VIP of posterior parietal cortex. MST and FST, in turn, are connected (although not in a feedforward pattern) with VIP, LIP, and other unidentified areas of posterior parietal cortex. MST and FST project in a feedforward pattern to more rostral cortex in the superior temporal sulcus, which includes STP by location. Areas V3A and PO, which receive projections from striate cortex, also project to MST and FST.

Thus, details about visual cortex connections learned from macaque monkeys during the past 5 years support in general the two cortical systems model of Ungerleider and Mishkin (1982), but also show that pathways to posterior parietal and inferior temporal cortex are not dichotomous. In fact, because some areas participate in both pathways (albeit, in the instances examined, via separate populations of cells) and connections are not strictly 'parallel' in form, it seems inappropriate to continue using the term 'parallel' to describe the relay of information from striate to posterior parietal and inferior temporal cortex.

The organization of visual cortex in owl monkeys

Next to macaque monkeys, our understanding of primate visual cortex is most complete for New World owl monkeys. For studies of visual cortex, owl monkeys offer the advantages of having a relatively smooth neocortex and of being nocturnal. This latter feature simplifies visual mapping experiments, because nocturnal animals lack the overemphasis on central vision found in diurnal animals. Over the past 15 years, an extensive series of electrophysiological and anatomical studies in the owl monkey have elucidated much of the organization of its visual cortex. Thus, the owl

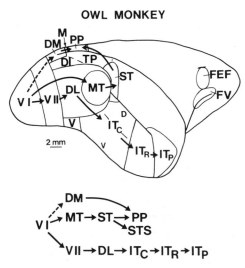

Fig. 2. Subdivisions of visual cortex of owl monkeys and some of their connections. Areas V I, V II, DL, MT, DM, and M were defined in physiological mapping studies (Allman and Kaas 1971, 1974a,b, 1975, 1976); for delineation of other areas, see text. The location of M is indicated where it would be found on the medial wall. A dashed line crosses IT_C where it appears subdivided into dorsal (D) and ventral (V) areas (Weller and Kaas 1987). Not shown are the feedforward projections of ST to the caudal sylvian fissure and IT_M. DI, dorsointermediate area; DL, dorsolateral area; DM, dorsomedial area; FV, frontal visual area; IT_C, IT_R, and IT_P, the caudal, rostral, and polar subdivisions of inferior temporal cortex (only IT_C and IT_R are coextensive with architectonic area TE of von Bonin and Bailey 1947); M, medial area, PP, posterior parietal cortex; ST, superior temporal area; V, ventral areas (ventroposterior and ventroanterior). Other abbreviations and conventions as in Fig. 1.

monkey is currently the best subject in which to evaluate whether the processing streams defined in macaques exist in other primates.

The subdivisions of visual cortex of owl monkeys are shown in Fig. 2. Electrophysiological mapping techniques were used to define six visual areas in the cortex of the owl monkey. These areas are V I, V II, MT, the dorsolateral area (DL), the dorsomedial area (DM), and the medial area (M; Allman and Kaas 1971, 1974a,b, 1975, 1976; for review, see Weller and Kaas 1981). In addition to these areas, other subdivisions of visual cortex have also been identified. Some areas (the dorsointermediate area, DI; the posterior parietal area, PP) were found to be visually responsive, but no maps were derived for them (Allman and Kaas 1976). The ventral areas (ventroposterior and ventroanterior) were defined by limited mapping data and patterns of callosal connections (Newsome and Allman 1980). Other areas (the temporoparietal area, TP; superior temporal area, ST; subdivisions of inferior temporal cortex, IT) were identified as visual primarily on the basis of connections with other subdivisions of visual cortex (Weller et al. 1984; Weller and Kaas 1985, 1987). Additional subdivisions of visual cortex may also exist.

It should be apparent by the names given to subdivisions of visual cortex in owl monkeys that only some areas are definitely considered homologous to areas found in macaques. In particular, similarities in the organization of V I, V II (or V2), and MT across primates strongly support the view of these areas being considered the same (Weller and Kaas 1982). Similarities or possible homologies have also been pointed out between V4 and DL, PO and M, V3A and DM, MST-FST and ST, and IT_C-IT_R and IT or TE (Weller and Kaas 1985; Van Essen 1985; Ungerleider and Desimone 1986; Maunsell and Newsome 1987; Weller and Kaas 1987). However, we know less about these areas and it is thus more difficult to compare them across primates.

Connections of many of the subdivisions of visual cortex in owl monkeys are known. Some of these connections are shown in Fig. 2, following the convention of defining and indicating feedforward projections described above for Fig. 1. These connections provide evidence in owl monkeys of two pathways, similar to those found in macaques, which originate from striate cortex and relay to posterior parietal or inferior temporal cortex.

Striate cortex projects in owl monkeys primarily to areas V II and MT. It also sends weaker projections to the dorsomedial area, DM (Lin et al. 1982). All of these projections terminate in layer IV of cortex. The sole clearly 'feedforward' target of V II is DL (Kaas and Lin 1977; Weller and Kaas, unpublished observations). V II projects in a feedback laminar pattern to V I, and sends input of unknown laminar pattern to DM and perhaps also MT (Kaas and Lin 1977). Thus, V II of owl monkeys does not appear to project strongly to MT, unlike V2 of macaque monkeys (see above).

DL sends a dense, feedforward projection to caudal inferior temporal cortex, IT$_C$ (Weller and Kaas 1985). Although DL also projects to layer IV of another subdivision of inferior temporal cortex (IT$_M$), in the region of the macaque area TF, this projection is weak and inconsistently observed. DL also projects to TP, and these projections terminate in layer IV and layers above IV. It is interesting that DL projects to TP, because TP, like DL, relays to IT cortex (Weller and Kaas 1987). However, because the organization of TP is not well understood and the laminar pattern of its projection to IT$_C$ is unknown, the connections of TP are not included in Fig. 2. DL also projects to DM, DI, V, PP, MT, and V II, but these projections have a feedback laminar pattern (Weller and Kaas 1985). Terminations in the region of the frontal eye field have an 'intermediate' laminar pattern.

A serial relay of connections continues in inferior temporal cortex, with caudal IT (IT$_C$) projecting to more rostral cortex, IT$_R$, and IT$_R$ projecting to polar cortex (IT$_P$; Weller and Kaas 1985, 1987). The laminar patterns of these connections conform to the standard feedforward – feedback plan.

The other major target of striate cortex projec-

tions, besides V II, is MT. MT is involved in the pathway directed towards posterior parietal cortex. The single major target of MT that receives feedforward input is the superior temporal area, ST (Weller et al. 1984). MT sometimes also projects to the part of DL bordering MT in a feedforward pattern. MT sends projections with a feedback laminar pattern to V I, V II, DM, DI, V, and perhaps M. MT also sends a feedback type projection to posterior parietal cortex, but this projection is weak and only inconsistently observed.

The superior temporal area (ST) provides the major direct input to posterior parietal cortex (PP) in owl monkeys (Weller et al. 1984). This projection is focused in layer IV of cortex. Processing may continue in posterior parietal cortex, based on the observation that a single location in PP can project to more distant locations in PP (Kaas et al. 1977). Besides its projections to PP, ST also projects in a feedforward laminar pattern to cortex in more anterior portions of the superior temporal sulcus, to the sylvian fissure, and to IT$_M$ (Weller et al. 1984). These latter sites may be multimodal (see Weller et al. 1984). Of these projections, only those to the superior temporal sulcus are shown in Fig. 2 because limited evidence from macaque monkeys implicates this region in spatial perception (Bruce et al. 1981; Boussaoud et al. 1987). ST also projects to the region of the frontal eye field, and these projections include but are not restricted to layer IV. Finally, ST provides a diffuse, feedback pattern of input to MT.

In addition to its projections to V II and MT, striate cortex of owl monkeys also sends a sparse projection to DM (Lin et al. 1982). The connections of DM, in turn, suggest that DM is an alternative route along which visual information is relayed from striate to posterior parietal cortex. The major projection of DM is to PP, and this projection terminates strongly in layer IV of cortex (Wagor et al. 1975). DM also projects to MT, DL, the region of the medial area, and perhaps DI and ST. Terminations in MT and DL may include layer IV.

Additional support for the proposed roles of

MT in the parietal pathway and DL in the inferior temporal pathway is provided by results of single-unit studies in owl monkeys. Cells in MT respond well to rapidly moving targets and are usually directionally selective (Baker et al. 1981; Felleman and Kaas 1984). In contrast, cells in DL are relatively insensitive to such stimuli but are quite sensitive to the specific dimensions of a visual stimulus (Petersen et al. 1980; Baker et al. 1981). It is interesting that connections between the medial area (M) and DM, MT, and PP (Graham et al. 1979) suggest that M is also involved in the pathway directed toward parietal cortex, because neurons in M have certain stimulus preferences that are similar to those of neurons in MT (Baker et al. 1981).

In summary, subdivisions of visual cortex in the owl monkey are dominated by connections that form pathways emanating from striate cortex and terminating in posterior parietal or inferior temporal cortex. The pathway directed to inferior temporal cortex relays through V II and DL. The 'pathway' terminating in posterior parietal cortex actually involves two possible routes. One route consists of a relay from V I to MT, from MT to ST, and from ST to posterior parietal cortex. ST also projects to other areas, including cortex further rostral in the superior temporal sulcus. Although the identity of this cortex is unknown in owl monkeys, cortex in a comparable location in macaque monkeys has been suggested to be part of the cortical system for spatial perception (Boussaoud et al. 1987). Direct connections also exist in owl monkeys between MT and PP, but these are sparse, variably observed, and do not terminate in a feedforward pattern. The other route to posterior parietal cortex uses projections from V I to DM, and from DM to PP. In some respects, connections directed toward posterior parietal and inferior temporal cortex appear simpler in owl monkeys than those found in macaque monkeys. It is presently unclear whether this impression is valid, or whether the situation is due to the fact that some areas that exist in macaques are not present in owl monkeys, or that not all the connections of visual cortex are known in owl monkeys.

The organization of visual cortex in squirrel monkeys

We know much less about the organization of visual cortex in New World monkeys other than owl monkeys. Next to owl monkeys, however, our best understanding of visual cortex is in squirrel monkeys (Fig. 3). In squirrel monkeys, V I and the part of V II exposed on the surface of the hemisphere have been electrophysiologically mapped (Cowey 1964). Cortex in the caudal superior temporal sulcus in the location of MT is also known to be visually responsive (Doty et al. 1964), and a frontal eye field has been identified (Huerta et al. 1986). Other regions of cortex in squirrel monkeys are considered visual on the basis of their connections (see below).

Although current knowledge of the connections of visual cortex in squirrel monkeys is incomplete, the available information suggests that squirrel

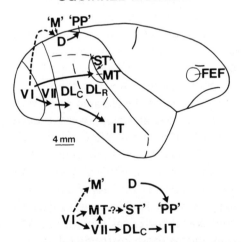

Fig. 3. Subdivisions of visual cortex of squirrel monkeys and some of their connections. The caudal (C) and rostral (R) subdivisions of DL are defined on anatomical grounds (Kaas and Cusick 1985; Cusick 1987a,b; see text for details). 'M', 'PP', and 'ST' are tentatively identified with the names of comparably located areas in owl monkeys on the basis of their patterns of cortical connections. The borders of IT shown are those of architectonic area TE (Weller, unpublished observations). The '?' in the wiring diagram at bottom indicates that the laminar pattern of the MT to 'ST' projection is not known. Other conventions and abbreviations as in Figs. 1 and 2.

monkeys may also possess the two cortical systems found in macaque and owl monkeys. These systems begin at the cortical level with the projections of striate cortex. Striate cortex has two major targets in squirrel monkeys, V II and MT, similar to results described for owl monkeys (Spatz et al. 1970; Tigges et al. 1973, 1981; Wong-Riley 1978). Projections to V II and MT terminate in layer IV of cortex. Parts of striate cortex in the calcarine fissure, which represent peripheral vision, also project to a third area, located in the parieto-occipital sulcus on the medial wall of the hemisphere (Martinez-Millán and Holländer 1975). This medial projection zone is in the location of the medial area of owl monkeys, which has an expanded representation of peripheral vision. Thus, this striate-receptive region on the medial wall of squirrel monkeys may be homologous to the medial area of owl monkeys.

Lateral V II projects in a feedforward pattern to cortex just rostral to it (Tigges et al. 1974, 1981; Wong-Riley 1978, 1979). Initially, it was not clear whether this V II projection zone was part of a band-like V3, such as found in cortex rostral to V II in macaques, or whether the zone comprised a DL-like area, such as found in cortex rostral to lateral V II in owl monkeys (Tigges et al. 1974). This uncertainty existed because only the projections of the part of V II on the exposed portion of cortex, representing central vision, were studied (e.g., Tigges et al. 1974; Wong-Riley 1978). This lateral part of V II could be expected to project to rostrally bordering cortex for either a V3- or DL-like area. However, results of later studies have suggested that dorsal V II does not project to strictly adjacent dorsal cortex, as though to a V3, but projects instead to more rostrolateral cortex, as though to a DL-like area (Kaas and Cusick 1985). Thus, the V II projection zone in squirrel monkeys is called DL (Kaas and Cusick 1985; Cusick 1987a,b).

Projections from exposed parts of V II to 'DL' never extend to the border of MT (Tigges et al. 1974; Kaas and Cusick 1985). Although the possibility exists that this rostral part of DL is connected with parts of V II representing the visual periphery, this and other differences in connections and architectonic appearance were used to suggest that two subdivisions, caudal (DL_C) and rostral (DL_R), exist in the region of DL in squirrel monkeys (Kaas and Cusick 1985; Cusick 1987a,b).

Besides projecting to caudal DL, V II also projects in a feedforward pattern to MT. Thus, V II of squirrel monkeys is involved in both inferior temporal and posterior parietal pathways, as found for V II in macaque monkeys, but not owl monkeys. V II of squirrel monkeys also projects sparsely to a small, unidentified region in the caudal end of the sylvian fissure and to the frontal eye field (Tigges et al. 1974, 1981; Wong-Riley 1978). Finally, V II projects in a feedback manner to V I (Tigges et al. 1974, 1981; Wong-Riley 1978, 1979).

Caudal DL of squirrel monkeys provides a major projection to inferior temporal cortex (Cusick, personal communication). This input terminates mainly in layer IV of cortex. Other connections of caudal DL are with MT, ventral temporal cortex, the frontal lobe, and perhaps foveal V I (Cusick 1987a,b). The laminar patterns of these connections are presently unknown. Projections from caudal DL to V II conform to a feedback pattern (Tigges et al. 1974, 1981).

The connections of MT have been recently described in squirrel monkeys (Krubitzer and Kaas 1987). MT has connections with V I, V II, a region similar in location to ST of owl monkeys, cortex further rostral in the superior temporal sulcus, rostral DL, an unidentified dorsomedial region, the frontal eye field and cortex below it, and cortex in the ventral temporal lobe. Most of these connections are similar to those of MT in owl monkeys, the only differences being the presence in squirrel monkeys, but not owl monkeys, of connections between MT and V II and rostral locations in the superior temporal sulcus. The laminar patterns of the connections of MT are as yet unknown. However, it seems significant that MT of squirrel monkeys has connections with an area that may be homologous to ST of owl monkeys, and with a region of dorsomedial cortex that may be homologous to DM of owl monkeys. Both of these areas, of course, relay to posterior parietal cortex in owl monkeys.

We have identified a new visual area in squirrel monkeys that provides input to posterior parietal cortex. This is the dorsal area, D (Weller et al. 1987). We are presently calling the dorsal area by a name different from those of areas in the owl monkey because we are unsure of its homology with owl monkey areas. The dorsal area is located rostral to dorsal V II and lateral to the caudal end of the sylvian fissure. It can be distinguished from DL by its connections; it receives little or no input from adjacent parts of V II, and it sends a projection that is minor, at best, to inferior temporal cortex (Weller et al. 1987).

The existence of the dorsal area was first suggested by patterns of connections with rostral DL (Cusick 1987a,b). D also has connections with adjacent posterior parietal cortex (Weller et al. 1987). These projections have a feedforward laminar pattern. The dorsal area also has connections with MT, cortex of the ventral occipitotemporal lobe, and an area in the location of ST. Because the laminar patterns of connections between D and areas such as MT and rostral DL are not yet known, it is not currently obvious what areas are providing D with feedforward cortical input. The fact that the medial wall area receives input from striate cortex only when peripheral parts of the visual field are involved (Martinez-Millán and Holländer 1975) suggests that it may be part of the posterior parietal pathway, which in macaques emphasizes peripheral rather than central vision (see earlier). However, the projections of the 'medial area' of squirrel monkeys are presently unknown.

In summary, there is compelling anatomical evidence to suggest that squirrel monkeys have, in general, the same serial relay of visual information from striate cortex to inferior temporal cortex as described for other primates (Fig. 3). Striate cortex projects to V II, V II projects to (caudal) DL, and (caudal) DL projects to IT cortex. Anatomical data in squirrel monkeys is less strong in support of a pathway from striate cortex to posterior parietal cortex, but suggestive. V I projects to MT. MT has connections with cortex in the region of ST and with dorsomedial cortex close to parietal cortex. The laminar patterns of these connections are unknown, as are the projections of 'ST'. I have speculated in Fig. 3 that MT may provide a 'feedforward' projection to 'ST'. 'ST', in turn, may provide the driving input to posterior parietal cortex. The involvement of the dorsal area in the parietal pathway is easier to support, because D provides a feedforward projection to posterior parietal cortex. However, the source of the dorsal area's cortical input is presently unclear; both MT and rostral DL can be considered as potential afferents.

The organization of visual cortex in other New World monkeys

The only other New World monkey in which connections of visual cortex have been investigated to any extent is the marmoset. Reciprocal striate cortex and MT connections have been described in this primate (Spatz 1975, 1977). MT also projects to V II, to cortex adjacent to MT that may correspond to areas DL or ST or both, to cortex on the medial wall in the location of M, to two locations in parietal cortex perhaps homologous to DM and PP, and to the frontal lobe (Spatz and Tigges 1972). Unlike results described so far for other primates, many of the targets of MT in marmosets receive projections focused in layer IV of cortex. Thus, there exists in marmosets a serial relay of information from V I to MT, and from MT to a number of areas that potentially could provide input to posterior parietal cortex. There may also be direct projections from MT to posterior parietal cortex.

The organization of visual cortex in prosimians

Two subdivisions of visual cortex, MT and a dorsal area, have been electrophysiologically defined in the prosimian bushbaby (galago), and V I and V II are known to exist on anatomical grounds

(Allman et al. 1973, 1979; Tigges et al. 1973; for review, see Weller and Kaas 1982; Fig. 4). Although the representation of the visual field in the dorsal area of galago is similar to that of the medial area in owl monkey, the dorsal area has no clearly established homology with any area in New World monkeys. Patterns of callosal connections have been used to argue that galagos also possess a ventral pair of areas, ventroposterior and ventroanterior, and a DL-like area, similar to areas identified in owl monkeys (Newsome and Allman 1980; Cusick and Kaas 1986).

In galagos, striate cortex projects in a feedforward pattern to V II and MT (Tigges et al. 1973; Symonds and Kaas 1978). Sparse and variable projections to additional areas also exist, but these were not specified (Symonds and Kaas 1978). Thus, it remains possible that galagos possess more

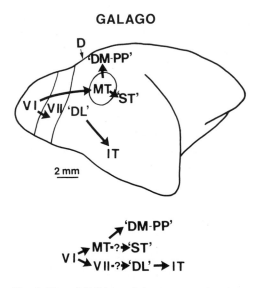

GALAGO

Fig. 4. The subdivisions of visual cortex of galagos and some of their connections. The location of a dorsal area (D) on the dorsal surface is indicated by the small arrow. Projections from V II to 'DL' are hypothesized only. MT projects to much of bordering cortex. Because it is not clear whether any of these projections are to an ST-like area, projections from MT to ST are indicated at bottom with a question mark. Another of the feedforward targets of MT, 'DM-PP', may consist of two areas, both of which receive input from MT (Wall et al. 1982). Conventions and abbreviations as in previous figures. See text for details.

than two striate cortex projection zones, as found in other primates.

The projections of V II have not been directly investigated in galagos. Injections of retrograde tracers in V I, however, have shown that V II projects to V I in a feedback laminar pattern (Symonds and Kaas 1978). Cortex rostral to V II, roughly between V II and MT, projects to inferior temporal cortex (Wall et al. 1982; Weller and Kaas, unpublished observations). In this respect, cortex rostral to V II in galagos is similar to DL of owl monkeys. The pathway from this potential 'DL' to inferior temporal cortex has a feedforward laminar pattern (Wall et al. 1982).

MT projects to many areas in the bushbaby. These include V I, V II, cortex bordering various aspects of MT, and a region of cortex that includes both dorsomedial and posterior parietal cortex in location (Wall et al. 1982). The projections from MT to V I are clearly of the feedback type. Most other targets of MT projections receive terminations that extend from layers II to IV of cortex. Thus, MT projects to many areas in galagos, as in marmosets, in a feedforward pattern. The projections from MT to cortex bordering MT may include those to an area comparable to ST. Input to dorsomedial and posterior parietal cortex is usually in the form of two foci. This result suggests that two areas exist in this region, perhaps comparable to DM and PP of owl monkeys (Wall et al. 1982).

Based on these limited results, galagos also appear to have subdivisions of visual cortex that are connected in pathways relaying (via MT) to posterior parietal cortex and (via a DL-like area) to inferior temporal cortex. MT may project directly in a feedforward pattern to PP, and perhaps also relay to PP through an ST-like area. Whether galagos also possess an additional pathway to posterior parietal cortex, which involves striate cortex targets besides V II and MT, remains to be determined.

Conclusions

Ungerleider and Mishkin (1982) suggested that two

major, diverging pathways exist in visual cortex of macaque monkeys. Both originate from striate cortex and terminate in either the posterior parietal lobe or the inferior temporal lobe. The results of more recent studies of cortical connections in macaque monkeys, when compared with those from three different species of New World monkeys and one Old World prosimian primate, suggest the hypothesis that processing streams directed toward posterior parietal and inferior temporal cortex exist in all primates. The significance of this hypothesis is that it suggests that these pathways arose early in the evolution of primates. Although the broad plan of these pathways is similar in the five primates examined, some details are species variable.

In all primates examined, the relay from striate cortex to inferior temporal cortex involves synapses in at least V II and DL (V4). Additional areas, such as TP in owl monkeys and V3 and TEO in macaques, may also be involved. The relay from striate cortex to posterior parietal cortex involves a pathway through MT and its targets ('ST', MST and FST) in all primates. A species variable feature of this pathway appears to be whether MT projects directly and/or indirectly (via an ST-like area) to posterior parietal cortex. At least one other route to posterior parietal cortex is clearly established in primates other than prosimians. This route begins with striate cortex projections to areas other than V II and MT. These additional striate-receptive areas, such as PO in macaque monkeys and DM in owl monkeys, project directly or indirectly to posterior parietal cortex. Thus, the 'two cortical visual systems' common to primates are the broad termination zones in the posterior parietal and inferior temporal lobes, not the actual number of routes visual information travels through cortex to these zones.

Acknowledgements

Comments on an earlier version of the chapter were kindly provided by Jim Cox, Cassie Cusick, Jon Kaas, Tom Norton, Gregg Steele, and Leslie Ungerleider. Supported in part by UAB Faculty Research Grant 212319 and NIH Grant R29 EY07147.

References

Allman, J., Campbell, C.B.G. and McGuinness, E. (1979) The dorsal third tier area in *Galago senegalensis. Brain Res.*, 179: 355 – 361.

Allman, J.M. and Kaas, J.H. (1971) A representation of the visual field in the caudal third of the middle temporal gyrus of the owl monkey *(Aotus trivirgatus). Brain Res.*, 31: 85 – 105.

Allman, J.M. and Kaas, J.H. (1974a) The organization of the second visual area (V II) in the owl monkey: A second order transformation of the visual hemifield. *Brain Res.*, 76: 247 – 265.

Allman, J.M. and Kaas, J.H. (1974b) A crescent-shaped cortical visual area surrounding the middle temporal area (MT) in the owl monkey *(Aotus trivirgatus). Brain Res.*, 81: 199 – 213.

Allman, J.M. and Kaas, J.H. (1975) The dorsomedial cortical visual area: A third tier area in the occipital lobe of the owl monkey *(Aotus trivirgatus). Brain Res.*, 100: 473 – 487.

Allman, J.M. and Kaas, J.H. (1976) Representation of the visual field on the medial wall of occipital-parietal cortex in the owl monkey. *Science*, 191: 572 – 575.

Allman, J.M., Kaas, J.H. and Lane, R.H. (1973) The middle temporal visual area (MT) in the bushbaby *(Galago senegalensis). Brain Res.*, 57: 197 – 202.

Baker, J.F., Peterson, S.E., Newsome, W.T. and Allman, J.M. (1981) Visual response properties of neurons in four extrastriate visual areas of the owl monkey *(Aotus trivirgatus)*: A quantitative comparison of medial, dorsomedial, dorsolateral, and middle temporal areas. *J. Neurophysiol.*, 45: 397 – 416.

Bolster, B. and Crowne, D.P. (1979) Effects of anterior and posterior inferotemporal lesions on discrimination reversal in the monkey. *Neuropsychologia*, 17: 11 – 20.

Boussaoud, D., Ungerleider, J.G. and Desimone, R. (1987) Cortical pathways for motion analysis: Connections of visual areas MST and FST in macaques. *Soc. Neurosci. Abstr.*, 13: 1625.

Bruce, C.J., Desimone, R. and Gross, C.G. (1981) Visual properties of neurons in a polysensory area in superior temporal sulcus of the macaque. *J. Neurophysiol.*, 46: 369 – 384.

Colby, C.L., Gattass, R., Olson, C.R. and Gross, C.G. (1983) Cortical afferents to visual area PO in the macaque. *Soc. Neurosci. Abstr.*, 9: 152.

Cowey, A. (1964) Projection of the retina on to striate and prestriate cortex in the squirrel monkey, *Saimiri sciureus. J. Neurophysiol.*, 27: 366 – 393.

Cragg, B.C. and Ainsworth, A. (1969) The topography of the afferent projections in the circumstriate visual cortex of the monkey studied by the Nauta method. *Vision Res.*, 9: 733 – 747.

Cusick, C.G. (1987a) Cortical connections of the dorsolateral visual area in squirrel monkeys. *Anat. Rec.*, 218: 30A.

Cusick, C.G. (1987b) Evidence from patterns of cortical connections for subdivisions within the dorsolateral visual cortex of squirrel monkeys. *Neurosci. Suppl.*, 22: S122.

Cusick, C.G. and Kaas, J.H. (1986) Interhemispheric connections of visual cortex of owl monkeys *(Aotus trivirgatus)*, marmosets *(Callithrix jacchus)*, and galagos *(Galago crassicaudatus)*. *J. Comp. Neurol.*, 230: 311 – 336.

Desimone, R., Albright, T.D., Gross, C.G. and Bruce, C. (1984) Stimulus-selective properties of inferior temporal neurons in the macaque. *J. Neurosci.*, 4: 2051 – 2062.

Desimone, R., Fleming, J. and Gross, C.G. (1980) Prestriate afferents to inferior temporal cortex: an HRP study. *Brain Res.*, 184: 41 – 55.

Desimone, R. and Gross, C.G. (1979) Visual areas in the temporal cortex of the macaque. *Brain Res.*, 178: 363 – 380.

Desimone, R. and Schein, S.J. (1987) Visual properties of neurons in area V4 of the macaque: sensitivity to stimulus form. *J. Neurophysiol.*, 57: 835 – 868.

Desimone, R. and Ungerleider, L.G. (1986) Multiple visual areas in the caudal superior temporal sulcus of the macaque. *J. Comp. Neurol.*, 248: 164 – 189.

DeYoe, E.A. and Van Essen, D.C. (1985) Segregation of efferent connections and receptive field properties in visual area V2 of the macaque. *Nature*, 317: 58 – 61.

Doty, R.W., Kimura, D.S. and Mogenson, G.J. (1964) Photically and electrically elicited responses in the central visual system of the squirrel monkey. *Exp. Neurol.*, 10: 19 – 51.

Felleman, D.J. and Kaas, J.H. (1984) Receptive field properties of neurons in the Middle Temporal Visual Area (MT) of owl monkeys. *J. Neurophysiol.*, 52: 488 – 513.

Felleman, D.J. and Van Essen, D.C. (1983) The connections of Area V4 of macaque monkey extrastriate cortex. *Soc. Neurosci. Abstr.*, 9: 153.

Felleman, D.J., Knierim, J.J. and Van Essen, D.C. (1986) Multiple topographic and non-topographic subdivisions of the temporal lobe as revealed by the connections of Area V4 in macaques. *Soc. Neurosci. Abstr.*, 12: 1182.

Graham, J., Wall, J. and Kaas, J.H. (1979) Cortical projections of the medial visual area in the owl monkey, *Aotus trivirgatus. Neurosci. Lett.*, 15: 109 – 114.

Gross, C.G., Rocha-Miranda, C.E. and Bender, D.B. (1972) Visual properties of neurons in inferotemporal cortex of the macaque. *J. Neurophysiol.*, 35: 96 – 111.

Hendrickson, A.E., Wilson, J.R. and Ogren, M.P. (1978) The neuroanatomical organization of pathways between the dorsal lateral geniculate nucleus and visual cortex in Old World and New World primates. *J. Comp. Neurol.*, 182: 123 – 136.

Huerta, M.F., Krubitzer, L.A. and Kaas, J.H. (1986) The frontal eye field as defined by intracortical microstimulation in squirrel monkeys, owl monkeys, and macaque monkeys. I. Subcortical connections. *J. Comp. Neurol.*, 253: 415 – 439.

Hyvärinen, J. and Poranen, A. (1974) Function of the parietal associative area 7 as revealed from cellular discharges in alert monkeys. *Brain*, 97: 673 – 692.

Jones, E.G. and Powell, T.P.S. (1970) An anatomical study of converging sensory pathways within the cerebral cortex of the monkey. *Brain*, 93: 793 – 820.

Kaas, J.H. and Cusick, C.G. (1985) Cortical connections of area 18 in squirrel monkeys. *Soc. Neurosci. Abstr.*, 11: 1011.

Kaas, J.H. and Lin, C.-S. (1977) Cortical projections of area 18 in owl monkeys. *Vision Res.*, 17: 739 – 741.

Kaas, J.H., Lin, C.-S. and Wagor, E. (1977) Cortical projections of posterior parietal cortex in owl monkeys. *J. Comp. Neurol.*, 171: 387 – 408.

Krubitzer, L.A. and Kaas, J.H. (1987) Connections of modular subdivisions of cortical visual areas 17 and 18 with the middle temporal area, MT, in squirrel monkeys. *Soc. Neurosci. Abstr.*, 13: 3.

Kuypers, H.G., Szwarcbart, M.K., Mishkin, M. and Rosvold, H.E. (1965) Occipitotemporal corticocortical connections in the rhesus monkey. *Exper. Neurol.*, 11: 245 – 262.

Levine, D.N. (1982) Visual agnosia in monkey and in man. In D.J. Ingle, J.W. Mansfield and M.A. Goodale (Eds.), *Advances in the Analysis of Visual Behavior*, MIT Press, Cambridge, MA, pp. 629 – 670.

Lin, C.-S., Weller, R.E. and Kaas, J.H. (1982) Cortical connections of striate cortex in the owl monkey. *J. Comp. Neurol.*, 211: 165 – 176.

Martinez-Millán, M. and Holländer, H. (1975) Cortico-cortical projections from striate cortex of the squirrel monkey *(Saimiri sciureus)*, A radioautographic study. *Brain Res.*, 83: 405 – 417.

Maunsell, J.H.R. and Newsome, W.T. (1987) Visual processing in monkey extrastriate cortex. *Ann. Rev. Neurosci.*, 10: 363 – 401.

Maunsell, J.H.R. and Van Essen, D.C. (1983a) Functional properties of neurons in the middle temporal visual area (MT) of the macaque monkey. I. Selectivity for stimulus direction, speed and orientation. *J. Neurophysiol.*, 49: 1127 – 1147.

Maunsell, J.H.R. and Van Essen, D.C. (1983b) The connections of the middle temporal visual area (MT) and their relationship to a cortical hierarchy in the macaque monkey. *J. Neurosci.*, 3: 2563 – 2586.

Mishkin, M. (1966) Visual mechanisms beyond the striate cortex. In R. Russell (Ed.), *Frontiers in Physiological Psychology*, Academic Press, New York, NY, pp. 93 – 119.

Mishkin, M. (1972) Cortical visual areas and their interactions. In A.G. Karzmar and J.C. Eccles (Eds.), *Brain and Human Behavior*, Springer, Berlin, pp. 187 – 208.

Mishkin, M. and Ungerleider, L.G. (1982) Contribution of striate inputs to the visuospatial functions of parietopreoccipital cortex in monkeys. *Behav. Brain Res.*, 6: 57–77.

Mountcastle, V.B., Lynch, J.C. and Georgopoulos, A. (1975) Posterior parietal association cortex of the monkey: command functions for operations within extrapersonal space. *J. Neurophysiol.*, 38: 871–908.

Newsome, W.T. and Allman, J.M. (1980) Interhemispheric connections of visual cortex in the owl monkey, *Aotus trivirgatus*, and the bushbaby, *Galago senegalensis. J. Comp. Neurol.*, 194: 209–233.

Newsome, W.T. and Wurtz, R.H. (1982) Identification of architectonic zones containing visual tracking cells in the superior temporal sulcus (STS) of macaque monkeys. *Invest. Ophthalmol. Vis. Sci. Suppl.*, 22: 238.

Petersen, S.E., Baker, J.F. and Allman, J.M. (1980) Dimensional selectivity of neurons in the dorsolateral visual area of the owl monkey. *Brain Res.*, 197: 507–511.

Pohl, W. (1973) Dissociation of spatial discrimination deficits following frontal and parietal lesions in monkeys. *J. Comp. Physiol. Psych.*, 82: 227–239.

Rockland, K.S. and Pandya, D.N. (1979) Laminar origins and terminations of cortical connections of the occipital lobe in the rhesus monkey. *Brain Res.*, 179: 3–20.

Saito, H., Yukie, M., Tanaka, K., Hikosaka, K., Fukada, Y. and Iwai, E. (1986) Integration of direction signals of image motion in the superior temporal sulcus of the macaque monkey. *J. Neurosci.*, 6: 145–157.

Seltzer, B. and Pandya, D.N. (1978) Afferent cortical connections and architectonics of the superior temporal sulcus and surrounding cortex in the rhesus monkey. *Brain Res.*, 149: 1–24.

Shipp, S. and Zeki, S. (1985) Segregation of pathways leading from area V2 to areas V4 and V5 of macaque monkey visual cortex. *Nature*, 315: 322–325.

Spatz, W.B. (1975) An efferent connection of the solitary cells of Meynert. A study with horseradish peroxidase in the marmoset *Callithrix. Brain Res.*, 92: 450–455.

Spatz, W.B. (1977) Topographically organized reciprocal connections between areas 17 and MT (visual area of superior temporal sulcus) in the marmoset *Callithrix jacchus. Exp. Brain Res.*, 27: 559–572.

Spatz, W.B., Tigges, J. and Tigges, M. (1970) Subcortical projections, cortical associations and some intrinsic interlaminar connections of the striate cortex in the squirrel monkey *(Saimiri). J. Comp. Neurol.*, 140: 155–174.

Spatz, W.B. and Tigges, J. (1972) Experimental anatomical studies on the 'Middle Temporal Visual Area (MT)' in primates. I. Efferent corticocortical connections in the marmoset, *Callithrix jacchus. J. Comp. Neurol.*, 146: 451–464.

Spiegler, B.J. and Mishkin, M. (1981) Evidence for the sequential participation of inferior temporal cortex and amygdala in the acquisition of stimulus-reward associations. *Behav. Brain Res.*, 3: 303–317.

Symonds, L.L. and Kaas, J.H. (1978) Connections of striate cortex in the prosimian, *Galago senegalensis. J. Comp. Neurol.*, 181: 477–512.

Tigges, J., Spatz, W.B. and Tigges, M. (1973a) Reciprocal point-to-point connections between parastriate and striate cortex in the squirrel monkey *(Saimiri).* J. Comp. Neurol., 148: 481–490.

Tigges, J., Tigges, M. and Kalaha, C.S. (1973b) Efferent connections of area 17 in *Galago. Am. J. Phys. Anthro.*, 38: 393–398.

Tigges, J., Spatz, W.B. and Tigges, M. (1974) Efferent cortico-cortical fiber connections of area 18 in the squirrel monkey *(Saimiri). J. Comp. Neurol.*, 158: 219–236.

Tigges, J., Tigges, M. and Perachio, A.A. (1977) Complementary laminar terminations of afferents to area 17 originating in area 18 and the lateral geniculate nucleus in squirrel monkey. *J. Comp. Neurol.*, 176: 87–100.

Tigges, J., Tigges, M., Anschel, S., Cross, N.A., Letbetter, W.D. and McBride, R.L. (1981) Areal and laminar distribution of neurons interconnecting the central visual cortical areas 17, 18, 19, and MT in squirrel monkey *(Saimiri). J. Comp. Neurol.*, 202: 539–560.

Ungerleider, L.G. and Mishkin, M. (1978) Interactions of striate and posterior parietal cortex in spatial vision. *Soc. Neurosci. Abstr.*, 4: 649.

Ungerleider, L.G. and Mishkin, M. (1979) The striate projection zone in the superior temporal sulcus of *Macaca mulatta*: location and topographic organization. *J. Comp. Neurol.*, 188: 347–366.

Ungerleider, L.G. and Mishkin, M. (1982) Two cortical visual systems. In: D.J. Ingle, J.W. Mansfield and M.A. Goodale (Eds.), *Advances in the Analysis of Visual Behavior*, MIT Press, Cambridge, MA, pp. 549–586.

Ungerleider, L.G. and Desimone, R. (1986) Cortical connections of visual area MT in the macaque. *J. Comp. Neurol.*, 248: 190–222.

Ungerleider, L.G., Gattass, R., Sousa, A.P.B. and Mishkin, M. (1983) Projections of area V2 in the macaque. *Soc. Neurosci. Abstr.*, 9: 152.

Ungerleider, L.G., Desimone, R. and Moran, J. (1986) Asymmetry of central and peripheral field inputs from area V4 into the temporal and parietal lobes of the macaque. *Soc. Neurosci. Abstr.*, 12: 1182.

Van Essen, D.C. (1979) Visual areas of the mammalian cerebral cortex. *Ann. Rev. Neurosci.*, 2: 227–263.

Van Essen, D.C. (1985) Functional organization of primate visual cortex. In A. Peters and E.G. Jones (Eds.), *Cerebral Cortex, Vol. 3*, Plenum Press, New York, pp. 259–329.

Van Essen, D.C., Newsome, W.T., Maunsell, J.H.R. and Bixby, J.L. (1986) The projections from striate cortex (V1) to areas V2 and V3 in the macaque monkey: asymmetries, areal boundaries, and patchy connections. *J. Comp. Neurol.*, 244: 451–480.

Von Bonin, G. and Bailey, P. (1947) *The Neocortex of Macaca Mulatta*, University of Illinois Press, Urbana, IL.

Wagor, E., Lin, C.-S. and Kaas, J.H. (1975) Some cortical projections of the dorsomedial visual area (DM) of association cortex in the owl monkey, *Aotus trivirgatus. J. Comp. Neurol.*, 163: 227 – 250.

Wall, J.T., Symonds, L.L. and Kaas, J.H. (1982) Cortical and subcortical projections of the middle temporal area (MT) and adjacent cortex in galagos. *J. Comp. Neurol.*, 211: 193 – 214.

Weller, R.E. and Kaas, J.H. (1981) Cortical and subcortical connections of visual cortex in primates. In C.N. Woolsey (Ed.), *Cortical Sensory Organization, Vol. 2*, Humana Press, Clifton, New Jersey, pp. 121 – 155.

Weller, R.E. and Kaas, J.H. (1982) The organization of the visual system in *Galago*: Comparisons with monkeys. In D.E. Haines (Ed.), *The Lesser Bushbaby (Galago) as an Animal Model: Selected Topics*, CRC Press, Boca Raton, Florida, pp. 107 – 135.

Weller, R.E. and Kaas, J.H. (1983) Retinotopic patterns of connections of Area 17 with visual areas V-II and MT in macaque monkeys. *J. Comp. Neurol.*, 220: 253 – 279.

Weller, R.E. and Kaas, J.H. (1985) Cortical projections of the dorsolateral visual area in owl monkeys: The prestriate relay to inferior temporal cortex. *J. Comp. Neurol.*, 234: 35 – 59.

Weller, R.E. and Kaas, J.H. (1987) Subdivisions and connections of inferior temporal cortex in owl monkeys. *J. Comp.*

Neurol., 256: 137 – 172.

Weller, R.E., Wall, J.T. and Kaas, J.H. (1984) Cortical connections of the Middle Temporal Visual Area (MT) and the superior temporal cortex in owl monkeys. *J. Comp. Neurol.*, 228: 81 – 104.

Weller, R.E., Steele, G. and Cusick, C.G. (1987) Cortical connections of a dorsal visual area in squirrel monkeys. *Soc. Neurosci. Abstr.*, 13: 626.

Wong-Riley, M. (1978) Reciprocal connections between striate and prestriate cortex in the squirrel monkey as demonstrated by combined peroxidase histochemistry and autoradiography. *Brain Res.*, 147: 159 – 164.

Wong-Riley, M. (1979) Columnar corticocortical interconnections within the visual system of the squirrel and macaque monkeys. *Brain Res.*, 162: 201 – 217.

Zeki, S.M. (1969) Representation of central visual fields in prestriate cortex of monkey. *Brain Res.*, 14: 271 – 291.

Zeki, S.M. (1971) Cortical projections from two prestriate areas in the monkey. *Brain Res.*, 34: 19 – 35.

Zeki, S.M. (1978) The cortical projections of foveal striate cortex in the rhesus monkey. *J. Physiol. (Lond.)*, 277: 227 – 244.

Zeki, S.M. (1980) A direct projection from area VI to area V3A of rhesus monkey visual cortex. *Proc. R. Soc. Lond. Ser. B.*, 207: 499 – 506.

T.P. Hicks and G. Benedek (Eds.)
Progress in Brain Research, Vol. 75
© 1988 Elsevier Science Publishers B.V. (Biomedical Division)

CHAPTER 28

Extrageniculo-striate visual mechanisms: compartmentalization of visual functions*

O.D. Creutzfeldt

Department of Neurobiology, Max-Planck-Institute for Biophysical Chemistry, P.O.B. 2841, D-3400 Göttingen-Nikolausberg, F.R.G.

After the foregoing series of lectures on various aspects of extrageniculo-striate visual mechanisms, I would like to discuss some more general ideas related to this subject. We have learned over the last 20 years or so, that a large part of the whole neocortex is excitable by visual stimuli and that this visually excitable cortex can be compartmentalized anatomically and functionally into various visual areas. Although the definition of a 'visual area' is not always clear, it is supposed that each of them represents specific aspects of visual stimuli. The anatomical connectivity and location of the various areas suggests a grouping of these distributed visual field representations into various visual subsystems. Thus, according to their different afferent organization, two visual systems, a retino-geniculo-striate and a retino-collicular-extrastriate visual system were distinguished (Trevarthen 1968; Sprague et al. 1973) (see Fig. 1A). According to their different involvement in cognitive processes, the extrastriate visual cortex was divided into a more object-related and a more space-related system (in the temporal and parietal association cortex, respectively) (Ungerleider and Mishkin; 1980; Weller at this meeting) (see Fig. 1B). These two schemes also stand for two alternative mechanisms of information flow in the cor-

tex, the first one for the model of parallel representation and the second for sequential processing. However, this latter alternative should not simply be related to one or the other of the more anatomically biased divisions, as the parallel and the sequential models are not necessarily tied to only one anatomical mechanism. In the following, I shall comment on some aspects related to such models. At the end, we will discuss yet an alternative way of how to look at the problem of the multiplicity of visual areas.

Two visual systems

The division into a geniculo-striate and an extrageniculate visual system was originally proposed for the cat. It was based on the observation that visual functions in the cat may be largely preserved after ablation of area 17 (Doty 1973; Sprague et al. 1977) and that a large part of the visual cortex, especially the cortex within and around the suprasylvian sulcus (Clare-Bishop area) receives visual afferents from the superior colliculi and the pretectum via the nucleus lateralis posterior thalami (Graybiel and Berson 1980). Neurons in this region do indeed still respond to visual stimuli after ablation of the striate cortex (Spear and Baumann 1979; Guedes et al. 1983; Spear, at this meeting). They even preserve some rather specific functional properties such as movement and direc-

---

* Dedicated to Prof. János Szentágothai on occasion of his 75th birthday, on October 31, 1987.

tion sensitivity. It is still a matter of debate and it was discussed here, which properties actually change after ablation of area 17. Neurons in the intermediate part of the nucleus lateralis posterior, which project to the cortex around the lateral suprasylvian sulcus show similar properties as their cortical target neurons (Benedek et al. 1983). Neurons of the cat's infero-temporal visual cortex (the anterior ectosylvian visual area, AEV, and the insular visual cortex) clearly respond to visual stimuli to which neurons of the striate cortex or any extrastriate area do not respond at all (e.g., very fast moving stimuli) (see Mucke et al. 1982). On the other hand, the suprasylvian visual cortex receives also input from area 17 through association fibres, and we heard an interesting approach at this meeting from H. Sherk about how to demonstrate them. We therefore have to face the fact that we do not know to what extent and how the association fibres interact in cortex with activities elicited by the specific thalamic afferent input. This applies to all extrastriate regions of the cat and even to V2 (area 18) except that this area belongs in this scheme also to the retino-geniculate system because of its afferents from the lateral geniculate body.

In primates and especially in man we assume that the extrastriate visual cortex is functionally more dependent on the striate cortex in that neurons in the prelunate and inferotemporal cortex are reported to become visually inexcitable after ablation or cooling of the striate cortex (Gross 1973; Schiller and Malpeli 1977) and in that area 17 lesions in monkey and man appear to be more devastating to visual behavior than in lower mammals. It is premature, however, to conclude from the few observations and the few areas from where recordings were taken after area 17 lesion that in monkeys all visual or visually related input to extrastriate visual areas comes through area 17. Would it be so, primates would differ significantly from other mammals in that they would have only one single, that is a geniculo-striate cortical visual system. The pulvinar, on the other hand, would become a sort of appendix of the brain involved

perhaps in some general non-localized functions such as attention or so, as occasionally has been suggested. I cannot believe this, knowing that the

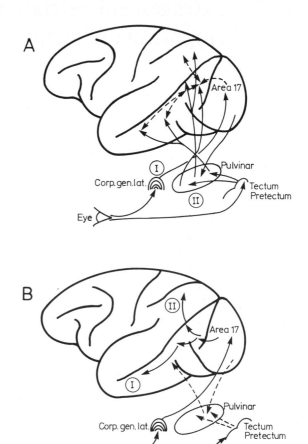

Fig. 1. Two concepts of 'two visual systems' (A) Here, a retino-geniculo-striate (I) and a retino-tecto-thalamo-extrastriate (II) system are distinguished. The second system also depends on the retino-geniculo-striate system in that area 17 sends efferents also to a sector in the LP-pulvinar-complex, and from there into a circumscribed region of the extrastriate visual cortex. Interconnections between the two visual systems through association fibres (broken arrows) are subordinate in this model. (B) Here, all essential visual information reaches the cortex through the retino-geniculo-striate pathway and is transmitted to the extrastriate cortex through a cascade of intercortical association connections. These connections are later divided into two main streams, one responsible for object recognition in the temporal association cortex (I), one for localization in space in the parietal association cortex (II). The retino-tecto-thalamo-cortical input plays, in this scheme a subordinate, modulatory role (broken lines).

relative size of the pulvinar increases significantly in primates like that of the parietal and temporal association areas, and knowing from our ongoing experiments the lively, visually related and visuo-motor related activity in the pulvinar of awake monkeys. Whatever the answer to this question will be, there is the fact that the intercortical connections between the various areas are bidirectional. From the anatomical point of view it is impossible to decide, e.g., for the prelunate visual association cortex (V4) whether the cortical input from the superior temporal sulcus, from the inferior parietal lobule and from the frontal eye field are more important than those from area 18. Or, whether the infero-temporal or parietal cortex receives or sends information to V4 (Fig. 2). We clearly have not yet sufficiently understood the functional significance of the intricately bidirectional connections between cortical areas via association fibres.

It is a fact, on the other hand, that each part of the neocortex − except perhaps of the temporal pole − receives a thalamic input. The principal organization of this thalamo-cortical input is the same in all parts of the cortex. The functional properties of a piece of cortex depends largely on the type of thalamic afferents which it gets (Creutzfeldt 1983). This was demonstrated again by the impressive experiments of Frost (1981) and those of Sur and colleagues presented at this meeting, where visual geniculo-cortical afferents were made to grow into a piece of cortex which normally would have become the auditory cortex. Such projections preserved their retinotopy and neurons in this wrongly innervated cortex showed properties similar or even equal to those normally known from the visual cortex. There is no anatomical or neurophysiological reason to assume that the effect of input from a thalamic association nucleus on its target in a piece of association cortex should be principally different from that of a sensory relay nucleus on its target in a primary sensory area. This then would give also the pulvinar a central role for the functional organization of extrastriate visual areas, including the temporal and the parietal association cortices.

We know very little about the pulvinar except that it contains several representations of the visual field (Gattas et al. 1978; Bender 1982) and that, in the behaving monkey its neurons tend to discharge preferentially in connection with eye movements (Perryman et al. 1980). We also know that it receives a massive input from the tectum opticum, the pretectum and from area 17 in topographically separate sections (Benevento et al. 1975, 1977) and that it projects in a topically organized manner to the various parts of the extrastriate visual and the parietal and temporal association cortex. From my own experience in the acute and the chronic monkey I know that neurons in the pulvinar may − in addition to what I mentioned earlier − show quite peculiar functional properties indeed, including rather specific responses to meaningful stimuli, to faces, etc. Reports on similar observations begin to accumulate also from other laboratories (see e.g., this year's Abstracts of the Society for Neuroscience). Thus, we would be ill-advised to neglect completely the specific thalamic input to the extrastriate visual cortex.

Many visual areas

If confronted with the many visual areas now described in the extrastriate visual cortex and beyond, one may first ask for the criteria of a visual area and then ask what is represented in each of them. One of the criteria to delineate a visual area is that it represents the visual field in a retinotopic order. Another criterion is that its neurons respond specifically to particular aspects of a visual stimulus such as contours, orientation, movement, colour, or even complex forms such as faces, etc. In other words, one expects them to be filters for certain stimulus aspects, partially preserving their retinotopic position, partially generalizing for the meaning at the expense of spatial information. As a consequence, each of these areas should not only be involved but also be necessary for representation and for cognition of a certain aspect of a visual stimulus (Zeki 1978).

None of these criteria is completely fulfilled for the different extrastriate visual areas, although some may apply more or less to one or the other area. Even V2 does not represent the whole visual field (Tusa et al. 1979) and contains various holes (or scotomas) (Albus and Beckmann 1980; Albus 1987). The rather crude retinotopy with very large receptive fields, large scatter of receptive field positions of nearby neurons and wide-ranging overlap in all 'retinotopic' extrastriate areas including V2 in cat and monkey clearly indicates that in such areas no real image could be represented by activity patterns across the visual field. Furthermore, in none of the extrastriate areas are specific features so exclusively represented that one could conclude that certain perceptual aspects of visual stimuli are represented only in one or the other of them. An exception may be to some extent area

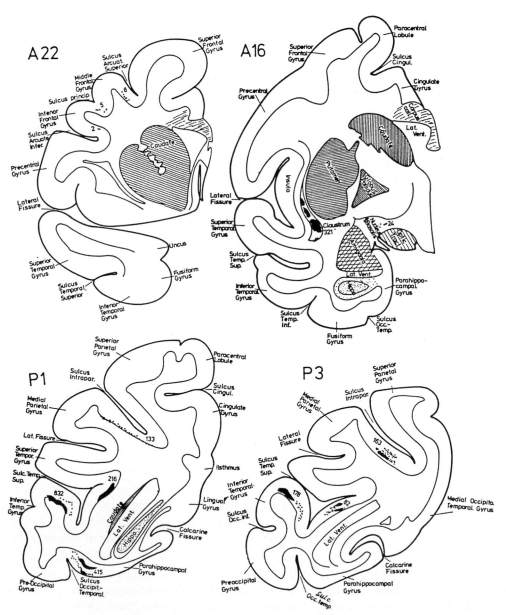

Fig. 2.

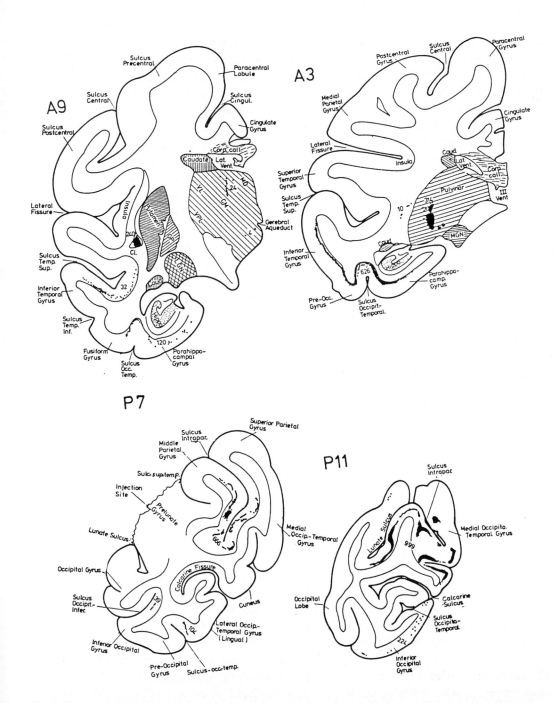

Fig. 2. Retrogradely labelled cells in various brain structures after injection of horseradish peroxidase (HRP) into the prelunate visual association area V4. *Macacca fascicularis*. Samples of coronal section are shown with labelled cells indicated as dots. The numbers next to a dot population are numbers of labeled cells found in this location and this section. The coronal level anterior (A) and posterior (P) to the interaural plane is given in mm. Cortical afferents to V4 come from the frontal eye field (A 22), the superior temporal sulcus (A 9, P 1, P 3), the intraparietal sulcus (P 7) and from peristriate cortex (P 11). Subcortical afferents can be traced from the claustrum (A 16, A 9), the nucleus basalis of Meynert (A 16) and the pulvinar (A 3) (from Creutzfeldt and Tanaka, unpublished).

MT in which most neurons appear to share the property of movement sensitivity (Movshon et al. 1985). However, movement sensitivity is found also in other extrastriate visual areas and area MT alone does not appear to be necessary for movement perception as lesion experiments indicate (Newsome et al. 1985). On the other hand, it is certainly involved in such a function and may even play a dominant role.

In following up the idea of the representation of certain stimulus aspects in one of the extrastriate areas one would have to assume that co-activation of one or the other of the extrastriate visual areas would put a 'label' on the specific and detailed representation of a visual stimulus in area 17: "This is blue, that moves, this is a face", etc. Thus, the prelunate visual association area (V4) is supposed to be specifically involved in colour perception (Zeki 1980). However, it also contains neurons which are not sensitive to spectral properties or to the colour of a stimulus, but to oriented textures, contours, movement and other properties (Zeki 1978; Schein et al. 1982; Tanaka et al. 1986; Desimone and Schein 1987). In fact, the distribution of spectrally sensitive and non-spectral cells is about the same as in area 17 (Creutzfeldt et al. 1987). Lesion of the prelunate gyrus produces, in monkeys, an impairment of cognition of form (orientation) and colour 'resembling a mild achromatopsia with associated apperceptive agnosia for objects and patterns' (Heywood and Cowey 1987). This demonstrates that area V4 is to some extent involved in such functions as colour and object recognition, and may be even necessary for unfailing functions in these respects, but appears not to be involved alone and is not sufficient for such functions.

We may finally take, as another example, the visually responsive zones in the supratemporal sulcus where cells are found which are particularly responsive to faces (Gross 1973; Perret et al. 1982). Cells with such properties are rare in such areas (about 5%), the specific responses can be elicited only in unanesthetized, behaving monkeys and the cells do not much or not at all discriminate be-

tween individual faces. Their peculiar responsiveness to the appearance of faces is certainly remarkable and is as yet the only example of a Gestalt-specific response. Yet, what do such responses indicate? If anything, they can put the label 'face' on a complex visual stimulus and alert the rest of the visual system to analyze it. The cortical output of this region to area V4, inter alias, may be brought in connection with such a function. On the other hand, one may ask, why are there only so relatively few such cells in this region and is it really justified to call this area a 'face area'? Could it not be that activation of such cells as well as of others, which may be responsive to other features or Gestalt aspects of living objects, just represents the response of the subject or a readiness to respond (MacKay 1970) to such objects *after* they had been identified by other parts of the visual system rather than being identified *by* the 'face' neurons? Could their activation not just indicate to the limbic system that something belonging to an animal is present and thus mediates a signal for emotional alertness without specification of what exactly it is? Whatever it is that the activation of such neurons may signify, the task of the analysis of details and identification is all back in that part of the visual system which is capable of analyzing the details of such a complex stimulus, and that is only area 17. Whichever way one likes to see it, it is clear that if specific aspects of visual stimuli are represented predominantly in other extrastriate visual areas, they are meaningless without the detailed information on such stimuli as is only and exclusively represented in the primary visual cortex.

I shall mention here only in passing the question of homologies between different extrastriate visual areas in different species as I have discussed this aspect in detail elsewhere (Creutzfeldt 1985). It should be mentioned, however, that the general organization of the extrastriate thalamo-cortical system is in fact comparable in different mammals, especially in cat and monkey. The quantitative and qualitative differences are due to the almost explosive increase of the number of retinal ganglion cells in monkeys (by a factor of 10 relative to the cat), and the emergence of a massive system for spectral discrimination (due to an increase in cone density in the retina). On the other hand, the recent demonstration of 'face neurons' also in the infero-temporal cortex of sheep (Kendrick and Baldwin 1987) near (or within?) the anterior ectosylvian visual area (AEV) demonstrates that even responses to such complex Gestalt aspects are not a privilege of monkeys and are found in the same topographic region of the cortex which we therefore may call homologous.

Behavior related activities in the extrastriate visual cortex

We have reminded ourselves that the extrastriate cortex receives a topographically organized afferent input from the pulvinar and is in this respect no exception to other cortical areas. We will now have a short look at its efferents. Also in this respect, the extrastriate areas do not differ, in principle, from other cortical areas including area 17 or the motor cortex in that the cortico-fugal fibres originate from cells in layer V. Association fibres (from layer III and V), callosal fibers (from across nearly the whole cortex), cortico-thalamic and cortico-claustral fibres (from layer VI) will not be considered, as their targets are either going to other cortical regions (assocation and callosal fibres) or to places of origin of afferent fibres to the same cortical regions from which they receive their cortical input (thalamus and claustrum). Only the efferents from the Vth layer pyramidal cells leave the cortical system and they actually go all into different motor control systems (the caudate nucleus, the various layers of the superior colliculi, the pontine nuclei, the mesencephalic reticular nucleus). Some of these target structures do not only send efferents on into more peripheral motor executive structures such as the supranuclear oculomotor command system of the midbrain, motor nuclei of the medulla and of the spinal cord, but also back to the cortex such as the collicular-pulvinar, the ponto-cerebellar or the caudate-thalamic recurrent loops to extrastriate, motor and premotor areas, respectively. The pattern of output from the various visual areas differs in that, for example, the efferents from the striate cortex terminate mainly in the superficial layers, those from extrastriate areas in deeper layers, of the superior colliculi. Area 17 (Kawamura et al. 1974) sends only few efferents to the pontine nuclei, while the extrastriate areas send many (Brodal 1978). Unfortunately, our knowledge of the detailed output pattern from the various visual areas is as yet rather limited and we have to leave it for the moment with such a sketchy picture (for review, see Creutzfeldt 1983).

However, this anatomical organization indicates that excitation of any area or, more precisely, of any point of the visually excitable cortex leads also to activation of its efferent neurons into the respective motor control systems thus either modifying or directly eliciting motor responses for eye, head or body movements. Not all such commands need to be excitatory and not all need to be executed. They are in fact not when execution is temporarily occupied or blocked by other control systems such as the motor or the prefrontal cortex, respectively, or during other behavioral involvement. However, one can well imagine that these combined outputs from the various sensory representations produce a motor model of appropriate responses to such an input. Donald MacKay has emphasized this all along and taught us to consider neuronal activities even in sensory areas not so much as explicit representations of the sensory stimulus but rather as a 'readiness to respond' to a certain stimulus configuration. The sensory message may be contained implicitly in this neuronal message (MacKay 1986). However one is inclined to lean to one or the other side, to the sensory or the action representation; the anatomical situation clearly suggests a model of the cortex such as sketched in Fig. 3, as a series of parallel input/output loops (Fig. 3A) laterally interconnected and interacting through short (intracortical) and long (association fibre) connections (Fig. 3B) (Creutzfeldt 1983). The inputs of one or the other area may be closer or fur-

314

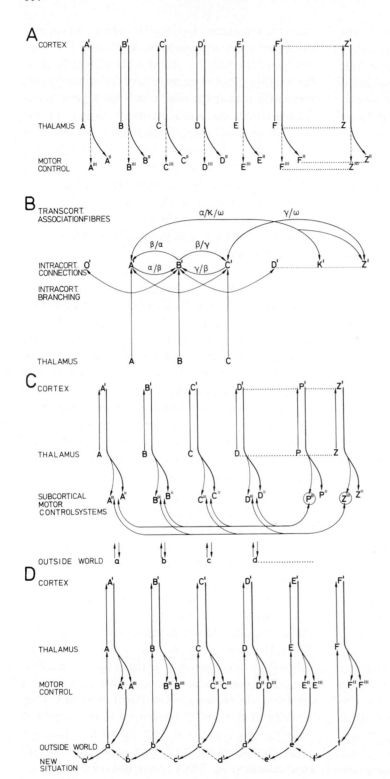

Fig. 3.

ther away from a sensory organ and the outputs may more or less directly relate to the final common path of motor command. The extremes in this respect are the primary sensory and the precentral motor cortical areas, respectively. At the lower executive levels of motor control, these outputs are brought together and may interact here in various ways (Fig. 3C). It should be realized that in such a scheme the brain is an 'open loop' system closed through the interactions of the individuum with the outside environment, the external loop. Any change in the relationship between the subject and his environment induced by action (output) will also change the sensory representation of the world within the system (input) (see Fig. 3D).

It is evident from this that the representation of function by neuronal activities can be fully revealed only in a behaving subject. Thus, in the prelunate visual association area (V4) of the awake monkey neurons may not only be driven by visual stimuli, but may discharge before an eye movement, or to a visual stimulus when it becomes the target for an eye movement (Fischer and Bloch 1981), or they discharge more when a stimulus has behavioral significance (Moran and Desimone 1985; Haenny et al. 1988). Neurons in the lateral part of the prelunate gyrus may discharge only when a monkey attends to a stimulus (Tanaka et al. 1986). In the medial segment of the prelunate gyrus (area DP) neurons respond in close connections with saccadic eye movement or with visual pursuit movements (Li, Tanaka, Creutzfeldt, unpublished results). Such eye movement related activations are only seen when the monkey is in a

visual task, but are not present when his gaze just jumps around, without looking at a specific visual target. Most of them discharge strongly only when the monkey fixates and explores a visual object with attention, especially if this involves an emotional response such as threatening or submission, e.g. to a human face (Fig. 4). One may ask, of course, where such activations come from. In DP it is clear, that saccade-related neurons receive a non-visual input, as saccade-related activations begin between 10 and 20 msec after the start of the saccade, that is at a latency as expected from a visual response. Visual latencies in V4 in the prelunate gyrus are between 60 and 80 msec (Tanaka et al. 1986).

Representations of various subject-object relations in extrastriate visual areas

We will now try to combine these various observations into a model of the visual cortex. The anatomical organization with its multiple and parallel input-output loops suggests that each visual area and in fact each point in the striate and extrastriate visual cortex represents a functional relation between a visual object and the subject. By that I mean that the excitation pattern across the whole visual cortex, striate and extrastriate, does not only represent the presence of a certain visual object but also the intended or actual response of the subject to such an object, be it an eye, head or body movement, an explorative or a more complex behavioral response. Each point contributes differently to such a response, the output from each

◀ Fig. 3. A schematic representation of the parallel representation of parallel input-output loops across the cerebral cortex. (A) Each 'point' in the cortex (A′ . . . Z′) receives an input from a thalamic 'point' (A . . . Z). This leads to an output from the respective cortical points corresponding structures at the motor control level which change their state from A′′ → A′′′ . . . Z′′ → Z′′′. (B) Cortical 'points' are in fact integrated to larger volumes because of the scatter and aborization of thalamo-cortical afferent fibres (A, B, C), bidirectional intracortical connections ($\alpha/\beta, \beta/\alpha$; $\beta/\delta, \delta/\beta$). Each of these systems has a similar modular dimensions across the whole cortex. Different regions of the cortex are related to each other through transcortical association fibres ($\alpha/\kappa/\omega$; δ/ω). (C) Integration of the efferent signals to coordinated movement commands takes place in subcortical motor control systems (A′′ . . . Z′′) which are again bidirectionally connected with each other. (D) Each signal from the outside world (a . . . f) elicits a response or the intention to respond which sets the subject into a new situation relative to the outside world (a′ . . . f′) (from Creutzfeldt 1983).

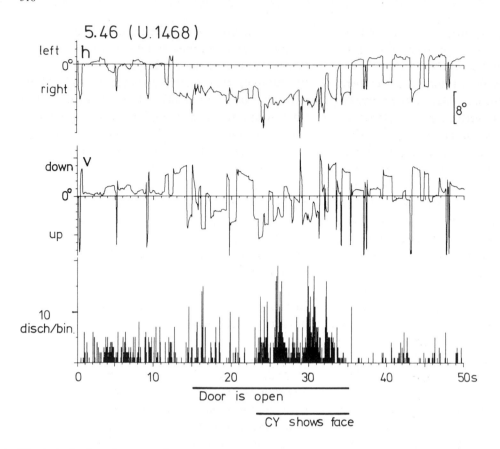

Fig. 4. Activation of a neuron in area DP on the dorsal segment of the prelunate gyrus while visually exploring a face. When the door to the experimental cage is opened, the monkey looks towards the open door on the right (upper eye movement record, h) and explores the opening with vertical up and down eye movements (second eye movement record, v). The neurons' discharge rate (lower record) is slightly depressed during this exploration period (sec 16.5 – 23). Then the experimenter shows his face in the door slit. The monkey still explores by moving the eyes up and down but with smaller excursions concentrating mainly on the face, while the horizontal gaze position does not change significantly. The neuron now discharges vigorously. This neuron could not be driven by flashing or moving lights within 30 – 40° around the fixation point during a fixation task (from Lichao-yi, Tanaka and Creutzfeldt, unpublished).

point has a different function depending on the target level of its output fibres in subcortical structures of action control, and the weighting of each output can be controlled by other regions of the cerebral cortex or other levels of the brain. The outputs from all striate and extrastriate visual areas may then be understood as a cooperative or synergistic response to a visual object, its position or variation in space. The object cannot be reconstructed directly from this activation pattern, however, if the function of the individual output

and of its target neurons within the subcortical integrating action system is not known.

What I mean may be explained by the example of cooperative action (I have adapted this term from Foerster (1936)) of the motor cortical areas: only output from the precentral motor cortex reaches the motoneurons directly, while many efferents from the same precentral as well as all efferents from the various premotor areas terminate at various levels of the motor control systems: the spinal reflex pathways, the mesencephalic motor nuclei or the corpus striatum (see Kuypers 1985). Thus, activation of somatotopically corresponding points in the precentral and the premotor areas have each different effects according to where the terminals end in the various subcortical integrating levels of movement control. In addition, the representation of the motor apparatus differs in the various motor areas. The precentral motor cortex has a more elaborate representation of distal muscles and therefore a more precise effect on motoneurons innervating muscles of hand and fingers, while the representation of proximal and trunk muscles is relatively larger in premotor areas. As a consequence, fine movements of the fingers depend on the functioning of the precentral motor cortex, while coordinated movements of the limbs and body including postural movements for supporting hand and limb movements involve the premotor areas (including the supplementary motor area) as well. The actual movement results from the temporally adjusted coactivation of the various motor areas.

Now let us return to the visual system. Visual perception is closely related to active visual exploration of visual objects. This implies fixation, saccadic and pursuit movements of eye and head, and of course other body movements. Commands to fixate, to let go or to pursue probably come from different parts of the visual system including the frontal eye fields, and depend on various evaluation criteria. Perception breaks down, when the retinal image is stabilized and the intended explorative action or response is thus made ineffective. We may say that the external loop between the subject and the object in terms of the model of Fig. 4 is interrupted. Perception also breaks down to some extent, if intended movements and the position of the object do not match as, e.g., during intermittent stroboscopic illumination.

As mentioned earlier, object recognition is impaired after lesion of the prelunate visual association cortex, where neuronal responses have been found to be related not only to visual stimuli but also to responses to visual stimuli, i.e., appropriate eye movements and fixation. More complex forms of object recognition (agnosias) are seen after parietal lesions. It is well demonstrated that neurons in the parietal association cortex are activated by sensory stimuli and/or during responses to such sensory stimuli (Mountcastle 1976; Hyvärinen 1982; Andersen 1987). We may interpret the effects of lesions in the prestriate visual as well as in the parietal association cortex as an incomplete and insufficient representation of a model for action (or behavioral response) to a visual stimulus. We usually say: "The subject does not recognize or identify this object". However, we may also say: "The subject does not know what to do with that visual object, he cannot work it out appropriately, he is not able to translate the visual stimulus into an object for action; i.e., for appropriate eye, head and limb movements".

An appropriate response to a visual object also involves an appropriate 'emotional' evaluation, i.e., whether the object means a reward (in a conditioning situation), whether it is a living being or a part thereof, a face, an animal in attack or flight, etc. Such emotional responses very probably involve the limbic system. The main output of the inferotemporal cortex goes, in fact, into the limbic system (the amygdala and the temporo-basal cortex) (for review see Creutzfeldt 1983). Bilateral temporal lobe ablation leads to an 'indiscriminative' visual behavior (Klüver-Bucy syndrome), in which any visual object be it neutral, edible or potentially dangerous (e.g., a snake), is orally explored. We say that the meaning of an object is not appropriately recognized. However, we may also, and I think more appropriately, say that the object is not signalled to the emotional system. Therefore, the subject does not know what the object is good for. The subject does not know whether the object is good or bad within the frame of his behavioral repertoire. Neuronal responses to faces in the superior temporal sulcus (see above) are found only in behaving monkeys (in fact, no eye movement recordings are yet available in the literature which could indicate whether the monkeys or sheep actually look at the faces when these neurons respond). On the other hand, neurons in the infero-temporal cortex may discriminate between a rewarded and a non-rewarded stimulus (Rolls et al. 1977). In AEV of the infero-temporal cortex of cats neurons may respond preferentially to very fast moving stimuli (Mucke et al. 1982), which could correspond to objects of prey (flying or running animals) in a free behavioral situation. Activation of such neurons cannot give any information about where to look (the receptive fields are too large) or what to do (they have no direct access to the motor system), but they could alert the system to look or to respond.

Let us finally go back to area 17. None of the extrastriate visual areas could give sufficient information about the exact position of a contour or corner, a colour or texture border, on which to fixate the gaze when exploring a visual object. Also the location of a small moving object in the visual field would be rather vague if the subject would have to rely on information from extrastriate movement-sensitive areas such as area MT or the Clare-Bishop area. Patients with a scotoma due to circumscribed area 17 lesions, who are still able to turn their eyes to a visual target (blind sight) do this, in fact, only very approximately. Thus, the decision on where exactly to fixate next during visual exploration or where exactly to look if a fly or a mouse moves in the peripheral visual field, must come from area 17 and its output into the gaze-controlling visuo-motor system.

Conclusion

These examples may suffice to illustrate what I mean in saying that the activation of neurons in the striate and extrastriate visual cortex represents various components of the relation between the subject and the visual object. We do not know the sequences of events which finally lead from one step to the next in any type of visual behavior. Thus we do not know the decision and command structure for visual behavior in the visual cortex. It looks as if the sequence of events and thus the command structure changes depending on the type of visual behavior and on the demands of the

visual environment and the subject. Thus, there is no simple hierarchy of visual behavior. And there is also no simple hierarchy of cognitive visual processes, although we like to believe in such hierarchies from introspective analysis of cognitive processes.

Instead, the well-timed but sufficiently synchronous activations (latencies from area 17 to infero-temporal neurons vary by less than 100 msec) of various combinations of different afferent-efferent cortical loops or, in terms of these presentations, of the different representations of object-subject relations represent the correct meaning of a stimulus in terms of a possible or actual behavioral response. A correct response is, of course, all we know about when we test 'perception' or 'cognition' in animals, but also neuropsychological tests in human patients usually test only the performance. The outcome of recognition tests in animal and man may be interpreted in 'cognitive' categories, which are, however, not measured. The synthesis of the activities of the parallel object-subject relating loops of the striate and extrastriate visual areas to a cooperative action takes place in the subcortical action controlling system. We have a long way to go to understand and disentangle this in detail. However, it is conceivable, in principle. Some of these subcortical mechanisms were demonstrated during the first part of this meeting, where subcortical mechanisms of visuo-motor control were discussed. If we want to distinguish two visual systems, we should do it at this point and draw the dividing line at the level between a subcortical and a cortical visuo-motor system, which mutually interact with each other.

Even if one is ready to accept what I have tried to outline in this essay — and I am aware that many will not accept it — there remains the difficulty of understanding how visuo-motor action and perception are integrated over time. What we see in anatomical studies are connections, the significance of which we do not fully understand yet. What we record in neurophysiological experiments are responses to temporally and spatially defined visual stimuli, activities during, preceding or following eye, head or visually elicited limb movements, during attentive behavior, etc., but we have difficulties to conceive how they could possibly be combined to a unified action or perception over time, no matter whether they are contained in these neural responses, explicitly or implicitly.

References

Albus, K. (1987) A neuronal subsystem in the cat's area 18 lacks retinotopy. *Brain Res.,* 410: 199 – 203.

Albus, K. and Beckmann, R. (1980) The second and the third visual areas of the cat: interindividual variability in retinotopic arrangement and cortical location. *J. Physiol.,* 299: 247 – 276.

Andersen, R.A. (1987) Inferior parietal lobule function in spatial perception and visuomotor integration. In: Mountcastle, V.B., Plum, F. and Geiger, S.R. (Eds.), *Handbook of Physiology, The Nervous System, Vol. 5,* Am. Physiol. Soc., Baltimore, MD, pp. 483 – 518.

Bender, D.B. (1982) Receptive field properties of neurons in the macaque inferior pulvinar. *J. Neurophysiol.,* 1: 1 – 16.

Benedek, G., Norita, M. and Creutzfeldt, O.D. (1983) Electrophysiological and anatomical demonstration of an overlapping striate and tectal projection to the lateral posterior pulvinar complex of the cat. *Exp. Brain. Res.,* 52: 157 – 169.

Benevento, L.A. and Fallon, J. (1975) The ascending projections of the superior colliculus of the rhesus monkey (*Macacca mulatta*). *J. Comp. Neurol.,* 160: 339 – 362.

Benevento, L.A., Rezak, M. and Santos-Andersen, R. (1977) An autoradiographic study of the projections of the pretectum in the rhesus monkey (*Macaca mulatta*): Evidence for sensorimotor links to the thalamus and oculomotor nuclei. *Brain Res.,* 127: 197 – 217.

Brodal, P. (1978) The cortico-pontine projection in the rhesus monkey. Origin and principle of organization. *Brain Res.,* 10: 251 – 283.

Creutzfeldt, O.D. (1983) *Cortex Cerebri. Leistung, strukturelle und funktionelle Organisation der Hirnrinde,* 484 pp. Springer-Verlag, Berlin, Heidelberg, New York, Tokyo.

Creutzfeldt, O.D. (1985) Comparative aspects of representation in the visual system, In: Chagas, C., Gattass, R. and Gross, C. (Eds.), *Pattern Recognition Mechanisms, Exp. Brain. Res. Suppl. 11*, pp. 53 – 81.

Creutzfeldt, O.D., Weber, H., Tanaka, M. and Lee, B.B. (1987) Neuronal representation of spectral and spatial stimulus aspects in foveal and parafoveal area 17 of the awake monkey. *Exp. Brain. Res.,* 68: in press.

Desimone, R. and Schein, S.T.J. (1987) Visual properties of neurons in area V 4 of the macaque: Sensitivity to stimulus form. *J. Neurophysiol.,* 57: 835 – 867.

Doty, R.W. (1973) Ablation of visual areas in the central nervous system. In: Jung, R. (Ed.), *Handbook of Sensory Physiology,* Vol. VII/3B, Springer-Verlag, Berlin, Heidelberg, New York, pp. 483 – 543.

Fischer, B. and Bloch, R. (1981) Enhanced activation of neurons in prelunate cortex before visually guided saccades of trained rhesus monkeys. *Exp. Brain Res.,* 44: 129 – 137.

Foerster, O. (1936) Motorische Felder und Bahnen. In: Bumke, O. and Foerster, O. (Eds.), *Handbuch der Neurologie,* Bd 6, Springer, Berlin, Heidelberg.

Frost, D.O. (1981) Orderly anomalous retinal projections to the medial geniculate, ventrobasal, and lateral posterior nuclei of the hamster. *J. Comp. Neurol.,* 203: 227 – 256.

Graybiel, A.M. and Berson, D.M. (1980) Histochemical identification and afferent connections of subdivisions in the lateralis posterior-pulvinar complex and related thalamic nuclei in the cat. *Neuroscience,* 5, 115 – 123.

Gattas, R.E., Oswaldo-Cruze and Sousa, A.P.B. (1978) Visuotopic organization of the Cebus pulvinar. *Brain Res.,* 152: 1 – 16.

Gross, C.H.G. (1973) Visual functions of infero-temporal cortex. In: Jung, R. (Ed.), *Handbook of Sensory Physiology, Vol. VII/3B: Visual Centers in the Brain,* Springer-Verlag, Berlin, Heidelberg, New York, pp. 451 – 482.

Guedes, R., Watanabe, S. and Creutzfeldt, O.D. (1983) Functional role of associative fibres for a visual association area: The posterior suprasylvian sulcus of the cat. *Exp. Brain Res.,* 49: 13 – 27.

Haenny, P.E. and Schiller, P.H. (1988) State dependent activity in the monkey visual cortex. I. Single cell activity in V1 and V4 on visual tasks. *Exp. Brain Res.,* 69: 225 – 244.

Haenny, P.E., Maunsell, J.H.R. and Schiller, P.H. (1988) State dependent activity in the monkey visual cortex. II. Retinal and extraretinal factors in V4. *Exp. Brain Res.,* 69: 245 – 259.

Heywood, C.A. and Cowey, A. (1987) On the role of cortical area V4 in the discrimination of hue and pattern in macaque monkeys. *Neuroscience,* 174 – 218.

Hyvärinen, J. (1982) (Ed.), *The Parietal Cortex of Monkey and Man.* Springer-Verlag, Berlin, Heidelberg, New York.

Kawamura, S., Sprague, J.M. and Niimi, K. (1974) Corticofugal projections from the visual cortices to the thalamus, pretectum and superior colliculus in the cat. *J. Comp. Neurol.,* 158: 339 – 362.

Kendrick, K.M. and Baldwin, B.A. (1987) Cells in temporal cortex of conscious sheep can respond preferentially to the sight of faces. *Science,* 236: 448 – 450.

Kuypers, H.G.J.M. (1981) Anatomy of the descending pathways. In: Brookhart, J.M., Mountcastle, V.B., Brooks, V.B. and Geiger, St. R. (Eds.), *Handbook of Physiology, The Nervous System. Chapter 13, Part 1.* Am. Physiol. Soc., Bethesda, MD, pp. 597 – 666.

Lin, C.S. and Kaas, J.H. (1978) The inferior pulvinar complex in the owl monkeys: Architectonic subdivisions and patterns of input from the superior colliculus and subdivisions of the visual cortex. *J. Comp. Neurol.,* 187: 655–678.

MacKay, D. (1970) Perception and brain function. pp. 303–316. In: F.O. Schmitt et al. (Ed.), *The Neurosciences, Second Study Program,* Rockefeller University Press, New York.

MacKay, D. (1986) Vision – the capture of optical covariation. In: Pettigrew, J.D., Sanderson, K.J., Levick, W. (Eds.), *Visual Neuroscience,* Cambridge University Press, pp. 487–500.

Moran, J. and Desimone, R. (1985) Selective attention gates visual processing in the extrastriate cortex. *Science,* 229: 782–784.

Mason, R. (1981) Differential responsiveness of cells in the visual zones of the cat's LP-pulvinar complex to stimuli. *Exp. Brain Res.,* 43: 25–33.

Mountcastle, V.B. (1976) The world around us. Neural command functions for selective attention. *Neurosci. Res. Progr. Bull.,* 14: Suppl.

Movshon, J.A., Adelson, E.H. Gizzi, M.S. and Newsome, W.T. (1985) The analysis of moving visual patterns. In: Chagas, C., Gattas, R. and Gross, C. (Eds.), *Pattern Recognition Mechanisms, Exp. Brain Res. Suppl.* 11, pp. 117–152.

Mucke, L., Norita, M., Benedek, G. and Creutzfeldt, O.D. (1982) Physiologic and anatomic investigation of a visual cortical area situated in the ventral bank of the anterior ectosylvian sulcus of the cat. *Exp. Brain Res.,* 46: 1–11.

Newsome, W.T., Wurtz, R.H., Dürstler, M.R. and Mikami, A. (1985) Deficits in visual motion processing following ibotenic acid lesions of the middle temporal visual area of the macaque monkey. *Neuroscience,* 5: 825–840.

Perret, D.I., Rolls, E.T. and Caan, W. (1982) Visual neuron responses to faces in the monkey temporal cortex. *Exp. Brain Res.,* 47: 329–342.

Perryman, K.M., Lindsley, D.F. and Lindsley, D.B. (1980) Pulvinar neuron responses to spontaneous and trained eye movements and to light flashes in squirrel monkeys. *Electroenceph. clin. Neurophysiol.,* 49: 152–161.

Robinson, D.L., Baizer, J.S. and Dow, B.M. (1980) Behavioral enhancement of visual responses of prestriate neurons of the rhesus monkey. *Invest. Ophthalmol. Vis. Sci.,* 19: 1120–1123.

Rolls, E.T., Judge, S.J. and Sanghera, M.K. (1977) Activity of neurons in the alert monkey. *Brain. Res.,* 130: 229–238.

Schein, S.J., Marrocco, R.T. and de Monasterio, F.M. (1982) Is there a high concentration of color-selective cells in area V4 of monkey visual cortex? *J. Neurophysiol.,* 47: 193–213.

Schiller, P.H. and Malpeli, J.G. (1977) The effect of striate cortex cooling on area 18 cells in the monkey. *Brain Res.,* 126: 366–369.

Spear, P.D. and Baumann, T.P. (1979) Receptive field characteristics of neurons in lateral suprasylvian visual area of the cat. *J. Neurophysiol.,* 38: 1403–1420.

Sprague, J.M., Berlucchi, G. and Rizzolatti (1973) The role of the superior colliculus and pretectum in vision and visually guided behavior. In: Jung, R. (Ed.), *Handbook of Sensory Physiology, Vol VII/3,* Springer-Verlag Berlin, Heidelberg, New York, pp. 27–101.

Sprague, J.M., Levy, J.D., Di Bernadino, A. and Berlucchi, G. (1977) Visual cortical areas mediating form discrimination in the cat. *J. Comp. Neurol.,* 172: 441–488.

Tanaka, M., Weber, H. and Creutzfeldt, O.D. (1986) Visual properties and spatial distribution of neurones in the visual association area on the prelunate gyrus of the awake monkey. *Exp. Brain Res.,* 65: 11–37.

Trevarthen, C.B. (1968) Two mechanisms of vision in primates. *Psychol. Forsch.,* 31: 299–337.

Tusa, R.J., Rosenquist, A.C. and Palmer, L.A. (1979) Retinotopic organization of areas 18 and 19 in the cat. *J. Comp. Neurol.,* 185: 637–678.

Ungerleider, L.G. and Mishkin, M. (1980) Two cortical visual systems. In: Ingle, D.J., Mansfield, R.J.W. and Goodale, M.A. (Eds.), *Advances in the Analysis of Visual Behavior,* MIT Press, Cambridge, MA.

Zeki, S.M. (1978) Uniformity and diversity of structure and function in rhesus monkey prestriate visual cortex. *J. Physiol.,* 277: 273–290.

Zeki, S.M. (1980) The representation of colours in the cerebral cortex. *Nature,* 284: 412–418.

Subject Index